OXFORD MEDICAL PUBLICATIONS

Oxford Handbook of
Palliative Care

Oxford Handbook list

Oxford Handbook of
Palliative Care

Max S. Watson
Locum Consultant in Palliative Medicine,
Northern Ireland Hospice,
Research Fellow,
Belfast City Hospital,
Belfast, UK

Caroline F. Lucas
Deputy Medical Director,
Princess Alice Hospice, Esher, Surrey;
Clinical Director,
North Surrey Primary Care NHS Trust;
Honorary Consultant in Palliative Medicine,
St Peter's Hospital, Chertsey, Surrey, UK

Andrew M. Hoy
Medical Director,
Princess Alice Hospice, Esher, Surrey;
Consultant in Palliative Medicine, Epsom and
St Helier NHS Trust, UK

Ian N. Back
Consultant in Palliative Medicine,
Holme Tower Marie Curie Centre, Penarth;
Consultant in Palliative Medicine,
Pontypridd and Rhonda NHS Trust,
Mid Glamorgan, UK

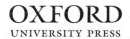

OXFORD
UNIVERSITY PRESS

OXFORD

UNIVERSITY PRESS

Great Clarendon Street, Oxford OX2 6DP

Oxford University Press is a department of the University of Oxford.
It furthers the University's objective of excellence in research, scholarship,
and education by publishing worldwide in

Oxford New York

Auckland Cape Town Dar es Salaam Hong Kong Karachi
Kuala Lumpur Madrid Melbourne Mexico City Nairobi
New Delhi Shanghai Taipei Toronto

With offices in

Argentina Austria Brazil Chile Czech Republic France Greece
Guatemala Hungary Italy Japan Poland Portugal Singapore
South Korea Switzerland Thailand Turkey Ukraine Vietnam

Oxford is a registered trade mark of Oxford University Press
in the UK and in certain other countries

Published in the United States
by Oxford University Press Inc., New York

British Library Cataloguing in Publication Data
Data available

Library of Congress Cataloging in Publication Data
Data available

Typeset by Newgen Imaging Systems (P) Ltd., Chennai, India
Printed in Italy
on acid-free paper by Legoprint S.p.A

ISBN 0-19-850897-2 (flexicover)
ISBN 0-19-856989-0 (Pbk, Part 1)
ISBN 0-19-856990-4 (Pbk, Part 2)

10 9 8 7 6 5 4 3 2 1

This book is dedicated to computer-abandoned families in Dungannon, Esher, Epsom, and Cardiff. Without their patience and understanding support, this project could never have been completed.

MW, CL, AH, IB

You matter because you are you. You matter to the last moment of your life and we will do all we can not only to help you die peacefully but to live until you die.

(Dame Cicely Saunders)

Foreword

Derek Doyle
*President Emeritus of the International Association for Hospice and
Palliative Care,*
*Vice President of the National Council for Hospice and Specialist
Palliative Care Services,*
*Medical Director/Consultant Physician St Columba's Hospice,
Edinburgh, UK (retired)*

Before his Cubist phase Picasso painted a moving scene, one that he had
perhaps witnessed as a boy. He entitled it *Science and Charity* (words that
will remind some readers of the motto of the Royal College of General
Practitioners). An old doctor, in what is clearly a poor home, is sitting
by the bedside of a dying patient. His expression is one of compassion and
deep thought as he leans on the bed looking at the patient he has perhaps
known for many years. It is impossible not to be moved by this image of a
general practitioner in 'the old days' and tempting to compare him with us
who care for the dying in a very different world.

Some will look at the painting and sigh with nostalgia for far-off days
when, as young GPs, they too made time to sit by a bedside. Today, even if
they wanted to, there is seldom sufficient time. They might smile to see so
few pieces of equipment—no syringe drivers and drips, nebulisers or
suction machines, or even catheter bags. Neither are there any nurses.
Many might be surprised to see someone who looks so young dying at
home—something that is getting less common in today's world in spite
of the expressed wishes of so many patients and the personnel and
resources being poured into community care.

Others will wonder if that old doctor ever felt as they often do today
when caring for the dying; lonely, sometimes a little frightened, less confident and competent than at any other time in their work, and, in our secu-
larized society, often at a loss to help with existential questions.

Junior hospital doctors (and, one would like to think, some consultants)
will perhaps look at the painting and give a wry smile. The old man may
have felt inadequate, poorly trained, and lonely but, they will ask themselves, is that any different from what they feel day in day out, caring for
the dying in the wards of our hospitals? Yes, they have had a few lectures
on palliative care and communication skills but their sense of inadequacy
in the face of a spectrum of suffering is little assuaged. They have had tutorials on ethical decision-making but in today's real world most responses
seem to be knee-jerk reactions made under pressure, not decisions talked
through with colleagues in the luxury of a mutually supportive team.

It is tempting to wonder what Picasso's doctor would have thought about
today's palliative care and this new book. We can be sure he would have
smiled with disbelief at something so much a part and parcel of every doctor's life being glorified with a name like *palliative care*. After all, he might
have asked, is that not what good care is all about; comforting, explaining,
and listening, being there when needed and especially when the days of
further tests and new therapies have long passed; sharing one's humanity

with all its frailties with someone on the loneliest journey of life. He might be shocked to learn why 'the principles of all clinical care' as he knew them, had to be dignified with such a title in the last decades of the 20th century.

Given a copy of this new *Handbook* he would have been amazed and, hopefully, a little envious. Amazed at the cornucopia of drugs and formulations available to today's doctors to ease suffering. Amazed at how much scientific research has uncovered and made possible. Amazed at how many, other than doctors, now share in this ministry of caring and in doing so bring a richness of skills and compassion. Envious that, to his surprise, it is now possible to have so much information and guidance at one's finger tips, in a book small enough for his desk or his bag. Surprised and thrilled, one hopes, that underpinning this handbook is a yet more comprehensive *Oxford Textbook of Palliative Medicine*, the resource for the specialists in palliative medicine—the specialists across the country, eager to take away some of the loneliness and sense of inadequacy our old doctor felt at that bedside.

No, there is nothing new about the principles of palliative care. They are the age-old principles of all good care but, as this *Handbook* so beautifully illustrates, now enhanced by new knowledge, new drugs, new approaches, new insights—all available to every doctor, nurse, chaplain, professional allied to medicine privileged to share themselves with someone on their final journey. What a challenge but what a privilege, as Picasso's doctor would surely have reminded us. Picasso seems to have chosen the right words for us—palliative care is, before all else, science and charity in action.

Edinburgh, September 2004

Preface

Most clinical professionals have been affected by caring for patients with palliative care needs. Such patients may challenge us at both a professional and at a personal level in areas where we feel our confidence or competence are challenged.

'I wanted to help her, but I just didn't know what to do or say'

As in every other branch of medicine, knowledge and training can help us extend our comfort zone, so that we can better respond to such patients in a caring and professional manner. However, in picking up this handbook and reading thus far you have already demonstrated a motivation that is just as important as a thirst for knowledge, the central desire to improve the care of your patients.

It was out of just such a motivation that the modern hospice movement began 40 years ago, and it is that same motivation that has fuelled the spread of the principles of palliative care—in fact the principles of ALL good care—across the globe: respect for the person, attention to detail, scrupulous honesty and integrity, holistic care, team caring, and consummate communications (often more about listening than telling and talking).

'I knew we couldn't cure him, but didn't know when or how to start palliative care'

Increasingly it is being recognized that every person has the right to receive high quality palliative care whatever the illness, whatever its stage, regardless of whether potentially curable or not. The artificial distinction between curative and palliative treatments has rightly been recognized as an unnecessary divide, with a consequent loss of the border crossings that previously signified a complete change in clinical emphasis and tempo.

Medical knowledge is developing rapidly, with ever more opportunities for and emphasis on curative treatment, to the point when any talk of palliative care can sometimes be interpreted as 'defeatist'.

Today the principles of palliative care interventions may be employed from the first when a patient's illness is diagnosed. Conversely, a patient with predominantly palliative care needs, late in their disease journey, may benefit from energetic treatments more usually regarded as 'curative'.

'I just felt so helpless watching him die. Surely it could have been better?'

Governments and professional bodies now recognize that every nurse and doctor has a duty to provide palliative care and, increasingly, the public and the media have come to expect—as of right—high quality palliative care from their healthcare professionals irrespective of the clinical setting.

Many of these palliative care demands can best be met, as in the past, by the health care professionals who already know their patients and families well. This handbook is aimed at such hospital or community-based professionals, and recognizes that the great majority of patients with palliative needs are looked after by doctors and nurses who have not been trained in specialist palliative care but who are often specialist in the knowledge of their patients.

'Even though I knew she had had every treatment possible, still, when she died I really felt that we had failed her and let her family down.'

Junior healthcare staff throughout the world have used the Oxford Handbook series as their own specialist pocket companion through the lonely hours of on-call life. The format, concise (topic-a-page), complete and sensible, teaches not just clinical facts but a way of thinking. Yet for all the preoccupation with cure, no healthcare professional will ever experience greater satisfaction or confirmation of their choice of profession, than by bringing comfort and dignity to someone at the end-of-life.

'I had never seen anyone with that type of pain before and just wished I could get advice from someone who knew what to do.'

The demands on inexperienced and hard-pressed doctors or nurses in looking after patients with palliative care needs can be particularly stressful. It is our hope that this text, ideally complemented by the support and teaching of specialist palliative care teams, will reduce the often-expressed sense of helplessness, a sense of helplessness made all the more poignant by the disproportionate gratitude expressed by patients and families for any attempts at trying to listen, understand and care.

'It was strange, but I felt he was helping me much more than I was helping him'

While it is our hope that the handbook will help the reader to access important information quickly and succinctly, we hope it will not replace the main source of palliative care knowledge: the bedside contact with the patient.

It is easier to learn from books than patients, yet what our patients teach us is often of more abiding significance: empathy, listening, caring, existential questions of our own belief systems and the limitations of medicine. It is at the bedside that we learn to be of practical help to people who are struggling to come to terms with their own mortality and face our own mortality in the process.

Readers may notice some repetition of topics in the handbook. This is not due to weariness or oversight on the part of the editors, but is an attempt to keep relevant material grouped together—to make it easier for those needing to look up information quickly.

It is inevitable that in a text of this size some will be disappointed at the way we have left out, or skimped, on a favourite area of palliative care interest. To these readers we offer our apologies and two routes of redress: almost 200 blank pages to correct the imbalances, and the OUP website, http://www.oup.co.uk/isbn/0-19-850897-2, where your suggestions for how the next edition could be improved would be gratefully received.

Acknowledgements

This Handbook could not have been completed without the whole-hearted involvement of a team of healthcare professionals who freely shared of their time and expertise in advising, editing and contributing various chapters or sections.

That such writing was completed on top of existing heavy clinical work loads is a testimony to these advisors, their capacity for hard work and commitment to sharing knowledge and expertise.

The costs of such extracurricular activities as contributing to handbooks like this is ususally also paid for by the families and partners of those whom we have trapped in their studies—thank you.

We particularly thank Catherine Barnes and Georgia Pinteau at Oxford University Press for their patience through the long birthing process of the handbook, and their ready supply of encouragement.

We are indebted to Ian Back both for permission to use some of the material contained in his excellent *Palliative Medicine Handbook* and for his input into the project despite several other major commitments.

The South West London and The Surrey, West Sussex and Hampshire Cancer Networks gave permission to use material contained in their Adult and Paediatric palliative care guidelines.

Jan Brooman at the Princess Alice Hospice Library was an invaluable help in the painstaking task of checking through the references.

The management and colleagues at the Princess Alice Hospice and the Northern Ireland Palliative Medicine Training Scheme have been very supportive of this project.

Handbooks, by their very nature, are distillations of accumulated and shared clinical knowledge. There is no claim to originality in these pages. We must accredit the hundreds of palliative care professionals who have observed, researched, recorded and written in journals and textbooks, to create the palliative care knowledge base which has been our primary text—a text which, almost unbelievably, did not exist in medical literature only 40 years ago.

MW
CL
AH
IB

We are indebted for permission to reproduce material within the Handbook from the following sources.

I. Back (2001) *Palliative Medicine Handbook*, 3rd edition. Cardiff: BPM Books.

E. Bruera and I. Higginson (1996) *Cachexia-Anorexia in Cancer Patients*. Oxford: Oxford University Press.

D. Doyle, N. Hanks, and N. Cherny (eds.) (2004) *Oxford Textbook of Palliative Medicine*, 3rd edition. Oxford: Oxford University Press.

J-H. R. Ramsay (1994) A King, a doctor and a convenient death. *BMJ*, **308**: 1445.

The South West London and the Survey West Sussex and Hampshire Cancer Networks. M. Watson and C. Lucas (2003) *Adult Palliative Care Guidelines*.

K. Thomas (2003) *Caring for the Dying at Home: companions on the journey*. Oxford: Radcliffe Medical Press.

R. Twycross, A. Wilcock, S. Charlesworth, and A. Dickman (2002) *Palliative Care Formulary*, 2nd edition. Oxford: Radcliffe Medical Press.

Winston's Wish: supporting bereaved children and young people. *www.winstonswish.org.uk*.

www.rch.org.au/rch_palliative; www.rch.org.au.

Contents

Advisors and contributors

Jennifer Barraclough
Former Consultant in Psychological Medicine
Sobell House
Churchill Hospital
Oxford

Pauline Beldon
Nurse Consultant Tissue Viability
Epsom and St Helier NHS Trust
Surrey

Jo Bray
Former Occupational Therapist
Project Director
Royal Marsden Hospital
Chelsea

Jan Brooman
Librarian
Princess Alice Hospice
Esher

David Cameron
Associate Professor of Family Medicine
University of Pretoria
South Africa

Beverly Castleton
Medical Director for Specialist Services and Consultant Physician
Care of the Elderly and the Young Physically Disabled
Surrey Heath and Woking NHS PCT
Chertsey

Robin Cole
Consultant Urological Surgeon
St Peter's Hospital
Chertsey

David Conkey
Clinical Oncology Department
Belvoir Park Hospital
Belfast

Simon Coulter
Specialist Registrar
Palliative Medicine Training Scheme
Belfast

Jill Cooper
Head Occupational Therapist
Royal Marsden Hospital
Sutton

Elizabeth Cruickshank
Speech and Language Therapist
South Glasgow University Hospitals
NHS Trust
Glasgow

Dwipaj Datta
Specialist Registrar
Palliative Medicine Training Scheme
South Thames
London

Judith Delaney
Haematology/Oncology Senior Pharmacist
Great Ormond Street Hospital for Children NHS Trust
London

Julie Doyle
Consultant in Palliative Medicine
Northern Ireland Hospice and Mater Hospital
Belfast

Martin Eatock
Consultant Medical Oncologist
Belfast City Hospital
Belfast

Patricia Enes
Formerly Research Nurse
Princess Alice Hospice
Esher

Gill Eyers
Senior Principal Pharmacist
Princess Alice Hospice, Esher
Kingston Hospital NHS Trust
Surrey

Craig Gannon
Consultant in Palliative Medicine
Princess Alice Hospice
Ashford and St Peter's Hospitals NHS Trust
Surrey

Louise Gibbs
Consultant in Palliative Medicine
St Christopher's Hospice
Lawrie Park Road
Sydenham, London

J. Simon Gibbs
Senior Lecturer in Cardiology
National Heart and Lung Institute at
Imperial College London, and
Honorary Consultant Cardiologist
Hammersmith Hospital, London

David Head
Former Chaplain
Princess Alice Hospice
Esher

Irene Higginson
Professor of Palliative Care and Policy
King's College School of Medicine and Dentistry
London

Jenny Hynson
Consultant Paediatrician
Victorian Paediatric Palliative Care Program
Royal Children's Hospital
Melbourne
Australia

David Hill
Consultant in Anaesthesia and Pain Management
Ulster Hospital
Honorary Senior Lecturer
Queen's University
Belfast

Allan Irvine
Consultant Radiologist
Ashford and St Peter's Hospitals NHS Trust
Surrey

Aleen Jones
Consultant Physician
Care of the Elderly
South Tyrone and Craigavon Area Hospitals
Craigavon

Emma Jones
Consultant in Palliative Medicine
Phyllis Tuckwell Hospice
Farnham

Carol Katté
Stoma Care Specialist Nurse
Ashford and St Peter's Hospitals NHS Trust
Surrey

Sian Lewis
Senior Dietician
Velindre Hospital
Cardiff

Victoria Lidstone
Specialist Registrar
Palliative Medicine Training Schemes
South Thames/South Wales
Cardiff

Mari Lloyd-Williams
Professor, Honorary Consultant in Palliative Medicine
Director of Primary Care
University of Liverpool
Liverpool

Jayne Macauley
Consultant in Palliative Medicine
Antrim Area Hospital and Northern Health Board
Antrim

Sarah McKenna
Consultant Medical Oncologist
Belfast City Hospital Trust
Belfast

Pamela MacKinnon
Formerly at the Department of Human Anatomy and Genetics
University of Oxford
Oxford

Sarah MacLaran
Specialist Registrar
Palliative Medicine Training Scheme
Myton Hamlet Hospice, Warwick

Dorry McLaughlin
Lecturer in Palliative Care
Northern Ireland Hospice Care
Belfast

Penny McNamara
Consultant in Palliative Medicine
Sue Ryder Care—St John's
Bedford

Elaine McWilliams
Clinical Psychologist
Harrow Primary Care Trust
Harrow

Anne Miller
Consultant Haematologist
Ashford and St Peter's Hospitals NHS Trust
Surrey

Dan Munday
Consultant in Palliative Medicine
Honorary Senior Lecturer Warwick University
Coventry Primary Care Trust
Warwick

Simon Noble
Specialist Registrar Palliative Medicine
All Wales Higher Training Programme
Cardiff

Victor Pace
Consultant in Palliative Medicine
St Christopher's Hospice
Lawrie Park Road
Sydenham, London

Sheila Payne
Professor in Palliative Care
Sheffield Palliative Care Studies Group
University of Sheffield
Sheffield

Margaret Reith
Social Worker Team Manager
Princess Alice Hospice
Esher

Joan Regan
Specialist Registrar
Palliative Medicine Training Scheme
Belfast

Patti Stevely
Day Hospice Manager
Senior Physiotherapist
Princess Alice Hospice
Esher

Robert Sudderick
Consultant in Otolaryngology and Head
and Neck surgery
Royal Surrey County Hospital
Guildford

Keri Thomas
GP, National Clinical Lead Palliative Care
Cancer Services Collaborative of NHS Modernisation Agency
Macmillan Gold Standards Framework Programme
Associate Clinical Director Community Palliative Care, Birmingham
Senior Clinical Lecturer, Warwick University

Patrick Trend
Consultant Neurologist
Royal Surrey County Hospital
Guildford

Jo Wells
Nurse Consultant in Palliative Care
Princess Alice Hospice
Kingston Hospital NHS Trust
Surrey

Andrew Wilcock
Macmillan Clinical Leader in Palliative Medicine and Medical Oncology
Nottingham University
Consultant Physician, Hayward House Macmillan
Specialist Palliative Care Unit
Nottingham City Hospital
Nottingham

Abbreviations

AF	atrial fibrillation
AIDS	acquired immune deficiency syndrome
Amp.	ampoule
b.d.	twice daily
BNF	British National Formulary
BP	blood pressure
Caps.	capsules
CD	controlled drug
CHF	congestive heart failure
CMV	cytomegalovirus
CNS	central nervous system
CO_2	carbon dioxide
COPD	chronic obstructive pulmonary disease
COX	cyclo-oxygenase
CSCI	continuous subcutaneous infusion
C/T	chemotherapy
CT	computerized tomography
CTZ	chemoreceptor trigger zone
CVA	cerebrovascular accident
DIC	disseminated intravascular coagulation
DN	District Nurse
DVT	deep vein thrombosis
ECG	electrocardiogram
EDDM	Equivalent Daily Dose of Morphine
FBC	full blood count
FEV_1	forced expiratory volume in one second
FNA	fine needle aspiration
g	gram
GERD	gastro-oesophageal reflux disease
GI	gastrointestinal
GP	General Practitioner
Gy	Gray(s) a measure of radiation
h	hour or hourly
HAART	highly active anti-retroviral therapy
HIV	human immunodeficiency virus
HNSCC	head and neck squamous cell carcinoma

ICP	intracranial pressure
i/m	intramuscular
Inj.	injection
i/r	immediate release
i/t	intrathecal
i/v	intravenous
IVI	intravenous infusion
IVU	intravenous urogram
KS	Kaposi's sarcoma
kV	kilovolt
l	litre
L/A	local anaesthetic
LFT	liver function tests
LVF	left ventricular failure
MAI	Mycobacterium avium intracellulare
MAOI	monoamine oxidase inhibitor(s)
max.	maximum
MeV	mega electronvolt
mcg	microgram
MND	motor neurone disease
m/r	modified release
MRI	Magnetic Resonance Imaging
MUPS	multiple unit pellet system
MV	megavolt
m/w	mouthwash
NASSA	noradrenergic and specific serotoninergic antidepressant
neb	nebuliser
NG	naso-gastric
NMDA	N-methyl-D-aspartate
nocte	at night
NSAID	non-steroidal anti-inflammatory drug
NSCLC	non small cell lung carcinoma
NYHA	New York Heart Association
o.d.	daily
o.m.	in the morning
OTFC	oral transmucosal fentanyl citrate
PCA	Patient Controlled Analgesia
PCF	Palliative Care Formulary
PCT	Palliative care team
PE	pulmonary embolism
PEG	percutaneous endoscopic gastrostomy

PET	positron emission tomography
PHCT	primary healthcare team
p.o.	by mouth
PPI	proton pump inhibitor
PR	per rectum
p.r.n.	when required
PSA	prostate-specific antigen
PV	per vagina
q.d.s.	four times daily
QoL	quality of life
RBL	renal bone liver (investigations)
RCT	randomized controlled trial
RT	radiotherapy
SALT	speech and language therapy
SC	subcutaneous
SCLC	small cell lung carcinoma
S/D	syringe driver (CSCI)
SE	side-effects
SERMs	selective oestrogen receptor modulators
SL	sublingual
soln.	solution
SPC	specialist palliative care
SR	slow or modified release
SSRI	selective serotonin reuptake inhibitor
stat	immediately
Supps.	suppositories
Susp.	suspension
SVC	superior vena cava
SVCO	superior vena cava obstruction
Tabs.	tablets
TB	tuberculosis
TBM	tubercular meningitis
t.d.s.	three times daily
TENS	transcutaneous electrical nerve stimulation
TIA	transient ischaemic attack
TSD	therapeutic standard dose
U&E	urea and elecrolytes
URTI	upper respiratory tract infection
UTI	urinary tract infection
VTE	venous thromboembolism
WHO	World Health Organization

Introduction

Palliative care definitions

Palliative care is the active, holistic care of patients with advanced, pro-gressive illness. Management of pain and other symptoms and provision of psychological, social and spiritual support is paramount. The goal of palliative care is achievement of the best quality of life for patients and their families. Many aspects of palliative care are also applicable earlier in the course of the illness in conjunction with other treatments.[1]

Palliative care:
- Affirms life and regards dying as a normal process
- Provides relief from pain and other symptoms
- Integrates the psychological and spiritual aspects of patient care
- Offers a support system to help patients live as actively as
  possible until death
- Offers a support system to help the family cope during the patient's
  illness and in their own environment.

Principles of palliative care

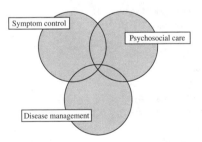

No single sphere of concern is adequate without considering the relation-ship with the other two. This usually requires genuine interdisciplinary collaboration.[2]

General palliative care is provided by the usual professional carers of the patient and family with low to moderate complexity of palliative care need. Palliative care is a vital and integral part of their routine clinical practice which is underpinned by the following principles:
- Focus on quality of life which includes good symptom control
- Whole person approach taking into account the person's past life
  experience and current situation

- Care which encompasses both the person with life-threatening illness and those that matter to the person
- Respect for patient autonomy and choice (e.g. over place of care, treatment options)
- Emphasis on open and sensitive communication, which extends to patients, informal carers and professional colleagues

Specialist palliative care

These services are provided for patients and their families with moderate to high complexity of palliative care need. The core service components are provided by a range of NHS, voluntary and independent providers staffed by a multidisciplinary team whose core work is palliative care.[2]

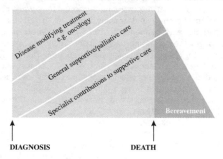

DIAGNOSIS   DEATH

Supportive care is that which helps the patient and their family to cope with cancer and treatment of it—from pre-diagnosis, through the process of diagnosis and treatment, to cure, continuing illness or death and into bereavement. It helps the patient to maximize the benefits of treatment and to live as well as possible with the effects of the disease. It is given equal priority alongside diagnosis and treatment.

The principles that underpin supportive and palliative care are broadly the same.

Hospice and hospice care refer to a philosophy of care rather than a specific building or service and may encompass a programme of care and array of skills deliverable in a wide range of settings.

Terminal care is an important part of palliative care and usually refers to the management of patients during their last few days, weeks or months of life from a point at which it becomes clear that the patient is in a progressive state of decline.

1 World Health Organization (1990) *Cancer Pain Relief and Palliative Care*. Geneva: WHO: 11 (World Health Organization technical report series: 804)

2 National Council for Hospice and Specialist Palliative Care Services (2002) *Definitions of Supportive and Palliative Care*. London: NCHSPCS (Briefing Bulletin 11)

History of palliative medicine as a specialty

The specialty of palliative medicine as a specific entity dates from the mid 1980s. However, medical activity related to terminal care, care of the dying, hospice care and end-stage cancer is of course as old as medical practice itself.[1] Palliative medicine is the medical component of what has become known as palliative care.

The history of the hospice movement during the nineteenth and twentieth centuries demonstrates the innovations of several charismatic leaders. These practitioners were enthusiasts for their own particular contribution to care of the dying, and they were also the teachers of the next generation of palliative physicians. Although they were products of their original background and training, they all shared the vision of regarding patients who happened to be dying as 'whole people'. They naturally brought their own approaches from specific disciplines of pharmacology, oncology, surgery, anaesthetics or general practice. This whole person attitude has been labelled as 'holistic care'. Comfort and freedom from pain and distress were of equal importance to diagnostic acumen and cure. However, rather than being a completely new philosophy of care, palliative medicine can be regarded more as a codification of existing practices from past generations.

Histories of the development of palliative medicine illustrate the thread of ideas from figures such as Snow, who developed the Brompton Cocktail in the 1890s, to Barrett who developed the regular giving of oral morphine to the dying at St Luke's, West London, to Saunders who expanded these ideas at St Joseph's and St Christopher's Hospices. Worcester, in Boston, was promoting the multidisciplinary care of whole patients in lectures to medical students at a time when intense disease specialization was very much the fashion as it was yielding great therapeutic advances.[2] Winner and Amulree, in the UK in the 1960s, were promoting whole person care particularly for the elderly, first challenging and then re-establishing the ethical basis for palliative medicine.

The early hospice movement was primarily concerned with the care of patients with cancer who, in the surge of post-war medical innovation, had missed out on the windfall of the new confident and increasingly optimistic medical world.

That this movement was responding to a need perceived across the world, has been evidenced by the exponential growth in palliative care services throughout the UK and across the globe since the opening of St Christopher's hospice in south-east London in 1967.

The expansion is set to increase further, as the point has now been reached where patients, doctors and governments alike are calling for the same level of care to be made available to patients suffering from non-malignant conditions as for those with cancer.

If this new challenge is to be met, healthcare professionals from early in their training will need to be exposed to palliative care learning which can be applied across the range of medical specialities.

The essence of such palliative medicine learning both for generalists and specialists remains that of clinical apprenticeship. Alfred Worcester, in the preface to his lectures, notes that:

The younger members of the profession, although having enormously greater knowledge of the science of medicine, have less acquaintance than many of their elders with the art of medical practice. This like every other art can of course be learned only by imitation, that is, by practice under masters of the art. Primarily, it depends upon devotion to the patient rather than to his disease.[2]

1 Saunders C. (1993). Introduction—history and challenge. In C. Saunders, N. Sykes (eds) *The Management of Terminal Malignant Disease. 3rd edition*, pp. 1–14. London: Edward Arnold.

2 Worcester A. (1935) *The Care of the Aged the Dying and the Dead.* London: Bailliere & Co.

The death of Harold Shipman

" Dr Harold Shipman died on 13 January in Wakefield Prison. He hanged himself on the day before his 58th birthday. He was convicted in January 2000 of the murder of 15 people. However, it is estimated that he killed at least 215 mainly elderly people. As well as being the UK's most prolific serial killer, what is most shocking is that his victims were his patients. They looked up to him as a trusted GP and friend. What significance does this have for those concerned with palliative care in both the UK and beyond?

All medical practice, but particularly palliative care, relies on the establishment of a relationship of trust between patients and their healthcare professional advisors. This trust is threatened by dishonesty on the part of doctors or nurses. For this reason, the palliative care movement has embraced the philosophy of truthful disclosure of clinical information to patients if that is what is asked for. This philosophy is sometimes confused with total disclosure of every last documented outcome and complication of a proposed management plan, whether or not the recipient of the information is in an emotional or intellectual state to process it. This offloading of detail may be advocated as part of the process of obtaining informed consent, or it may be the result of defensive practice to protect against future litigation. Neither is in the patient's best interest. Furthermore, frank disclosure does not imply brutal use of stark prognostic details, without first listening carefully to the patient's informational requests. So honesty and truthfulness are prerequisites for trust. Trust in turn is essential to prevent advice from becoming paternalistic.

Harold Shipman used opioids to kill his victims. We will never know the details of dose and methods, but it is safe to assume that he gave very large doses to opioid-naïve patients. This fact has not always been reported to the public, with the unfortunate consequence that there is now increasing suspicion of strong opioids even when such drugs would relieve severe pain. This makes palliative care more difficult and results in increased suffering especially for the vulnerable.

Although Shipman showed no remorse or inclination to collaborate in establishing his motives, while he was still alive there was still the chance that we might eventually have gained some insight into his psychopathology. Now he has killed himself, we are simply left to speculate that in death as in life his motive was the need to exert control over all those around him.

The popular press has named his activity as 'euthanasia without consent'. This term is unfortunate for several reasons. We do not have evidence that all his victims died peacefully and without anguish. They were certainly not given any opportunity to complete unfinished business with family and friends. In the immediate aftermath of Shipman's death, anger and resentment among relatives has increased not diminished. There would seem to be no sense of closure which either understanding or remorse might have brought. The use of the word euthanasia only muddies the water in a debate which is difficult in any event. Finally, although death can be viewed as the inevitable relinquishment of autonomy, at least in a physical sense, choices can be exercised before such relinquishment. Shipman removed consent, choices and therefore all autonomy and self-determination. His activity was murder with or without an understandable motive.

Since the conviction four years ago, there has been an exhaustive judicial inquiry of current law and regulations relating to death registration, monitoring of single-handed general practice, prescription, availability and supply of controlled drugs. The Prime Minister has already said that the recommendations of this review will be implemented in full. There is, however, considerable anxiety that this may result in a straitjacket for sensible community palliative care. It would be doubly tragic if Shipman's legacy of murder resulted in the frustration of good palliative care. An exceptional case makes for bad law. "

Reproduced with kind permission from the *European Journal of Palliative Care*.

Communication

Effective symptom control is impossible without effective communication

Buckman 2000

Communication is fundamental to good palliative care, but difficulties can arise that need to be understood and addressed.

Society's attitudes towards death and dying can hinder open communication. Health professionals may be uneasy with issues of death and dying: they may wish to protect themselves and others, and feel a sense of discomfort with strong emotions.

It is easy for the busy health professional to use a variety of blocking tactics which inhibit communication, such as hiding behind task-focused practice. An additional hazard may arise if the setting is not conducive to privacy with space and time to listen.

Information-giving can take the place of hearing the underlying feelings and emotions. The essence of good communication is not what we say, but how we listen. The quality of listening empathically to patients should not be underestimated if patients are to feel understood and cared for.

Communication in palliative care is necessary to achieve accurate assessment of patients' physical, emotional and psychosocial needs. If we are to be able to find ways of supporting patients and families facing change and uncertainty, we as health professional needs to find out about the patient's expectations and goals.

Enabling people to make informed choices and to make future plans involves careful listening and sensitive responses. Attending to cultural and language issues, and helping people face some of the strong emotions aroused by their situation such as anger, denial, depression and fear, are essential in providing holistic PALLIATIVE CARE.

Buckman, R. (2000) Communication in palliative care: a practical guide.
In D. Dickenson, M. Johnson and J. S. Katz (eds.) *Death, Dying and Bereavement*, 2nd edn.
pp 146–73. London: Sage.

Prognostication in end-of-life care

The natural history of disease has been documented over many years. This has become increasingly less relevant as successful therapies have developed. In present day palliative medicine, prognosis frequently relates to chronic progressive disease in patients with multiple co-morbidities, and not to the recovery prediction of a young adult with an acute illness, as was more common in the nineteenth century.

The reasons for making an attempt at predicting how long a patient with incurable disease might live include:

- Providing information about the future to patients and families so that they can set goals, priorities and expectations of care
- Helping patients develop insight into their dying
- Assisting clinicians in decision-making
- Comparing like patients with regard to outcomes
- Establishing the patient's eligibility for care programmes (e.g. hospice) and for recruitment to research trials
- Policy-making regarding appropriate use and allocation of resources and support services
- Providing a common language for healthcare professionals involved in end-of-life care.

Prognostic factors in cancer

There is a good literature on the probability of cure for the different cancers.

- Although individual cancers behave differently, as a generalization, predictions relate to tumour size, grade and stage
- Other factors include hormonal status (for hormone-dependent tumours such as cancer of the breast and prostate)
- Age
- Biochemical or other markers
- The length of time taken for the disease to recur.

In palliative care such prognostic indices may not be so relevant.

Factors such as physical dependency (due to e.g. weakness, low blood pressure), cognitive dysfunction, paraneoplastic phenomena (e.g. anorexia–cachexia, cytokine production), certain symptoms (weight loss, anorexia, dysphagia, breathlessness), lymphopaenia, poor quality of life and existential factors (either 'giving up' or 'hanging on' for symbolically important times) may be more important.

Some patients may survive for a long time (months and years) with a seemingly high tumour load, while others succumb within a short time (days) for no obviously identifiable reasons.

Several scores have been developed to aid prediction of survival. The Palliative Prognostic (PaP) score is predictive of short term survival and summarizes scores for dyspnoea, anorexia, Karnovsky performance status, the clinician's estimate of survival (in weeks), total white count, and percentage of lymphocytes.

Oncologists rely on prognosis assessments in order to predict which patients are likely to benefit from oncological interventions. Many of their decisions are based on the patient's functional status.

Patients with an ECOG score greater than two are usually deemed unsuitable for most chemotherapy interventions.

Eastern Co-operative Oncology Group (ECOG)

Fully active; able to carry on all activities without restriction	0
Restricted in physically strenuous activity but ambulatory and able to carry out work of a light or sedentary nature	1
Ambulatory and capable of all self care; confined to bed or chair 50% of waking hours	2
Capable of only limited self-care; confined to bed or chair 50% or more of waking hours	3
Completely disabled; cannot carry on any self care; totally confined to bed or chair	4

Prognostic factors in non-malignant disease

Predicting prognosis in patients with a non-cancer diagnosis is very difficult. These patients often remain relatively stable, albeit at a low level, only to deteriorate acutely and unpredictably. They are usually then treated acutely in hospital, and the disease course may consist of acute exacerbations from which recovery may take place.

One study showed that even in the last 2–3 days of life patients with congestive heart failure (CHF) or COPD were given a 80 per cent and 50 per cent chance respectively of living six months.

There are, however, general and specific indicators of the terminal stage approaching.

General predictors

Those predicting poorer prognosis include reduced performance status, impaired nutritional status (greater than 10 per cent weight loss over six months) and a low albumin.

Specific predictors

Congestive heart failure (CHF)
- More than 64 years old
- Left ventricular ejection fraction less than 20 per cent
- Dilated cardiomyopathy
- Uncontrolled arrhythmias
- Systolic hypotension
- CXR signs of left heart failure
- A prognosis of less than six months is associated with NYHA Class IV (chest pain and/or breathless at rest/minmal exertion) and already optimally treated with diuretics and vasodilators

Chronic obstructive pulmonary disease (COPD)
- Advanced age
- FEV_1 less than 30 per cent
- Pulmonary hypertension with cor pulmonale/right heart failure
- Other factors NHO sob at rest
- On 24 hour home O_2 with pO_2 less than 50 mm Hg and/or pCO_2 more than 55 mm Hg and documented evidence of cor pulmonale

Cortical dementias (Alzheimer's disease)
- Functional status—the onset of being unable to walk unaided
- Unable to swallow
- Unable to hold a meaningful conversation
- Increasing frequency of medical complications, e.g. aspiration pneumonia, urinary tract infections, decubitus ulcers

Stroke
- Impaired consciousness
- Lack of improvement within three months of onset
- Age
- Incontinence
- Cognitive impairment
- Dense paralysis

Communicating prognosis

Prognostication is a notoriously difficult task to perform accurately. The world abounds with stories of patients who have been told by their physicians that they have only a matter of months to live who twenty years later can recount in vivid detail the day they were given the news.

One of the reasons that prognostication is so difficult is that it is fraught with uncertainty and also with opportunities for misunderstandings between doctors and patients, who often have very different agendas as to what they want to get out of the interview.

> Mr. Jones listened carefully as the consultant went into great detail about the nature and the extensive spread of his metastatic prostate tumour. The explanations were detailed and scientific and long. Eventually the consultant stopped. 'Now Mr. Jones, do you have any more questions'
>
> 'Well, I didn't like to interrupt you but I was only asking how long I had before I needed to go down to get my X-Ray.'

Over the past 20 years there has been a huge shift in attitudes regarding disclosure of information to patents, and a culture of complete disclosure has now become the norm. Yet prognostication does not just involve passing on clinical details and predictions of disease progression; it also involves assessing:
- What does the patient actually want to know? (Giving too much information to a patient who does not want to have the exact details spelt out is as unprofessional as the patronising attitudes of 'best not to trouble the patient'
- How is the patient dealing with the information that is being given?

- How can the patient be helped to deal with the implications
  of the news?

  To pass on facts without regard for the implications of those facts is to increase the risk of dysfunctional communication taking place. (📖 See Chapter 2)

Risk and chance

While doctors are used to describing risk in terms of percentages, when such percentages are measuring out your own longevity it is hard to translate the mathematical chances into personal experience.

A doctor may feel that he has provided the patient with the clear facts when he states that in 100 patients with the particular malignancy, 36 will be alive after five years following treatment. Such sentences can be easily misunderstood, and the patient may hear something very different from what the doctor is saying.

Professional discomfort

Doctors are also particularly vulnerable to miscommunication at the time of passing on prognostic information.

- Society in the west is now death-denying, and if the prognosis is poor it can be uncomfortable for the doctor to pass on the information and confront the patent with their imminent death
- There is increasing fear of litigation, particularly if disease is not responsive to treatment, and any admission of failure may come across as an admission of guilt
- Doctors may feel uncomfortable in dealing with the emotional impact that their news may have on the patient, and develop techniques to protect themselves from this discomfort

Prognostic information can be extremely important to patients as it allows them to focus on tasks and goals which they want to achieve before their disease takes over: communicating such information effectively is a skill which all healthcare professionals should covet.

Paediatric palliative care

There can be no Doubt that a perfect Cure of the Diseases of Children is as much desired by all, as any thing else whatsoever in the whole art of Physick.

Walter Harris, 1698

Who needs paediatric palliative care?

The emergence of a new specialty

- Advances in the treatment of life-threatening neonatal and paediatric conditions have dramatically improved survival rates over recent years
- One of the most striking reductions in mortality has been achieved for children with malignant conditions, although there remain certain forms of cancer for which the prognosis remains extremely poor
- Similarly, there is a range of non-malignant conditions which continue to be life-limiting, despite the advances outlined above
- The patient population in paediatric palliative care is quite different from that encountered in adult practice. Approximately 40–50 per cent of children with palliative care needs have a malignancy
- The remainder have a variety of conditions including congenital abnormalities and neurodegenerative disorders
- Modern pharmacological and technical approaches now make it possible for some children, who would previously not have survived at all, to live longer, sometimes into adulthood. Many of these children have long illness trajectories which see them deteriorate slowly and inexorably toward a state of high dependency and disability
- It can be difficult to identify a point where treatment becomes exclusively palliative, and this presents a major challenge to service providers
- Many conditions are rare and the prognosis is often unpredictable, the child could die at any time or may live a number of years. These children often have multiple symptoms, requiring frequent medical intervention, in addition to complex psychological needs
- The parents and siblings of these children also need support in adjusting to the diagnosis and ongoing care of the child

Specialist paediatric palliative care services have recently been established in a number of centres throughout the world and focus variably on the three main care settings: home, hospice and hospital. Families will generally move between the various settings according to need but it has become clear that where home care is offered as a realistic option, most families will wish to care for their child at home. Children's home care teams and outreach nurses are becoming more common and are often able to take on a palliative care rôle providing support for children with life-limiting diseases and their families in their own homes.

In addition, children's hospices are also being established, providing an option for respite and terminal care. Specialist palliative care services for children in hospitals are not as widely available away from major centres, although adult palliative care teams are available for advice in many hospitals.

Much of the introductory material for this chapter has been produced by the Royal Children's Hospital, Melbourne Paediatric Palliative Care team.

The box below is taken from *A Guide to the Development of Children's Palliative Care Services* and lists numerous conditions that may affect the child in palliative care.[2]

---

1 Conditions for which curative treatment is possible but may fail. e.g. leukaemia.

2 Diseases where premature death is likely but intensive treatments may prolong good quality life e.g. cystic fibrosis, muscular dystrophy.

3 Progressive conditions where treatment is exclusively palliative and may extend for many years e.g. mucopolysaccharidoses, other neurodegenerative conditions.

4 Conditions, often with neurological impairment, causing weakness and susceptibility to complications e.g. non progressive CNS disease.

Background

Children in the terminal phase of illness are known to suffer significantly from inadequate recognition and treatment of symptoms, aggressive attempts at cure, fear and sadness. A child's death is experienced as a profound loss by parents, siblings, extended family and the wider community. Bereaved parents suffer intense grief and may be at increased risk of death themselves from both natural and unnatural causes.[1]

For those living in developed nations, child mortality has fallen to such an extent that the death of a child seems an utterly unnatural and devastating affront. It is now so uncommon as to create a sense of alienation for families who are caring for a dying child or whose child has died. This increases the importance of support for the family throughout the child's illness, from diagnosis and treatment through terminal care, to bereavement.

Prevalence of UK paediatric palliative care needs[2]

In a district of 250,000 people with a population of 50,000 children aged <19yrs, in one year:

- 5 are likely to die from a life-imiting condition of which 2 would be from cancer, 1 from heart disease and 2 from other life-limiting conditions.
- At the same time about 50 children would be suffering from a life-limiting condition and, of these, about half would have palliative care needs.[1]

---

1 Li J., Precht D. H., Mortensen P. B., Olsen J. (2003) Mortality in parents after death of a child in Denmark: a nationwide follow-up study. *Lancet*, **361**: 363–7.

2 Association for Children with Life-threatening or Terminal Conditions and their Families and the Royal College of Paediatrics and Child Health (2003) *A Guide to the Development of Children's Palliative Care Services*. 2nd edn. London: ACT.

Provision of paediatric palliative care

The provision of paediatric palliative care is patchy and the structure of specialist teams variable. Before thinking about service provision, it may be helpful to consider what and who surrounds a family in this situation.

A large number of agencies and individuals may be involved in supporting children and families and although this is appropriate, there is the potential for confusion, intrusion and replication of services. It is often helpful to nominate a *key worker* who can coordinate the various services involved and act as a first point of call for families. Through effective communication, including regular meetings, a comprehensive management plan can be created for the child in question. It is important that all the professionals involved are supported themselves, as this can be a demanding and unfamiliar area of practice. A specialist paediatric palliative care team can support the agencies and individuals involved in caring for the family. Such a team may include some or all of the following:

• Paediatric palliative care nurses (who may provide advice in both hospital and community settings)
• A specialist palliative care paediatrician
• Social worker
• Psychologist and or psychiatrist
• Chaplain

Sometimes, advice and support are needed from other teams or professionals with special expertise or knowledge regarding a particular condition. This is often necessary in cases where children have very rare conditions.

Differences between paediatric and adult palliative care

Developmental factors

An understanding of developmental issues is essential to the management of a child with palliative care needs. Infants and young children are completely dependent on the adults in their lives for care and protection. They also depend on others to make decisions on their behalf.

As children grow and develop, their capacity to care and decide for themselves increases. Indeed, the emergence of autonomy is a central developmental task of adolescence. In this way, care that is appropriate for a child of 11 may be inappropriate two years later as the need for independence, privacy and greater control grows. This can be difficult for both parents and healthcare professionals to accept. The natural desire to protect a child who is experiencing a devastating illness can lead to that child feeling stifled.

The relationship between development and illness is bidirectional. That is, the changing developmental status of the child influences the way in which they experience illness, and illness, in turn, influences the child's development. Chronic illness can delay development but the life experience it brings may also make a child seem old beyond their years.

The child's developmental level will influence all aspects of palliative care, but the following issues are worth highlighting:
- Communication of wishes, fears and symptoms
- Understanding of illness and death
- Assessment of symptoms
- Management of symptoms
- Decision-making
- Importance of play as a means of understanding the world
- Importance of kindergarten and school

Approach to consultation

Developmental level and cognitive ability will vary widely and are not necessarily related to age, so an appraisal of the child's level of understanding will need to be made early in the consultation. While not unique to the paediatric setting, the child and family's previous experience with medical procedures and staff will strongly influence their attitude to professionals. Honest communication and the development of trust early in the course of the illness will provide a solid foundation on which to face the challenges of palliative care. Conversely, long-term intense treatment involving repeated hospitalization and painful procedures may make a child wary of health professionals. Consultation and communication style therefore need to be highly flexible and adapted to each individual child and their family. A great deal of patience may be required.

Physiology/pharmacokinetics

These change as the child grows and develops. Neonates have a higher relative volume of distribution and lower clearance than adults, so the half-life of many drugs is prolonged. Conversely, infants and young children may metabolize certain drugs more quickly than adults. Children over six months of age, for example, may need higher doses of morphine than expected for their size.

Differences in family structure and function

Parents are socially and biologically invested with the responsibility of caring for and protecting their child. Consequently, the development of fatal illness in the child leads many parents to feel they have failed in this important rôle. Denial is a common reaction and despite advice to the contrary, parents may feel compelled to try everything and do anything to find a cure. This can be a difficult time for the child, the family, and the staff caring for them. Staff may feel the child is being subjected to overly burdensome treatment and may also worry that the child is not able to talk about the reality of what is happening. Maintaining hope and a supportive presence while advocating strongly for the child's needs are important elements in managing such situations. A 'hope for the best, prepare for the worst' approach is often helpful.

Whilst the management of the patient is foremost, involving the family in decisions and information sharing is extremely important. Families will often have a great deal of knowledge about their child's medical condition and in the case of a child with a rare disease, often know more about it than some professionals. In addition many parents will have already been heavily involved in treatment decisions, and will expect this level of involvement to continue.

The structure of families in the UK may now include the natural parents, step-parents, partners, foster parents and siblings not directly related to the child. Organizing effective communication amongst these groups is sometimes challenging but is extremely important, particularly towards the end-of-life.

Siblings require special consideration in paediatric palliative care. They are almost universally distressed, but often feel unable to share this with their parents. Negative outcomes such as developmental regression, school failure and behavioural problems may be seen if the needs of siblings are not adequately addressed (see Chapter 14).

School

The centre of a child's day-to-day life is school, and disruption of this routine can add to a child's sense of isolation and substantiate their feelings of being 'different' from their friends. Peer groups can be an enormous source of support for a child living with a life-limiting disease. For these reasons children often remain in school during treatment and even as death approaches. Keeping schools informed (with the permission of the parents/child) is important so that practical arrangements regarding the support required in school and flexibility of school hours can be discussed. Medical staff can facilitate school attendance by scheduling elective and semi-elective treatments appropriately. For example, the child with bone marrow suppression who really wants to be at school for art on Tuesdays might benefit from having their regular blood transfusion on Monday. As death approaches, the school staff may need support. A plan for supporting staff and pupils through bereavement may also be helpful.

Illness trajectory

This will vary with the particular diagnosis. Often the palliative phase of care in children is much longer than for adults. Indeed, it may extend from the time of diagnosis. There is also commonly a great deal of uncertainty surrounding the prognosis. Children in advanced states of disability and dependence are at high risk of dying from complications like respiratory infections but also have the potential to live many years. Families can find this extremely difficult to cope with, and they may experience negative thoughts and feelings about their situation and about their child.

Physical and emotional exhaustion, as well as concern for the child's suffering, may see them wishing it would all be over. Parents often feel alone with these thoughts, believing they are too terrible to share. The protracted nature of many illness trajectories presents challenges in planning support for the child and their family in terms of both symptom management and psychological support.

Ethical issues in paediatric palliative care

Medical ethics involves the application of ethical principles to medical practice and research.

As in adult palliative care, the most widely used framework for ethical decision-making involves the process of balancing four key principles:

1 **Autonomy**—the right to self-determination
2 **Non-maleficence**—the need to avoid harm
3 **Beneficence**—the ability to do good
4 **Justice**

In palliative care most dilemmas relate to end-of-life situations. In paediatric palliative care the inability of the child to act autonomously adds an extra dimension to the decision-making process.

Autonomy

- In order to act autonomously, one must act with intention and understanding and without controlling influences
- To act autonomously, individuals must demonstrate an understanding of their situation and the implications of their decisions
- They must also be able to communicate their decisions

Children represent a continuum in this regard, from the non-verbal infant to the adolescent striving for self-determination. A child's ability to make informed choices depends on his/her developmental level and life experience. For example, an eight-year-old child with a chronic illness may through his/her own experience and those of fellow patients be better positioned to participate in decision-making than an older child with no previous medical history.

Children may be able to make some decisions about their medical care even where major decisions are made by others. They may, for example, make choices regarding pain control and venepuncture sites. Empowering children in this way gives them a sense of control that impacts positively on their experience of care. Furthermore, even if not deemed sufficiently competent to act autonomously, a child's preferences and insights may guide decision-making by others and should be sought actively.

Decision-making in the palliative care setting requires

- The ability to understand one's illness in physiological terms and to conceptualize death as an irreversible phenomenon
- The capacity to reason and consider future implications (formal operations stage of cognitive development)
- The ability to act autonomously and not acquiesce to the authority of doctors and parents.[3]

The Royal College of Paediatrics and Child Health (UK) describes four levels of child involvement in decision-making:

1 Being informed
2 Being consulted
3 Having views taken into account in decision-making
4 Being respected as the main decision-maker[4]

Age is not necessarily a good measure of capacity although an arbitrary distinction is drawn for legal purposes.

Competence

Even young children have a right to be informed regarding decisions which affect their future. Both the Royal College of Paediatrics and Child Health and the American Academy of Pediatrics advocate strongly for the participation of children in decision-making to the extent that their ability allows.

Competence is assessed according to

- Cognitive ability. This may be reflected in young patients' ability to provide a clinical history as well as their understanding of the condition, treatment options and the consequences of choosing one option over another. Other factors to consider include level of schooling, verbal skills and demonstrated capacity to make decisions
- Presence or absence of disturbed thinking (eg. in the setting of psychiatric disorder)

Treatment should be discussed with parents and the child if appropriate, and ideally both will have an understanding of what is involved. Where this is not the case, providing more time for families to think about issues may help. In extreme circumstances a court of law can be asked to decide what is best.

Decision-making regarding life-sustaining treatment

'Doctors, children and informed parents share the decision; with doctors taking the lead in judging the clinical factors and parents the lead in determining best interests more generally.'[5]

Decisions are made on the grounds of benefits/burdens proportionality. In order to justify a particular intervention, the expected benefits of that intervention must outweigh the burdens.

End-of-life decision-making is a collaborative process. It should involve the child (where possible), the family, and all the health professionals involved in providing care to the child. An important underlying principle of the process is open communication between staff and families.

… 'physicians should do more than offer a 'menu' of choices—they should recommend what they believe is the best option for the patient under the circumstances and give any reasons, based on medical, experiential, or moral factors, for such judgements.'[6]

3 Leikin S. (1989) A proposal concerning decisions to forgo life-sustaining treatment for young people. *J Pediatrics*, **115**: 17–22.

4 Royal College of Paediatrics and Child Health (1997) *Withholding or Withdrawing Life-Saving Treatment in Children: a framework for practice*. London: RCPCH.

5 British Medical Association (2001) *Withholding and Withdrawing Life-prolonging Medical Treatment. Guidance for decision-making*. 2nd edn. London: BMJ Books.

6 American Academy of Paediatrics (1994) Guidelines on forgoing life-sustaining medical treatment. *Pediatrics*, **93**: 532–6.

The Royal College of Paediatrics and Child Health outlines five circumstances under which withholding or withdrawing curative medical treatment may be considered:

- The child has been diagnosed as brain dead according to standard criteria
- Permanent vegetative state. These children have 'a permanent and irreversible lack of awareness of themselves and their surroundings and no ability to interact at any level with those around them'[6]
- 'No chance situation': life-sustaining treatment simply delays death without providing other benefits in terms of relief of suffering
- 'No purpose' situation: the child may be able to survive with treatment but the degree of mental or physical impairment would be so great that it would be unreasonable to ask the child to bear it
- The 'unbearable' situation. In the face of progressive, irreversible illness, the burden of further treatment is more than can be borne

A practical approach to decision-making[7]—questions to be answered

- Is this intervention going to cure the disease?
- Is this intervention going to prevent progression of the disease?
- What impact will the intervention have on the child's quality of life?
- Will the intervention improve the child's symptoms?
- Will the intervention make the child feel worse?
- How long will the child feel worse for?
- What will happen without the intervention?
- How will the intervention change the outcome?

Disagreement

Society invests parents with the responsibility of acting on behalf of their children. There are occasions however, where parents insist on what staff may view as inappropriate treatment. Conversely, parents may refuse treatment that is of potential benefit to the child. It is important that the best interests of the child are advocated for and that decision-making is shared between the family and the healthcare team.

Families often need time to absorb and process difficult information and decision-making should be viewed as a process not an event. Most disagreements can usually be resolved by regular open and honest communication. Where conflict can not be resolved, it may be helpful to request a second opinion from an independent practitioner. It may also be beneficial to include other family members or cultural and religious leaders from the local community. In extreme circumstances where agreement can not be reached despite the above interventions, it may be necessary to seek legal judgement.

Advance directives

Where children have an existing condition, gradual or sudden deterioration may be anticipated. It is helpful for health professionals to assist families in planning for crises so that interventions considered unhelpful to the child are not initiated. Written documentation in the medical record as well as a letter for the family to have with them is required.

Advance directives should record:
- What has been discussed
- Who was present
- What decisions were made
- What the child and family's wishes are regarding various interventions
- Who should be called in case of crisis

Provision of hydration and nutrition
- Food and fluid should always be offered if the child is able to take it by mouth
- Most authors consider the provision of nutrition and hydration by artificial means to be a medical intervention subject to the same benefits/burdens assessment as any other
- The insertion of tubes into the gastrointestinal tract carries with it the burdens of discomfort and the potential for complications, and therefore needs to be justified on the grounds of the benefits it may provide to the patient
- Some argue, however, that the provision of food and fluid constitutes a basic component of humane care and can never be withdrawn or withheld
- In the paediatric setting, this concept is extended by the centrality of feeding to the parental rôle and the vulnerability of infants and small children
- Children in the terminal phase of illness will naturally cease eating and drinking as their requirements decrease, and it is not necessary in these circumstances to provide fluid and nutrition by artificial means

The situation faced by the family and staff is more problematic for children who have been kept alive for long periods prior to deterioration by gastrostomy or central venous feeding. Ethically there may be no difference between withdrawing treatment and not initiating potentially life saving treatment. Emotionally, however, it is often difficult for families not to feel guilty if they believe that by stopping artificial nutrition they are hastening their child's death. The effect of the provision or omission of artificial hydration and nutrition on the timing of death is uncertain. However, it is worth noting that dehydration may contribute to opioid toxicity, delirium and constipation and may require correction to alleviate these distressing clinical symptoms.

Medical ethics in different cultures
It is important to understand the limitations of Western ethics. The beliefs, values and conceptual frameworks used by other cultures must be considered when making decisions with families. The most appropriate source of information is the family itself, as there will be considerable variability within cultural groups.

---

7 Frager G. (1997) Palliative care and terminal care of children. *Child Adolescent Psychiatr Clin North Am*, **6**: 889–909.

Psychosocial needs in paediatric palliative care

Physical, emotional and spiritual needs cannot be addressed in isolation as each affects the other. For example, a child's pain can heighten parental anxiety and family distress may adversely affect pain control. A multidisciplinary approach to palliative care is required and there is therefore the potential for a large number of individuals and services to become involved in the care of the child. Coordination of these professionals and the services each is providing is essential to avoid the replication or omission of services, or disempowerment of the family. This can be achieved with regular communication between team members and the appointment of a key worker for each child. This person may be a general practitioner, paediatrician, nurse or an allied health worker.

> Providing emotional and psychological support for the sick child is as essential as providing relief of physical symptoms.

Communicating with children about death and dying

> A child can live through anything so long as he or she is told the truth and is allowed to share with loved ones the natural feelings people have when they are suffering..
>
> Herbert, 1997[8]

Parents may instinctively want to protect their children from 'bad news'. However, children very often know a great deal about their illness and prognosis. Children may not reveal what they know for fear of upsetting their parents, who then falsely assume their child knows very little. Children are very sensitive to discrepancies between verbal and non-verbal information. They readily sense distress in those around them and may feel anxious and isolated as a result. They may also generate fantasies to explain unusual behaviour in their parents (eg. 'I have been bad', 'Mummy and Daddy don't love me any more'). These notions may be more frightening than death and dying to a young child. This is particularly true of younger children, who are naturally egocentric and believe that the world revolves around them, and hence, personalize other people's emotional and behavioural reactions.

- Parents' reluctance to talk to their child about dying usually stems from an erroneous belief that their child's concept of death is similar to that of an adult's, and their consequent desire to protect them from emotional pain
- Younger childrens' greatest fear is usually around immobility and separation from loved ones during their illness and after. Opening up discussions about death can help allay these fears and provide reassurance to the child

- School-aged children frequently have worries about experiencing pain and can be greatly reassured by discussions about pain control. They may also ask questions about what will happen after their death, and can receive great comfort from religious or family beliefs about what will happen to them
- Just as parents and siblings need to plan the time they have left with the sick child in order to build memories and have as few regrets as possible, the dying child may also wish to prioritize the time left to do special activities or spend time with loved ones

Children very often ask staff questions about their illness and prognosis. When confronted by a difficult question, staff may be uncertain as to how best to respond. Questions often come unexpectedly, when the staff member is especially busy or distracted. Children generally know the answer to the question before they ask it. In this way the child who asks 'Am I dying?', may already know the answer. What they seek is a person who can be trusted to speak honestly with them. Responding with a question such as 'What makes you ask me that?' or 'What is it that makes you think you are going to die?' may elicit information on which to base a response. The real question may be something completely different. Of course children, just like adults, are very individual in how they respond, and while some children may ask plenty of questions and request lots of information, other children may wish to hear limited information. It is important to be guided by the child, and also to remind them that they can ask questions whenever they wish.

8 Herbert, M. (1996) *Supporting Bereaved and Dying Children and their Parents.* Leicester: BPS Books.

Supporting the sick child

These ideas mirror the supportive measures used in adult palliative care.
- Listen
  - Ask the child how he/she would like to be supported
  - Find out exactly what it is the child wants to know
  - Let the child set the pace
- Allow the child to make choices where possible
- Explain things in simple language appropriate to the child's development and cognitive ability
- Wherever possible answer questions honestly
- Answer the question that is being asked. Try not to burden the child with too much unsolicited information
- Children may find it easier to talk while drawing or doing some other activity. They may also find it helpful to talk in an abstract way eg. about a character in a story or during play with dolls
- Artwork, play, story writing, music and other creative activities may provide an outlet for emotion
- Normalize feelings of fear, anger and sadness
- Try not to dismiss a child's beliefs unless they are potentially damaging
- Model and encourage expression of emotion. Children need to know they can express their feelings without alienating those around them
- Provide physical contact and comfort
- Maintain routine to the greatest extent possible
- Involve the child's friends in visits. If this is not possible, encourage letters, photos, email, videos etc. Discourage social isolation but allow time for privacy

Recruit the child's school teacher to help—this may be helpful even where children are not able to attend school.[9]

9 Herbert, M. (1996) *Supporting Bereaved and Dying Children and their Parents.* Leicester: BPS Books.

Supporting parents

Communicating difficult information to parents

The way in which difficult information is communicated is important and sets the stage for the working relationship between professionals and family. Health professionals need to be aware of how their own feelings of anxiety, sadness and impotence may influence this process. Most parents desire a realistic appraisal of their child's condition delivered empathically and with a sense of hope. Realistic hope can be offered in terms of ongoing support from the team, attention to symptoms and help to maximize the child's quality of life. In situations where the family is pursuing curative treatment, hope can be maintained by 'hoping for the best but preparing for the worst'.

How should difficult news be delivered?

- Empathically
- In person, face-to-face
- Allow plenty of time
- Establish what the parents know or suspect e.g. 'How do you think things are going?'
- Allow the family to set the pace
- Respect silence and do not feel compelled to fill it
- Allow expression of emotion
- Avoid being evasive
- Offer to help inform other family members e.g. siblings, grandparents
- Offer to meet again soon

What information should be given?

- Honest accurate information devoid of technical jargon
- Try to determine what the family wish to know e.g. 'Are you the sort of person who likes to know everything or just the basic information?'
- Simple language—there will be time later to explore details
- Avoid ambiguous language such as 'we might lose the battle' or 'he's passed away'. The words death or dying should be used

A brief outline of the expected disease course should be given and expected symptoms mentioned. It may also be helpful for some families to understand what can be done for these symptoms. Many parents have not experienced the death of a relative or friend and may be frightened at the prospect of seeing someone die. Information about the bodily changes that accompany death may be helpful, and it is possible to be very reassuring about the process as, for most children who are managed carefully, it is very peaceful. Families may be worried about pain and distress or a final dramatic event. In most cases, however, the terminal phase is characterized by the progressive shut down of the various organ systems.

Parental reaction to bad news

Parents are often so shocked on being told that their child is dying, even if this is confirmation of their own suspicions, that they can not assimilate any other information at that moment. It is important to slow the process down, provide multiple opportunities to speak with the family, repeat information where necessary and provide written information. Following the initial shock, parents may feel confused and overwhelmed. They may be frightened that they will not be able to cope with the child's physical care or be able to control their emotions. Parents also experience feelings of uncertainty. They may have difficulty making sense of what is happening and are unsure of what to do first.

Denial occurs occasionally. For some parents it may be an adaptive defence and does not always need to be 'broken down'. In fact, great caution should be exercised in confronting denial. Where denial is impairing optimal care and family functioning, however, it may be helpful to gently challenge inconsistencies and explore underlying concerns. Asking a question like, 'Is there ever a time even for a few seconds where you worry things might not turn out the way you hope?' may provide a window of opportunity for the parent to work through the issues confronting them.

Anger may arise from fear and confusion, often as an expression of despair. Parents feel an enormous loss of power and control in their lives. Their sense of justice is rocked. The struggle to understand, make sense of the situation and control emotions can produce anger. This may be directed at staff. In managing angry parents, it is important:
• To acknowledge the anger e.g. 'I can see you're very angry'
• Not to take it personally
• Not to be defensive
• To allow ventilation of the anger 'Can you tell me more about what you're feeling?'
• Not to dismiss the complaint or try and explain the situation logically
• To set limits 'I can see you are angry and I am willing to speak with you about it but I can not let you damage property/threaten me etc.'

Guilt is another common reaction amongst parents of dying children. They may feel that they failed to recognize and respond effectively to the symptoms of the child's illness. They may feel responsible because the illness is inherited. They may experience 'survivor guilt', believing that children are not supposed to die before their parents. They may believe that their action or inaction somehow triggered the illness. Parents may externalize these feelings and blame others. Staff members occasionally find themselves unfairly blamed for a child's illness or death. This may feel hurtful, but it is important not to become defensive or allow this to impact on the care of the child. Any inclination to label the family as 'bad' should also be avoided.

What parents need to know
Explaining to parents that children often ask questions about their illness and prognosis provides a key opportunity for them to consider how they might deal with these themselves.

Planning in advance is helpful and a team approach, with parents forming part of the team, essential. Parents bring particular knowledge of their child as a unique individual. Staff bring knowledge of the literature in this area and experience with other families in similar circumstances.

Families need to know that:

- Children are generally more aware of their prognosis than those around them believe
- If a child does not ask questions or speak about his/her illness it does not mean that he/she is oblivious or indifferent. Children often protect parents by feigning ignorance— 'mutual pretence'
- The anxiety generated by misinformation is potentially more harmful than any arising from the truth. Children may have all sorts of worries and fantasies, many of which an adult might not expect. What will happen to the cat? Will my school friends forget me? Will somebody be with me? Are mummy and daddy breaking up? Are mummy and daddy cross with me? Did I get sick because I was bad? Will it hurt? To a young child, abandonment and withdrawal of their parent's love may be more frightening than the notion of death because they have not yet acquired a full understanding of death. An environment of honesty provides the child with opportunities to share these worries. They need to feel they can trust those around them
- A dying child may be better able to cope with news of their impending death than their parents
- They are important rôle models. Children look to their parents for cues regarding the appropriate way of reacting to a given situation. While courage and calm will help reassure a child, it is also reasonable for parents to show their sadness. It is helpful for children to understand why their parents are upset so that they do not make incorrect assumptions. An honest explanation may be reassuring

In extreme cases where parents still insist that information is withheld but the child is clearly distressed by this approach, the health professional's duty is to the child.

While, in general, honesty is the best approach, it is important to recognize that not all children benefit from detailed information and not all parents feel able to communicate openly with their child. The best interests of the child are what is important. Cultural factors also require careful consideration.

Parents' needs and the rôle of the health professional

Information: Parents generally want information so that they know what to expect. They may also want to discuss treatment options and plans for symptom control. Parents say that full information allows them to make decisions and helps them plan for the remaining time they have with their child. In general, it is best to be open and honest as a trusting relationship between parents and healthcare workers provides a solid foundation for the challenges of palliative care. It is also helpful to regularly check that families are not being overwhelmed with too much information (e.g. 'I know this is a lot of information for you to hear all at once. We can talk in more detail a little bit later on if you would prefer').

Time to be listened to: Many parents want to discuss their situation with the many healthcare workers involved in their child's care. They may need to speak about their concerns, fears, hopes, and expectations on numerous occasions to clarify and make sense of a world gone awry. The healthcare worker (whether it be a paediatrician, social worker, or nurse) needs to provide time and opportunities for parents to share these concerns. By listening to the concerns of parents, providing guidance, affirming their skills and resources and staying with them, staff can make a major difference to how a family copes. It is important to remember that some parents do not wish to have such discussions and individual coping styles should be respected.

Control: Parents talk of losing control of their lives. The healthcare worker can assist parents to regain a sense of control by providing them with information, including them in discussions regarding care, allowing them to decide who is allowed to visit and when, and so on. Making decisions for (rather than with) a family can be deskilling and destructive. Parents need to be viewed as competent partners in their child's care.

Emotional support: Parents with a sick child grieve for the 'normal' child they no longer have. With this grief comes a range of strong feelings and emotions which add to the task of caring. Parents need acknowledgement, compassion, empathy and non-judgemental understanding. Spiritual support may or may not be part of a family's support system when their child becomes sick. The child's illness may cause parents to question their faith, renew their faith or explore new avenues. Spirituality includes, but is not restricted to, religion. Local clergy, ministers of all faiths and other spiritual leaders are available to help during this confusing time.

Amidst major changes to their routines and view of the world, families may try to hang on to some sense of normality. Health professionals can facilitate this by scheduling treatment around important activities and school attendance, and encouraging the family to maintain routines and activities.

Practical support: Parents need advice and guidance from various professionals in order to learn what is available to help them. Most parents would not know where to begin if they have not had any previous experience. Liaison between the hospital and community team is a helpful step.

Medical equipment may be required as part of the child's care, either routinely or in an emergency. It is possible to have equipment items on loan from a hospital or community agency such as a palliative care service. Health professionals including social workers, occupational therapists and physiotherapists may be needed to make assessments of the child and family's needs.

Sibling needs

The needs of siblings are very similar to those of the dying child.[10]

Relationships within families and communication patterns are important factors in determining how siblings react to a brother or sister's illness. It may be easier for children to adapt to having a sick sibling in a family where it is usual to discuss matters openly and to share feelings and emotions.

Physical symptoms may develop such as nausea, vomiting, diarrhoea, constipation, headache and aching limbs. Symptoms similar to those experienced by the sick sibling may also be reported. Behavioural changes may occur including unusual aggression, temper tantrums or withdrawal from family or friends, rudeness, bullying and demanding attention. Regression in the form of thumb-sucking, enuresis, toileting problems or school refusal may occur. Sleeping problems include a fear of the dark, nightmares, waking in the night and wanting to sleep in the parents' bed. Older children and adolescents may withdraw completely or indulge in risk-taking behaviour.

It is important to note that some siblings will not experience any of the above.

Information—parents should be encouraged to be honest with siblings and to provide them with information at a level appropriate to their developmental stage. This might include facts about the illness, what treatment is being given, and what to expect. They may need reassurance that they and their parents are not likely to become ill and that nothing they did or said caused the illness. Siblings may have concerns regarding their own health and if they are reporting symptoms may benefit from the reassurance of a thorough physical examination by their doctor.

Routine

Whilst difficult to maintain at a time of such upheaval, familiar routines are important for a child's sense of security. This includes going to school, continuing with extracurricular activities and maintaining contact with his/her own peer group. Siblings may need to know that it is acceptable to have fun.

Emotional support—Siblings may try to protect their parents from added distress by not burdening them with their own worries. Many are known to suffer in silence. Unexpressed emotion may manifest as school failure, behavioural problems and physical symptoms. Siblings may also try to excel at school to 'cheer their parents up'. Feelings of resentment, jealousy, isolation, fear, guilt, anger and despair need to be explored, acknowledged and normalized. It is helpful if parents are able to dedicate special time to be with their well children. Some parents may need permission to do this as they feel guilty if they leave the sick child's side.

Contact with the sick child—Regular visits to the sick child in hospital allow siblings to see what is happening for themselves. It is important however that they are adequately prepared for what they might see e.g. 'John is very sleepy. He might not be able to talk to you but he will know you are there. He has medicine running into his body through a tube in his arm...this doesn't hurt etc.' In the rare circumstance where siblings cannot visit, regular updates, videos and photos can be helpful. Siblings can feel included by sending drawings, favourite toys, photos and videos to their brother or sister.

Inclusion in the care of the sick child—Siblings may benefit from the opportunity to be included in the care of the sick child and in the family's experience. Children can help by taking a drink to the child, changing the channel on the TV, reading a story, playing games, and taking the cat in to visit.

School—It is helpful if the sibling's school teachers are kept informed (with the family's permission) of the sick child's condition. Schools can also help by identifying one person to whom the sibling can go if they need help.

10 Goldman A. (1994) *Care of the Dying Child*. Oxford: Oxford University Press.

Community-based care

Most children who need palliative care will be looked after in, and by, their local community. It makes sense then that the community team is involved from early in the child's illness so that relationships are well established by the time the child's care needs increase. Resources available to families may include:

- General practitioner who will often know the child and family
- Community-based paediatrician
- Palliative care services
- Paediatric palliative care services
- Domiciliary nursing
- Respite
- Children's hospices
- Counselling
- Religious groups
- Family and friends
- Community agencies (which may offer family support and financial assistance)

Since children will often move between hospital and community settings, it is important that there is a collaborative approach to care and communication flows easily and appropriately. The use of a key worker can facilitate such communication.

The nature of the care available in a particular situation will vary a great deal depending on the particular community services available. Services are changing rapidly and it is important to check on current service availablity before planning community care. Non-evidence-based optimism or pessimism about the community service availability can cause much needless distress for the child and family.

Bereavement (📖 see Chapter 14)

Death and dying

- Most adult palliative care programmes become involved with patients towards the end-of-life
- In contrast children's programmes aim to identify children close to the time of diagnosis and provide services and support to the family as they progress through the disease process and eventual death
- Most children and their families wish to spend as much time at home as possible, and many hope to be able to care for their child during the terminal phase provided adequate support is available
- Some families will find this task extremely difficult and will wish to return to a hospital or hospice environment close to the time of death
- This should not be viewed as a failure of home care

The dying process

Taken from *A Practical Guide to Paediatric Oncology Palliative Care*, Royal Children's Hospital, Brisbane, 1999.

The actual dying process is usually an orderly and undramatic progressive series of physical changes which are not medical emergencies requiring invasive interventions. Parents need to know that these physical changes are a normal part of the dying process. It is very important that families are well supported at this time. If the child is dying at home, 24-hour support from experienced staff who they know and trust can make an enormous difference. Home visits by the GP, domiciliary nurse and oncology liaison nurse where appropriate, to assist with managing the child's symptoms, are greatly appreciated by the family. This is a very emotional and difficult time for the whole family.

Restlessness and agitation

Generally the child will spend an increasing amount of time sleeping, in part due to progressive disease and changes in the body's metabolism, but this may also be due to progressive anaemia or sedation from opioids required for pain relief.

Some children remain alert and responsive until the moment of death. Others may become confused, semiconscious or unconscious for several hours or days. Restlessness and agitation during the terminal phase is not uncommon and may be due to increasing pain, hypoxia, nausea, fear and anxiety. Agitation may be the child's only way of communicating distress. A calm peaceful environment and the presence of parents and family will assist in relieving the child's anxiety. Speech may become increasingly difficult to understand and words confused. Even though the child may not be able to communicate, they may be aware of people around them. Hearing may well be the last sense to be lost and the family should be encouraged to talk to the dying child. They may like to play their child's favourite music, read stories or just sit with and touch their child so the child knows they are not alone.

If agitation continues additional drugs may be needed (see medication section 'Agitation' and 'Terminal restlessness' pages for drugs and doses). Treatment is directed at inducing a degree of sedation appropriate for the individual child. At this stage oral medications may not be tolerated and alternative routes of medication are essential.

A continuous subcutaneous infusion of opioid and e.g. midazolam in a syringe driver is effective in controlling pain, agitation and restlessness. For the child dying at home it is important that the treating hospital/hospice has dispensed (or made provision for the general practitioner to organize) a home care pack containing drugs that may be required in the terminal phase of care. This ensures drugs are available in the home if and when the child requires them. Without a home care pack there may be a considerable delay in getting drugs required for symptom relief.

Doses of medication should be recorded for parents on a treatment sheet. Occasionally haloperidol is required when the benzodiazepines are unsuccessful. Regular monitoring of effectiveness of medication is essential. Additional drugs can be added to the syringe driver if needed.

Noisy/rattly breathing
Excessive secretions or difficulty in clearing pharyngeal secretions will lead to noisy breathing. Generally this occurs during the terminal phase of the child's illness and is associated with a diminished conscious state. It can also be problematic for children with neurodegenerative diseases or brainstem lesions where swallowing is impaired. Positioning on the side or slightly head down will allow some postural drainage and this may be all that is required. Reassurance and explanation to the family is essential as the noise of the gurgling can be very distressing to the family, while the child is usually unaware and untroubled by the noise and sensation.

Anticholinergic drugs can be used to reduce the production of secretions, and a portable suction machine at home may be of benefit for children with chronic conditions or those who are unconscious (see medication section 'Noisy breathing' for drugs and doses).

Incontinence
There may be a relaxation of the muscles of the gastrointestinal and urinary tracts, resulting in incontinence of stool and urine. It is important to discuss with parents this possibility and how they wish to manage incontinence. If the child is close to death parents are often reluctant for a catheter to be inserted to drain urine and may choose to use incontinence pads or disposable incontinence draw sheets. It is important for the family that their child's dignity is respected. Disposable draw sheets are also useful for incontinence diarrhoea.

Eye changes
The pupils of a dying person become fixed and dilated. The eyes may become sunken or bulging and glazed. Eye secretions can be removed with a warm damp cloth. If eyes are bulging, which can occur with neuroblastoma, the cornea should be protected and lubricated.

Circulatory and respiratory changes
As the heart slows and the heartbeat becomes irregular, circulation of blood is decreased to the extremities. The child's hands, feet and face may be cold, pale and cyanotic. The child may also sweat profusely and feel damp to touch. Parents may wish to change their child's clothes and keep them warm with a blanket. Respiration may be rapid, shallow and irregular

then may slow with periods of apnoea (Cheyne–Stokes breathing). This breathing pattern is distressing for parents and siblings to witness, and they need reassurance that it is a normal part of the dying process and that it is not distressing to the dying child.

It is important to inform parents that when death occurs the child may again be incontinent of urine and stool. There may also be ooze from the mouth and nose, particularly if they roll their child to undress and wash him/her. Parents who are not prepared will be distressed when this occurs.

In our efforts to achieve a peaceful death for the child, it is essential that symptoms are closely monitored and that there is ongoing assessment of effectiveness of therapeutic interventions. Early detection of symptoms and appropriate intervention is crucial to achieve a pain-free and peaceful death for the child.

Staff support

The death of a child is a relatively unusual event and the modern paediatrician is more familiar with cure and prevention than with death and dying. While advances in medicine have lead to happier outcomes for the majority of children, there remains a group for whom cure is impossible. The relative infrequency with which death occurs in childhood has implications for those caring for this group of children. Staff may feel a sense of failure and impotence. A lack of exposure to dying children may leave them feeling ill-equipped to support a child and family through this phase of their care. They may also have become very attached to the child and family and experience their own grief. All of these responses are normal but in the absence of adequate self-awareness and support, health professionals may, over time, become 'burnt out'.

Burn-out is 'the progressive loss of idealism, energy and purpose experienced by people in the helping professions as a result of the conditions of their work'.[11] This may manifest as excessive cynicism, a loss of interest in work and a sense of 'going through the motions'. Other features include fatigue, difficulty concentrating, depression, anxiety, insomnia, irritability and the inappropriate use of drugs or alcohol. The consequences for families are significant as staff affected in this way may:
• avoid families or blame them for difficult situations
• be unable to help families define treatment goals and make
  optimal decisions
• experience physical signs of stress when seeing families

The quality of care may be compromised and families may become disenchanted with the health professional and seek help elsewhere, sometimes from inappropriate sources.

Risk factors

There are a number of risk factors for the development of behaviours and responses which may impact upon patient care and these can be categorised in the following way:

- Clinician-related
  - Identification with the family or situation
  - Unresolved loss and grief in own past
  - Fear of death and disability
  - Psychiatric disorder
  - Inability to tolerate uncertainty
- Family-related
  - Anger, depression
  - Uncooperative families
  - Family member is a health professional
  - Complex or dysfunctional family dynamics
  - Well known to staff (e.g. friends, relatives, colleagues)
  - Intractable pain or difficult symptoms
- Situation-related
  - Family member/s are friends or relatives of the clinician
  - Uncertainty/ambiguity
- Disagreement about goals of care
  - Patient/clinician
  - Team
- Protracted hospitalization[12]

While it is common for health professionals to experience emotions such as anger and sadness in the course of clinical care, it is important that these do not result in behaviours which could compromise the quality of that care. Recognition of the emotion helps control it to some extent as does accepting the normality of experiencing emotion. It may also be helpful to seek out a trusted colleague to whom you can talk.

11 Edelwich J., Brodsky A. (1980) *Burn-out: Stages of disillusionment in the helping professions.* New York: Human Sciences PR.

12 Meier D. E., Back A. L., Morrison S. (2001) The inner life of physicians and care of the seriously ill. *JAMA*, **286**: 3007–14.

13 Vachon M. L. S. (1995) Staff stress in hospice/palliative care: a review. *Pall Med* **9**: 91–122.

Strategies for self care

Stress amongst staff who provide palliative care for children, in any setting, is likely to be great, and the stresses involved in providing palliative care for children may affect the caregiver's ability to provide care in a sensitive and professional manner. Regular supervision and access to professional expertise by staff in areas where long-term relationships with patients and families are built up are important, and should ideally be written into job descriptions.[14]

There are a number of ways in which staff may be supported:

- Formal support through regular team meetings reduces conflict between staff members as long as open discussion is encouraged. This is dependent on the structure of the team and the quality of facilitation.
- Formal support at an individual level is beneficial for some. It is particularly useful in circumstances where concerns can not be raised in the group context
- Informal peer support is generally regarded by staff as most effective[15]
- Support from family and friends
- Maintaining perspective through involvement in outside activities. Formal supervision may assist in developing the self-awareness necessary to achieve this
- Education provides staff with the skills they require to overcome feelings of impotence. In a recent survey of resident medical officers in the United Kingdom, lack of training in the breaking of bad news was identified as a serious deficiency in their education[16]

The care of the dying child presents enormous challenges but if done well, has the potential to bring lasting benefits to both the family and the health professional.

14 Association for Children with Life-threatening or Terminal Conditions and their Families and the Royal College of Paediatrics and Child Health (2003) *A Guide to the Development of Children's Palliative Care Services.* 2nd edn. London: ACT.

15 Woolley H., Stein A., Forrest G. C., Baum J. D. (1989) Staff stress and job satisfaction at a children's hospice. *Arch Dis Child,* **64**: 114–18.

16 Dent A., Condon L., Blair P., Fleming P. (1996) A study of bereavement care after a sudden and unexpected death. *Arch Dis Child,* **74**: 522–6.

The Association for Children with Life Threatening or Terminal Conditions and their Families (ACT) Charter

The diverse needs of children have led to the development of a national association, ACT (Association for the Care of Children with Life-threatening or Terminal Conditions and their Families).

As a service to such children and families ACT has developed the following charter.

1 Every child shall be treated with dignity and respect and shall be afforded privacy whatever the child's physical or intellectual ability.
2 Parents shall be acknowledged as the primary carers, and shall be centrally involved as partners in all care and decisions involving their child.
3 Every child shall be given the opportunity to participate in decisions affecting his or her care, according to age and understanding
4 Every family shall be given the opportunity of a consultation with a paediatric specialist who has a particular knowledge of the child's condition.
5 Information shall be provided for the parents, and for the child and the siblings, according to age and understanding. The needs of other relatives shall also be addressed
6 An honest and open approach shall be the basis of all communication which shall be sensitive and appropriate to age and understanding.
7 The family home shall remain the centre of caring whenever possible. All other care shall be provided by paediatric trained staff in a child-centred environment.
8 Every child shall have access to education. Efforts shall be made to engage in other childhood activities.
9 Every family shall be entitled to a named key worker who will enable the family to build up and maintain an appropriate support system.
10 Every family shall have access to flexible respite care in their own home and in a home from home setting for the whole family, with appropriate paediatric nursing and medical support.
11 Every family shall have access to expert, sensitive advice in procuring practical aids and financial support.
12 Every family shall have access to paediatric nursing support in the home, when required.
13 Every family shall have access to domestic help at times of stress at home.
14 Bereavement support shall be offered to the whole family and be available for as long as required.

Drugs and doses

The following section is divided into the common symptoms experienced by very ill children and outlines a management strategy for each.

- Agitation
- Anorexia
- Bleeding
- Breathlessness
- Constipation
- Convulsions
- Cough
- Gastro-oesophageal reflux
- Hiccup
- Infection
- Mouthcare
- Muscle spasm
- Nausea and vomiting
- Noisy breathing
- Pain
- Other pain syndromes
- Psychological issues
- Raised intracranial pressure
- Skin
- Sweating
- Terminal restlessness
- Emergency Drugs Summary

Introduction to drugs and doses

The approach to the care of a dying child and his/her family greatly influences the quality of their lives and the ability of the parents and siblings to cope with the child's death. Most symptoms are readily amenable to effective management. It is important, however, to adopt an individualized approach, taking into account the unique circumstances of each child and family.

Planning care

Medical assessment

- Make sure you are armed with as much information about the child and his family as possible
- Make sure you involve all the right people: this might include parents, siblings, grandparents and other carers. Whether you involve the child him/herself will depend on the child's age, understanding and state of health and the parents' wishes. It is often helpful to have another involved professional present, for example the district nurse in the community setting, so that someone else is fully aware of the discussion and can answer any questions the family might have after you have left
- Try and arrange things so that you are not in a hurry and are unlikely to be disturbed
- Be methodical: take a thorough history, and perform a full examination. Allow the child and parents time to voice their concerns as fully as possible

Explanations

- Explain symptoms and management
- Identify any misconceptions the child or family may have and address these (e.g. concerns about opioids causing addiction or hastening death)
- You may not have all the answers: if not, say so

Plans

- Identify, articulate and document the current goals of care
- Formulate a plan of action in consultation with the parents and/or child. Listen to any concerns that arise from this and be prepared to compromise on a management plan if the parents/child want something different
- Ensure there is a plan for the exacerbation of current symptoms and the development of new ones. Knowledge of the child's condition will be important here and expertise may be required from sub-specialists
- In most cases it is possible to **anticipate** either a worsening of current symptoms or the development of new symptoms, and it is vital that this is planned for so that appropriate medications and support are available
- Families need access to advice and support around the clock
- Run over the plan at the end of the consultation in language the parents and/or the child can understand
- It may be helpful to write the plan down and give a copy to the family

Review

Make a time/date when the management plan will be reviewed, and by whom.

Communication
- Make sure family members/carers know how to contact professionals, particularly out of normal working hours
- Liaise with relevant professionals and carers—leave clear written instructions in medical records or contact the community team to discuss directly—many different healthcare professionals may be involved particularly in the community, and it is important that everyone is aware of any changes in management
- It is often helpful to identify a key worker for the family

Routes for drug administration
According to the bioavailability of the drug and patient preference, different routes of administration should be considered for each drug prescribed. These include:
- Oral
- Sublingual
- Buccal
- Nasal
- Intravenous
- Subcutaneous
- Transdermal
- Rectal
- Epidural

The syringe driver
A syringe driver is a small portable battery driven infusion pump used to give continuous medication parenterally, usually over a 24h period. Syringe drivers can deliver medication intravenously (e.g. via a central venous catheter) or subcutaneously. This route of delivery is particularly suitable for children who are unable to tolerate oral medication or who require immediate control of difficult symptoms, which are resistant to oral medication. Although it is a common route by which to administer medication at the end-of-life, it can also be used for short periods prior to this to gain control of difficult symptoms or when the oral route is temporarily impractical (e.g. persistent vomiting).

Indications for using a syringe driver

- Unable to absorb or refusing oral medication
- Difficulty swallowing
- Persistent vomiting
- Bowel obstruction
- Not fully conscious
- Unsatisfactory response to oral medication

Advantages of using this delivery system are:
1 Continuous blood levels of medication
2 Less requirement for needles
3 Maintenance of mobility and independence
4 The ability to deliver complex drug combinations safely

Providing they are compatible, certain common combinations of drugs can be mixed together and given in the same syringe driver. In circumstances where high concentrations of drugs are required or the agents are unstable or incompatible, separate syringe drivers may be needed. As a general rule, it is advisable not to mix more than three drugs in any one syringe—check compatibility first.

A continuous infusion delivered via a Patient Controlled Analgesia (PCA) system is an alternative to the syringe driver and has been used effectively in the postoperative setting by children as young as 7yrs. This device provides a background continuous infusion and allows the patient to administer bolus p.r.n. doses of analgesia by pressing a 'boost' button. The dose and number of p.r.n. doses available is preset and the device has a 'lock-out' facility which prevents overdose.

Setting up a syringe driver (📖 see Chapter 6a)
Drug information
This document was written in January 2004. Whilst every effort has been made to ensure all information is accurate, it remains the responsibility of the prescriber to check this information against the most current available before administering any of the drugs in this document.

It is important to note that doses of the same medication may vary for different indications and this document should be consulted by symptom section rather than drug name.

Due to limitations of space, information regarding all side-effects and interactions for each drug are not included; further information regarding this should be sought from more detailed texts such as Royal College of Paediatrics and Child Health *Medicines for Children*[17] and the *British National Formulary*[18,19]. Many of the medications recommended in this text are not licensed for use in children or for the indications or by the routes for which they are suggested. This is a problem experienced not only by those who care for dying children but by paediatricians more generally. It is often necessary to prescribe medications 'off licence'. The recommendations that follow are based on evidence where it is available as well as the practice experience of clinicians working in paediatric palliative care and pain management. In the UK, unlicensed use is permitted at the discretion of the prescriber, and is the prescriber's responsibility.

17 Royal College of Paediatrics and Child Health (2003) *Medicines for Children*. 2nd edn. London: RCPH.

18 Prescribing for children (2004) *British National Formulary*. **48**: 12–13.

19 Prescribing in palliative care (2004) *British National Formulary*. **48**: 15–18.

Agitation/delirium

Consider the following causes:
- Terminal restlessness
- Uncontrolled pain
- Medication (e.g. benzodiazepines, polypharmacy)
- Gastro-oesophageal reflux
- Urinary retention
- Constipation
- Dehydration
- Sepsis
- Cerebral causes: raised intracranial pressure, intracranial bleed
- Hypoxia
- Environmental irritation: too hot/cold/bright light
- Fear/anxiety
- Nausea
- Positioning

Terminal restlessness

Restlessness and agitation are not uncommon in the terminal phase of illness. Families may need reassurance that these symptoms are part of the dying process and, although difficult to witness, may not be causing distress to the child. (📖 See section on Terminal restlessness, p. 546.)

Uncontrolled pain

Take a careful history and fully examine the child before excluding pain. Children in chronic pain may not be as demonstrative as those in acute pain. Indeed, they may appear quiet and withdrawn. In children unable to communicate, ask parents and carers how their child expresses pain. Look for facial expressions such as frowning and grimacing during examination and turning/mobilizing for clues.

In the setting of uncontrolled pain, sedation does not address the underlying problem. Indeed, it may render a child in pain unable to communicate this to those caring for them.

Urinary retention

Children with neurodegenerative disease or those on opioids may have problems with retention of urine. Constipation may exacerbate this problem. Retention predisposes to urinary tract infection, which will add to the discomfort. If a urinary tract infection is suspected, consider sending an appropriate sample for analysis. Antibiotic treatment is likely to reduce any discomfort caused by infection. Retention may be relieved by gentle bladder massage or a warm bath. Bethanechol or carbechol may also be helpful. Catheterization is only occasionally necessary and need not be a permanent solution.

Constipation

Common causes include analgesia (particularly opioids), dehydration and immobility. Poor diet may be contributing but may not be rectifiable. (📖 See section on Constipation, p. 492.)

Medication

Check drug chart for medications that may increase agitation.

Sepsis

Check temperature and examine for source of infection: wounds, Hickman lines and bladder are possible sites to consider. Swab/send samples as appropriate but first consider whether doing so will affect your management. Discuss whether treatment is appropriate/desirable with the child, their parents and other professionals involved. Sometimes treatment may be appropriate even in the terminal phase to control unpleasant symptoms. (📖 See section on Infection, p. 506.)

Cerebral causes

Raised intracranial pressure, intracranial bleeds.

History and careful neurological examination may help with this diagnosis. Consider whether investigation is in the best interests of the child and whether it will influence management.

Hypoxia

Invasive tests should be avoided. Pulse oximetry may be helpful.

Environmental irritation

Too hot/cold, bright light.

Fear/Anxiety

Discuss directly with the child if possible and appropriate. Children may have concerns that adults don't consider (e.g. they might be worried about pets or who's going to look after their parents). Explanations and reassurance are helpful if the child is able to identify and talk about what is worrying them. Children are often worried about being left alone, so make sure someone they trust is with them. Placing familiar objects near the child is also useful if they are not being nursed at home. Photos of family and friends, toys and stuffed animals are examples. Many children benefit from learning simple relaxation or guided imagery techniques. Anxiolytics may be necessary if other measures fail.

Nausea

Check history and drug chart for likely causes and treat/adjust medication as appropriate.

Gastro-oesophageal reflux/indigestion

Common in very disabled children. Also a possibility in children taking steroids or undergoing chemotherapy/radiotherapy. (📖 See section on Gastro-oesophageal reflux, p. 504.)

Positioning

The child may simply not be comfortable, and this may be frustrating for a child unable to turn himself. It may be worth adjusting the child's position if you suspect this may be a problem.

Delirium

Is characterized by:
- Disturbed consciousness and impaired attention
- Cognitive disturbances such as disorientation and memory impairment
- An acute or subacute onset and fluctuation throughout the day

Often there is a prodrome in the form of restlessness, sleep disturbance, irritability and anxiety. Early recognition and treatment are important.

Management

General measures
- Treat any reversible cause if possible and appropriate (make sure the child is not in pain)
- Nurse the child in a quiet and safe environment surrounded by familiar people and objects
- If other measures are unsuccessful, pharmacological intervention may be necessary
- Benzodiazepines are the most commonly used medication in this setting. Haloperidol may also be helpful, and is not too sedating
- Benzodiazepines are generally very effective but occasionally a paradoxical increase in irritability may be seen
- Families may need to understand that the child may not be as responsive once medication is given, but that the priority is the child's comfort

Medication

Benzodiazepines

The choice of benzodiazepine will depend on the circumstance for which it is being prescribed. Children experiencing brief periods of anxiety or panic attacks may benefit from a benzodiazepine with a very short half-life, such as midazolam, given buccally or subcutaneously. Sublingual lorazepam is another option for panic attacks or anxiety related to dyspnoea. Children needing a longer duration of action may do better with diazepam or clonazepam. Levomepromazine may be an appropriate agent for children who also have nausea and pain.

Lorazepam
- Short half-life
- Form:
  - Tablets: 1mg (scored), 2.5mg
  - Oral suspension: only available as 'special'
  - Injection: 4mg in 1mL, 1mL ampoule
- Dose (sublingual, oral): all ages: 25–50 mcg/kg (max. 4mg/24h in adults)
- Injectable form can be given sublingually
- Most children will not need more than 0.5–1mg for a trial dose. Well absorbed sublingually (good for panic attacks) and parent/child has control
- Contra-indications and warnings: severe pulmonary disease, sleep apnoea, coma, CNS depression. Caution in hepatic and renal failure
- Licence: tablets are licensed as premedication in children >5yrs. Injection not licensed in children <12yrs except for treatment of status epilepticus

Clonazepam
- Long half-life
- Form:
  - Drops: 2.5mg in 1mL (1 drop = 0.1mg), named patient basis
  - Tablet: 0.5mg, 2mg
  - Injection: 1mg in 1mL
  - Oral liquid: 500 mcg in 5mL, 2mg in 5mL 'specials'
- Dose (sublingual): all ages 0.01mg/kg/dose (max. 0.5mg) b.d./t.d.s.
- If necessary, increase by 10–25 per cent every 2–3 days to max.
  0.1–0.2mg/kg/day
- Prescribe as number of drops. Count drops onto spoon before
  administering. Irritability and aggression not uncommon in which case
  drug should be withdrawn
- Increased secretions may occur in infants and young children
- Licence: tablets and injections licensed for use in children but not for
  this indication

Midazolam
- Very short half-life
- Form:
  - Injection: 10mg in 2mL; 10mg in 5mL
  - Injection may be given orally, sublingually, intranasally, or rectally
  - Oral syrup 2.5mg in 1mL only available as 'special'
- **Single doses:**
  - Intravenous/subcutaneous:
    - >1month–18yrs: 100mcg/kg
  - Sublingual:
    - >1month–18yrs: 500mcg/kg (max. 10mg)
- Tastes bitter when given orally but can be mixed with juice or
  chocolate sauce
- Max. effect in 30–60mins. Duration 2 h
  - Intranasal:
    - >1month–18yrs: 200–300mcg/kg (max. 10mg)
- Intranasal route may be unpleasant but has a fast onset of action
  (5–15 minutes)
- **Important:** Drop dose into alternating nostril over 15 seconds
  - Rectal:
    - >1month–18yrs: 500–750 mcg/kg
  - Continuous intravenous/subcutaneous infusion:
    - >1month–18yrs: start at 2.5mg/24 h (note: this is not
      a per kg dose)
- Titrate to effect. There is considerable inter-individual variability in the
  dose required and doses of up to 40mg/24 h have been used in palliative
  care. If high doses are needed, consider trying a different agent
- Contra-indications and warnings: caution with pulmonary disease,
  hepatic and renal dysfunction (reduce dose), severe fluid/electrolyte
  imbalance and congestive cardiac failure
- Avoid rapid withdrawal after prolonged treatment
- Licence: injection licensed for sedation in intensive care, for induction of
  anaesthesia and conscious sedation in children. Other routes and
  indications not licensed

Diazepam
- Long half-life
- Form:
  - Tablets: 2mg, 5mg, 10mg
  - Oral solution: 2mg in 5mL and 5mg in 5mL
  - Injection (solution and emulsion): 5mg in 1mL
  - Suppositories: 10mg
  - Rectal tubes: 2mg in 1mL: 2.5mg tube, 5mg tube, 4mg in 1mL: 10mg tube
- Dose (oral):
  - 1 month–12yrs: 50–100mcg/kg/dose b.d.–q.d.s.
  - >12yrs: 2.5–5mg b.d.–q.d.s.
- Licence: rectal preparation is licensed for use in children >1yr with severe agitation. Other forms not licensed for agitation per se

Other medication

Haloperidol
- Form:
  - Tablets: 1.5mg, 5mg, 10mg, 20mg
  - Capsules: 500 mcg
  - Oral liquid: 1mg in 1mL, 2mg in 1mL. 1mg in 5 mL 'special'
  - Injection: 5mg in 1mL, 1mL ampoule; 10mg in 1mL and 2mL ampoules
- Dose (oral):
  - 2–12yrs: 10–25 mcg/kg b.d. (max. 10mg/24h)
  - >12yrs: 0.25–5mg b.d. (max. 30mg/24h)
- Dose (subcutaneous):
  - 2–12 yrs: 10–25 mcg/kg b.d. (max 10mg/24 h)
  - >12 yrs: 0.25–5mg b.d (max 30mg/24 h)
- Contra-indications and warnings: bone marrow suppression, phaeochromocytoma
- Licence: licensed for use in children

Levomepromazine
- Form:
  - Tablets: 25mg
  - Injection: 25mg in 1mL, 1mL ampoule
- Dose: (SC/i/v continuous infusion):
  - All ages: 0.5–1mg/kg/24 h then titrate to response (max. adult dose 300mg/24 h)
- Contra-indications and warnings: Parkinsonism, postural hypotension, antihypertensive medication, epilepsy, hypothyroidism, myasthenia gravis
- May reduce seizure threshold
- Sedating especially in SC doses exceeding 1mg/kg/24 h in children under 12 yrs or 25mg/24 h in children over 12 yrs
- Can be used subcutaneously but may cause inflammation at injection site
- Licence: Licensed for this indication in children

Anorexia

Poor appetite and weight loss are common in children with terminal illness, particularly towards the end-of-life. This causes a great deal of anxiety amongst many parents and carers because:

- They may consider one of their main caring roles is to keep their child well-fed
- They often perceive eating as a road to recovery
- Acceptance that their child doesn't want to eat may go hand in hand with acceptance that the terminal phase is approaching

Consider reversible causes

- Oral candidiasis
- Pain (in mouth or elsewhere)
- Nausea/vomiting
- Constipation
- Medication

Management

General measures

- Explanation and discussion with the family may be helpful. Listen to parents' concerns and reassure as appropriate. It may be helpful for families to understand that as the child becomes less mobile and as the body winds down, the child's need for fluid and food diminishes
- Provide small meals on small plates. The child may prefer to snack through the day rather than sit down to a meal
- Make food less effort to eat (e.g. by providing mashed meals or wholesome soups, ice cream and rice pudding)
- Offer 'favourite' meals
- Offer supplementary high calorie/high protein drinks
- Try not to make an issue out of meal times
- Low dose steroids will stimulate the appetite but will not change the course of the disease and may have harmful side-effects. They are almost never given for this indication

Bleeding

Management

General measures

- For children who are reasonably well but are thrombocytopenic and at risk of bleeding, regular platelet transfusions may be worthwhile
- If bleeding is likely, explain this to the parents and prepare a management plan
- If a significant bleed is a possibility benzodiazepines should be readily available (see below) and the use of red towels and blankets may be helpful. Consider a platelet transfusion if bleeding is problematic and related to low platelet count in a child with a reasonable prognosis where a transfusion would improve quality of life

Medication

Bleeding gums

Use a soft toothbrush if possible. If not, avoid brushes altogether. Consider gentle regular antibacterial mouthwash to prevent secondary infection.

Tranexamic acid
- Form:
    - Tablets: 500mg
    - Liquid: 500mg in 5mL 'special'
    - Injection: 100mg in 1mL. 5mL Amp.
- Dose (mouthwash): use undiluted preparation for injection and apply to bleeding point. Dilute preparation for injection 1:1 for oral use and use as mouthwash
- Dose (oral):
    - 1month–18yrs: 25mg/kg t.d.s.
- Caution: reduce dose in renal failure; do not use in children with haematuria because of the risk of clot retention
- Licence: licensed for use in children

Small bleeds

Tranexamic acid
See oral dose above

Topical adrenaline
- Form: 1:1000 solution
- Small external bleeds:soak gauze, apply directly to bleeding point

Sorbsan dressing
- Haemostatic dressing: apply directly to bleeding point

Catastrophic haemorrhage

An anxiolytic such as diazepam/midazolam is useful as a large haemorrhage is likely to be very frightening if the patient is conscious. If haemorrhage is likely an anxiolytic in a suitable form should be readily available, and carers/staff should be aware of how to administer it. A rapid onset of action may be desirable so provision should be made for parenteral administration. For example:

Midazolam
- Form:
  - Injection: 10mg in 2mL
- Dose (SC/i.v. stat):
  - All ages: 100–200 mcg/kg
- Dose may need to be repeated
- Haemorrhage is unlikely to be painful and the 'traditional' use of diamorphine in this instance may not be appropriate

Breathlessness

Dyspnoea, like pain, is a subjective symptom and may not correlate with objective signs.

Consider causes and treat reversible factors as appropriate:
- Anaemia
- Anxiety
- Ascites
- Cerebral tumours
- Congenital heart disease
- Cystic fibrosis
- Infection
- Raised intracranial pressure
- Respiratory muscle dysfunction e.g. neurodegenerative disorders
- Primary or secondary tumours
- Uraemia
- Pleural effusion/pneumothorax*/haemothorax
- Pulmonary fibrosis
- Superior vena cava (SVC) obstruction*
- Increased secretions
- Pain
- Pulmonary embolism
- Pericardial effusion

* These are medical emergencies and swift treatment of these conditions can significantly reduce symptoms; if suspected, urgent investigation and referral to appropriate specialist should be considered.

Management

General measures
- Anxiety is likely to be an associated feature. Try reassurance, relaxation techniques, distraction and anxiolytics where necessary
- Provide a flow of fresh air—fan/window
- Try not to overcrowd the room
- Optimise position
- Excess secretions may respond to gentle physiotherapy +/− suction

Oxygen
May be helpful in hypoxic patients but is not without consequences (e.g. wearing of mask can be uncomfortable and interfere with ability of child to be close to parents and carers. Equipment can also compromise mobility). The benefits of this intervention need to outweigh the burdens.

Children often refuse masks but may tolerate nasal specs. Consider humidifying oxygen which will dry the mouth less.

Caution is needed in circumstances where chronic hypercapnia has left the child dependent on hypoxic respiratory drive. Too much oxygen will result in hypoventilation, so titrate carefully.

Medication
The choice of medication will depend on the underlying cause. Bronchospasm will respond to a bronchodilator. Anxiety that is unresponsive to reassurance, distraction or relaxation techniques may require treatment

with a benzodiazepine. Excessive secretions may respond to physiotherapy and/or mucolytic agents. Opioids however, are generally very effective.

Bronchodilators
Salbutamol
May be helpful if bronchospasm present
- Form:
  - Nebulised solution 2.5mg/2.5mL. 5mg in 2.5mL
  - Inhaled form: 100mcg/dose
- Dose (nebulised):
  - 6 months—5yrs: 2.5mg t.d.s./q.d.s.
  - 5–12yrs: 2.5–5mg t.d.s./q.d.s.
  - >12 yrs: 5mg t.d.s./q.d.s.
- Dose (inhaled):
  - All ages: 1–2 puffs 4–6 times a day (a spacer device should be used to improve delivery)

There is some evidence that small babies do not respond to salbutamol because of receptor immaturity and it is advisable to use ipratropium first in those aged <1yr.
  Salbutamol may exacerbate anxiety.
- Licence: licensed for use in children

Ipratropium
May be helpful if bronchospasm present
- Form:
  - Nebulised solution: 250mcg in 1mL, 500mcg in 2mL
  - Inhaled form: 20mcg/dose and 40mcg/dose
- Dose (nebulised):
  - <1yr: 125mcg t.d.s.–q.d.s.
  - 1–5yrs: 250mcg t.d.s.–q.d.s.
  - 5–12yrs: 500mcg t.d.s.–q.d.s.
  - >12yrs: 500mcg t.d.s.–q.d.s.
- Dose (inhaled):
  - <6yrs: 20mcg/dose t.d.s.–q.d.s.
  - 6–12yrs: 20–40mcg/dose t.d.s.–q.d.s.
- Licence: licensed for use in children

Morphine
Effective in treating dyspnoea although there may be no measurable effect on respiratory rate or oximetry. Morphine reduces anxiety, pain, and pulmonary artery pressure. Begin with half the paediatric analgesic dose and titrate to effect (📖 See section on Pain, p. 520).

Benzodiazepines
Many children will be frightened by dyspnoea. Benzodiazepines may be helpful in addition to relaxation techniques and guided imagery. The choice of benzodiazepine will depend on the circumstance for which it is being prescribed. Children experiencing brief periods of anxiety or panic attacks in association with dyspnoea may benefit from a benzodiazepine with a very short half-life, such as midazolam, given buccally or subcutaneously. Sublingual lorazepam, is another option for panic attacks or anxiety related to dyspnoea. Children needing a longer duration of action may do better with diazepam, clonazepam or a subcutaneous midazolam infusion.

Diazepam
- Form:
  - Tablets: 2mg, 5mg, 10mg
  - Oral solution: 2mg in 5mL and 5mg in 5mL
  - Injection (solution and emulsion): 5mg in 1mL
  - Also available as Suppositories: 10mg
  - Rectal tubes: 2mg in 1mL: 2.5mg tube, 5mg tube
- Dose (oral): 4mg in 1mL: 10mg tube
  - 1 month–12 yrs: 50–100mcg/kg 6–12 h
  - >12yrs: 2.5–5mg 6–12 h
- Contra-indications and warnings: acute porphyria. Potential for dependency. Can affect respiration if given i/v or rectally
- Licence: not licensed for this indication in children

Lorazepam
- Form:
  - Tablets: 1mg (scored), 2.5mg
  - Oral suspension only available as 'special'
  - Injection: 4mg in 1mL, 1mL ampoule
- Dose (sublingual, oral):
  - All ages: 25–50mcg/kg (max. dose in adults 4mg/24h)
- Most children will not need more than 0.5–1mg for trial dose. Well absorbed sublingually (good for panic attacks) and child has control
- Contra-indications and warnings: severe pulmonary disease, sleep apnoea, coma, CNS depression. Caution in hepatic and renal failure children >5 years
- Licence: tablets licensed as premedication in children >5 yrs. Injection not licensed in children <12yrs except for treatment of status epilepticus

Clonazepam
- Form:
  - Drops: 2.5mg in 1mL (1 drop = 0.1mg). Named patient basis
  - Tablets: 0.5mg, 2mg
  - Injection: 1mg in 1mL
  - Oral liquid: 500 mcg in 5mL, 2mg in 5mL 'specials'
- Dose (sublingual):
  - All ages: 0.01mg/kg/dose (max. 0.5mg) b.d./t.d.s.
  - If necessary, increase by 10–25 per cent every 2–3 days to max. 0.1–0.2mg/kg/day
- Long half-life
- Prescribe as number of drops. Count drops onto spoon before administering
- Irritability and aggression not uncommon in which case drug should be withdrawn. Increased secretions may occur in infants and young children
- Offers the advantage of sublingual absorption and droplet administration
- Licence: tablets and injections licensed for use in children but not for this indication

Midazolam
- Form:
  - Injection: 10mg in 2mL; 10mg in 5mL
- Injection may be given orally, sublingually, intranasally, or rectally
- Oral syrup only available as 'special': 2.5mg in 1mL

- Single doses:
  - Intravenous/subcutaneous:
    - >1month–18yrs: 100mcg/kg
  - Sublingual:
    - >1month–18yrs: 500mcg/kg (max. 10mg)
- Tastes bitter when given orally but can be mixed with juice or chocolate sauce
- Max. effect in 30–60mins. Duration 2 h
  - Intranasal:
    - >1month–18yrs: 200–300mcg/kg (max 10mg)
- Intranasal route may be unpleasant but has a fast onset of action (5–15 minutes)
- Important:Drop dose into alternating nostril over 15 seconds
  - Rectal:
    - >1month–18yrs: 500–750 mcg/kg
  - Continuous intravenous/subcutaneous infusion:
    - >1month–18yrs: start at 2.5mg/24 h (note: this is not a per kg dose)
- Titrate to effect. There is considerable inter-individual variability in the dose required and doses of up to 40mg/24 h have been used in palliative care. If high doses are needed, consider trying a different agent
- Contra-indications and warnings:caution with pulmonary disease, hepatic and renal dysfunction (reduce dose), severe fluid/electrolyte imbalance and congestive cardiac failure. Avoid rapid withdrawal after prolonged treatment
- Licence: injection licensed for sedation in intensive care, induction of anaesthesia, and conscious sedation in children. Other routes and indications not licensed

Dexamethasone

May be helpful in circumstances such as bronchial obstruction, lymphangitis carcinomatosa, SVCO, and raised intracranial pressure. Administration needs to be carefully considered as steroids may produce potentially distressing side-effects in children if given for more than a few days. To avoid this, it is preferable to prescribe short courses (3–5 days) of steroids. These can be repeated if necessary.

- Form:
  - Tablets: 500mcg; 2mg
  - Oral solution: 2mg in 5mL
  - Injection: 4mg in 1mL, can be given orally
- Dose (oral):
  - <1yr: 0.5–1mg b.d.
  - 1–5yrs: 2mg b.d.
  - 6–11yrs: 4mg b.d.
  - >12yrs: 8mg b.d.
- Dose (SC/i/v)
  - Can be given in as single doses or as continuous infusion
- Higher doses may be needed in SVCO (consult paediatric oncologist)
- If no effect after 3–5 days, stop steroids (no need to tail off dose)
- Do not give after midday as can affect night time sleep
- Co-prescribing: consider antacids and anti-thrush treatment
- Contra-indications and warnings: caution in renal disease, cardiac disease or cystic fibrosis. Avoid in cardiac insufficiency
- Licence: not licensed for this indication in children

Constipation

Prophylaxis and early intervention are important in managing this distressing symptom. A laxative should always be prescribed when opioids are commenced.

- What are the child's usual bowel habits?—children vary a lot; what is constipation for one may be a normal pattern for another
- Has there been a change in the usual pattern?

Consider cause

- Inactivity
- Metabolic: dehydration; hypercalcaemia; hypokalaemia
- Cystic fibrosis
- Reduced oral intake
- Spinal cord/cauda equina compression
- Bowel obstruction
- Fear of pain on defaecation: secondary to hard stools, rectal/anal grazes and tears
- Drugs: opioids; anticholinergics; anticonvulsants; vincristine chemotherapy
- Social: shy about using toilets away from home, not knowing where the toilets are etc. Liaise with parents

Management

General measures

- Check for bowel obstruction, faecal impaction and rectal/anal grazes/tears (conduct a rectal examination only if absolutely necessary)
- Consider the underlying cause and address it if appropriate/possible
- Increase fluid intake where possible and appropriate
- Increase mobility if possible
- Optimise access to the toilet
- Encourage regular toileting especially after meals
- Try oral medication first, then proceed to rectal preparations if necessary

Medication

It is generally helpful to use a combination of a stimulant laxative (e.g. senna, bisacodyl, docusate or sodium picosulphate) and a softening agent (e.g. magnesium hydroxide). Combined preparations are available (e.g. co-danthramer and co-danthrusate) for use in palliative care. Prokinetic agents such as metoclopramide and domperidone may be helpful second line agents (□ See section on Nausea and vomiting, p. 512 for doses). Domperidone is less effective than metoclopramide but is less likely to cause dystonic reactions. If constipation is morphine-related and resistant to the usual measures, it may be helpful to change to an alternative opioid such as fentanyl.

Bisacodyl

- Form:
  - Tablets: 5mg
  - Suppository: 5mg, 10mg

- Dose (oral/rectal):
  - Give tablets at night, suppositories in the morning
  - 1month–10yrs: 5mg o.d.
  - >10yrs: 10mg o.d.
- Higher doses may be necessary
- Acts in 12h orally, in 20–60 minutes rectally
- Stimulant laxative

Senna
- Form:
  - Syrup: 7.5mg in 5mL
  - Tablets: 7.5mg
  - Granules: 15mg in 5mL
- Dose (oral):
  - <2yrs: Syrup 0.5mL/kg o.d.
  - 2–6yrs: Syrup 2.5–5mL o.d.
  - 6–12yrs: Syrup 5–10mL or 1–2 tablets o.d.
  - >12yrs: Syrup 10–20mL or 2–4 tablets o.d.
  - For granules use $^{1}/_{2}$ syrup dose
- Stimulant laxative
- Acts in 8–12h
- Often used in combination with lactulose
- Licence: Syrup licensed in children >2yrs, tablets not recommended in children <6yrs

Co-danthramer
- Form:
  - Suspension: dantron 25mg/poloxamer 200mg in 5 mL; dantron 75mg/poloxamer 1g in 5 mL (Forte)
  - Capsule: dantron 25mg/poloxamer 200mg; dantron 37.5mg/poloxamer 500mg (Forte)
- Dose (oral):
  - Only for use in terminally ill children
  - <12yrs: 2.5–5mL of the 25/200mg strength suspension or 1–2 (25/200mg strength) capsules o.d.–b.d.
  - >12yrs: 5–10mL of the 25/200mg strength suspension or 1–2 (25/200mg strength) capsules o.d.–b.d., titrate as needed
- Combined stimulant (dantron)/softener (poloxamer) laxative
- Acts in 8–12h
- Makes urine red (inform carers)
- Can cause superficial burns in children who are incontinent/in nappies
- Avoid in acute respiratory depression, paralytic ileus, liver disease and moderate to severe renal impairment
- Licence: only licensed for use in terminally ill children

Docusate sodium
- Form:
  - Elixir: 12.5mg in 5mL; 50mg in 5mL. Dilute with milk or orange juice
  - Capsule: 100mg
  - Enemas: Fletchers' enemette: 90mg in 5mL; Norgalax microenema: 120mg in 10g
- Dose (oral):
  - 6 months–12yrs: 2.5mg/kg t.d.s.
  - >12yrs: 100mg t.d.s.

- Dose (rectal):
  - <3yrs: 2.5mL Fletchers' enemette
  - >3yrs: 5mL Fletchers' enemette
- Softener and stimulant
- Acts in 24–48h
- Licence: capsule not licensed for children. Norgalax enema licensed for children >12yrs. Fletchers enemette licensed for children >3yrs

Lactulose
Lactulose is not very effective in opioid-induced constipation.
- Form:
  - Solution: 300mg lactose/550mg galactose in 5mL
- Dose (oral):
  - <1yrs: 2.5mL b.d.
  - 1–5yrs: 5mL b.d.
  - 5–10yrs: 10mL b.d.
  - >10yrs: 15mL b.d.
- Mild osmotic laxative, which is very sweet to taste, and can cause bloating
- Acts in 48h
- May cause colic
- Titrate dose up as required
- Can be disguised in fruit juice, milk or water

Magnesium hydroxide
Stool softener
- Form:
  - Liquid: 415mg in 5mL
- Dose (oral):
  - <3yrs not recommended
  - >3yrs 5–10mL nocte
    (adult 30–45mL nocte)

Sodium picosulfate
- Form:
  - Sachet: 10mg sachets contain sodium picosulfate 10mg + magnesium citrate powder
  - Sodium picosulfate liquid: 5mg in 5mL
- Dose (oral) sachet:
  - 1–2yrs: 1/4 sachet o.d.
  - 2–4yrs: 1/2 sachet o.d.
  - 4–9yrs: (1/2)–1sachet o.d.
  - >9yrs: 1 sachet o.d.
- Dose (oral) liquid:
  - 2–5yrs: 2.5mL nocte
  - 5–10yrs: 2.5–5mL nocte
  - >10yrs: 5–15mL nocte
- Effective within 2–3 h
- Drink plenty of water before and after administration
- Warning: can cause dehydration and electrolyte disturbance
  Caution in children with impaired renal or cardiac function

Arachis oil enema
- Form:
  - Enema 130mL arachis oil BP

- Dose (rectal):
  - 3–7yrs: (1/3)–(1/2) enema
  - 7–12yrs: (1/2)–(3/4) enema
  - >12yrs: (3/4)–1 enema
- Use as required
- Faecal softener
- Contra-indications and warnings:hypersensitivity to arachis oil or peanuts.
- Licence: licensed for children >3 yrs

Sodium citrate enema
- Form:
  - Micro-enema 450mg sodium citrate/75mg sodium laurylsulphate/5mg sorbic acid in 5mL (Relaxit). Other combinations available, but not licensed for children under 3yrs
- Dose (rectal):
  - 1 enema (when using in children <3yrs insert only half nozzle length)
- Osmotic laxative
- Licence: licensed for children >3 yrs

Phosphate enema
- Form:
  - enema sodium acid phosphate 21.4g/sodium phosphate 9.4g in 118mL (Fleet)
  - other combinations available
- Dose (rectal):
  - 3–7yrs: (1/3)–1/2 enema
  - 7–12yrs: (1/2)–3/4 enema
  - >12yrs: (3/4)–1 enema
- Osmotic laxative
- Licence: licensed for children >3 yrs

Convulsions

Convulsions are most commonly seen in the palliative care setting in children with neurodegenerative disorders or intracranial malignancies.

Children with neurodegenerative disorders will often already be on multiple anticonvulsant medications and their parents/carers will be knowledgeable about recognizing and treating fits. For these children fits are often variable in type and may become frequent, severe and more difficult to control towards the end-of-life.

Children with intracranial malignancy will not necessarily develop fits. However, for those who do, it is a frightening new symptom for the child and carers to learn how to manage. If fits are likely, prophylactic anticonvulsants should be considered and parents warned about what to expect. They should be given a clear plan of what to do in the event of a convulsion. The mainstay of medical treatment, diazepam, should be readily available with clear instructions as to how and when it should be administered.

Not all fits are grand mal: more subtle behaviours may also represent seizure activity. These may not require treatment if they are not troubling the child.

Investigation and treatment of persistent fitting should be tailored to the child's stage of illness and will require discussion with senior doctors and family.

Consider causes and treat as appropriate

The emergence of, or increasing frequency/severity of fits may be caused by worsening disease but other potentially reversible factors should be considered:

- Hypoglycaemia
- Electrolyte imbalance
- Sub-therapeutic anticonvulsant medication
- Infection e.g. UTI
- Raised intracranial pressure/other intracranial pathology

Management

- The choice of anticonvulsant depends on the type of fit. Advice from the paediatric unit where the child is being managed should be sought
- Single agent therapy is ideal. Where children are already on multiple medications, reducing the number of different anticonvulsants may improve seizure control
- Withdrawal or addition of anticonvulsants should be done cautiously as most agents need to be tailed off or titrated down
- Relatively higher doses of anticonvulsants are required for children <3yrs because of a higher metabolic rate and more efficient drug clearance
- Not all fits require treatment

The management of seizures will depend on the goals of care at the time. A child who is enjoying a reasonable quality of life and is in the early stages of a life-limiting illness should be treated as any other. Children in the terminal phase of illness should be kept comfortable and this will generally entail reasonable efforts to abort the seizure.

Acute management

In circumstances where the goals of care are to keep the child comfortable:
- Place the child on his/her side in a place where he/she cannot fall or be injured
- If the fit lasts longer than five minutes, prepare to give rectal diazepam (diazepam should not be given SC or i/m)

Diazepam
- Dose (rectal):
  - <1yr: 2.5–5mg
  - 1–5yrs: 7.5mg
  - 5–10yrs: 10mg
  - >10yrs: 10–15mg
- If the fit shows no signs of abating once the diazepam has been fetched and prepared, give the required dose
- Wait five minutes
- If the fit continues, the dose may be repeated
- If the fit continues after two doses of rectal diazepam, phenytoin, phenobarbital or rectal paraldehyde will be required

Alternatives
Midazolam
- Dose (buccal):
  - 500mcg/kg (max. 10mg)
- Dose (intranasal):
  - 200–300mcg/kg (dropped into alternating nostrils over 15 seconds). (Max. 10mg)

Clonazepam
- Form:
  - Drops: 2.5mg in 1mL (1 drop = 0.1mg). Only available as named patient
- Dose (sublingual):
  - All ages: 0.01mg/kg/dose (max 0.5mg)
- Prescribe as number of drops. Count drops onto spoon before administering
- Titrate up according to response
- Irritability and aggression are not uncommon in which case drug should be withdrawn. Increased secretions may occur in infants and young children.

Maintenance treatment

Medications used for emergency management of seizures do not have a prolonged effect, and if fitting is likely to be an ongoing problem, maintenance treatment is indicated. Control can usually be achieved even in the home environment but most agents will cause drowsiness. Phenytoin, phenobarbital and carbamazepine may be helpful for children able to take oral medication. For those who are unable to tolerate oral medication, phenobarbital given by subcutaneous infusion is an effective alternative. A continuous infusion of midazolam is another option. Rectal paraldehyde may also be helpful.

Provision should be made for breakthrough seizures, which may be managed with rectal diazepam, buccal intranasal or subcutaneous midazolam, or rectal paraldehyde.

Midazolam
- Form:
  - Injection: 10mg in 2mL; 10mg in 5mL
  - Injection may be used for oral, sublingual, rectal, and intranasal routes
- Dose (continuous intravenous or subcutaneous infusion):
  - Start at 5mg/24 h (note: this is not a per kg dose) and titrate to effect

Phenobarbital
Can be given orally or as a continuous subcutaneous infusion and has anticonvulsant and anxiolytic properties.
- Form:
  - Injection 60mg in 1mL. 200mg in 1mL available as 'special'
- Dose (i/v loading dose):
  - >1 month: 15mg/kg over 5 minutes. Single dose or loading dose, no faster than 1mg/kg/min
- Maintenance dose (i/v /SC continuous infusion or as oral doses):
  - Commence 24 h after loading dose
  - 1 month–12yrs: 5–10mg/kg/24h
  - >12yrs: 600mg/24h
- Review dose after one week as drug induces its own metabolism
- Requires separate syringe driver (does not mix)

Paraldehyde
- Form:
  - Injection 100 per cent (5mL ampoule) also available as already diluted 'special'
- Dose (rectal):
  - All ages: 0.3mL/kg/dose (max 10mL) 4–8h
  - Dilute twofold with olive oil or sunflower oil or dilute 1:10 with 0.9% sodium chloride
- Incompatible with most plastics so use immediately
- Do not give intramuscularly
- Licence: not licensed for use in children

Cough

Consider causes and treat reversible factors if appropriate:
- Infection
- Bronchospasm
- Gastro-oesophageal reflux
- Aspiration
- Drug induced (e.g. ACE inhibitors)/treatment related (e.g. total body irradiation)
- Malignant bronchial obstruction/Lung metastases
- Heart failure
- Secretions
- Cystic fibrosis

Management

General measures
- Keep child as upright as possible
- Raise head of bed:Use blocks under head end of cot/bed or pillows
- Consider physiotherapy +/– suction for children with secretions. Modified physiotherapy is the mainstay of treatment for children with thick secretions
- Consider a trial of humidified air/oxygen

Medication
The choice of medication will depend upon the underlying cause. A dry throat may respond to simple linctus. Bronchospasm will respond to bronchodilator therapy. If the underlying cause cannot be reversed, a suppressant such as an opioid will be required

Simple linctus
This may be helpful if the cough is exacerbated by a dry throat.
- Form:
  - Linctus: paediatric preparation (0.625 per cent citric acid monohydrate); adult preparation (2.5 per cent citric acid monohydrate)
- Dose (oral):
  - 1 month–12yrs: paediatric preparation 5–10mL t.d.s.–q.d.s.
  - >12yrs: adult preparation 5–10mL t.d.s.–q.d.s.
- Licence: licensed for children and adults (appropriate preparation)

Codeine linctus
- Form:
  - Linctus: paediatric preparation: codeine phosphate 3mg in 5mL; adult preparation: 15mg in 5mL
- Dose (oral):
  - 1–5yrs: 5mL paediatric preparation t.d.s.–q.d.s.
  - 5–12 yrs: 2.5–5mL adult preparation t.d.s.–q.d.s.
- Licence: not licensed for use in children under 1yr
- Very constipating: laxatives should always be prescribed

Dihydrocodeine tartrate
* Form:
  * Tablet: 30mg
  * Liquid: 10mg in 5mL
* Dose (oral):
  * 1–4yrs: 500mcg/kg 4–6h
  * 4–12yrs: 500mcg–1mg/kg 4–6h
  * >12yrs: 30mg 4–6h
* Very constipating:laxatives should always be prescribed
* Contra-indications and warnings:avoid or reduce dose in moderate/ severe renal failure, chronic liver disease and hypothyroidism. Avoid in respiratory depression, cystic fibrosis, head injury and raised intracranial pressure
* Licence: licensed for moderate to severe pain in children >4yrs

Morphine linctus
* Form:
  * Solution: 10mg in 5mL
* Start with half the paediatric analgesic dose (📖 See section on Pain, p. 520) and titrate to effect

Bronchodilators
Cough can be a manifestation of hyperreactive airways and a trial of nebulised salbutamol/ipratropium may be helpful.

Salbutamol
* Form:
  * Nebuliser solution:2.5mg in 2.5mL, 5mg in 2.5mL, 5mg in 1mL. (other preparations available, see appropriate text)
  * Inhaled form:100mcg/dose
* Dose (nebulised):
  * 6months–5yrs: 2.5mg t.d.s.–q.d.s.
  * 5–12yrs: 2.5–5mg t.d.s.–q.d.s.
  * >12yrs: 5mg t.d.s.–q.d.s
* Dose (inhaled):
  * All ages: 1–2 puffs 4–6 times a day (a spacer device should be used to improve delivery)
* May induce mild tachycardia, nervousness, tremor or hypokalaemia
* Interactions: see appropriate text
* Licence: licensed for use in children

Ipratropium bromide
* Form:
  * Nebuliser solution: 250mcg/mL. 500mcg in 2mL
  * Inhaled form: 20mcg/dose and 40mcg/dose
* Dose (nebulised):
  * <1yr: 125mcg t.d.s.–q.d.s.
  * 1–5yrs: 250mcg t.d.s.–q.d.s.
  * 5–12yrs: 500mcg t.d.s.–q.d.s.
  * >12yrs: 500mcg t.d.s.–q.d.s.

- Dose (inhaled):
  - <6 yrs: 20mcg/dose t.d.s.–q.d.s.
  - 6–12yrs: 20–40mcg/dose t.d.s.–q.d.s.
  - Licence: licensed for use in children

Mucolytics

May be helpful if secretions are thick. Agents like acetylcysteine and dornase alfa may be used in patients with cystic fibrosis who have thick secretions. Their use should be discussed with the child's paediatrician.

Normal saline

- Dose (nebulised):
  - All ages: 2.5–5mL p.r.n.
- May induce cough reflex in some cases

Gastro-oesophageal reflux

Many neurologically impaired children suffer with gastro-oesophageal reflux. Consider reflux if the child refuses food, vomits, has dysphagia, or is irritable when supine.

Management

General measures

- Check for overfeeding
- If nasogastric/gastrostomy fed, consider changing regimen from large bolus to smaller, more frequent volumes. Continuous feeding is another option
- Thicken feeds
- Ensure optimal posture for feeds
- Adjust posture overnight to keep child more upright: use blocks under cot/bed, or pillows
- Surgery can be considered in children with a longer prognosis. Gastrostomy and fundoplication is effective in 80 per cent but is not without complications
- Postpyloric tube feeding is also an option

Medication

Antacids

To be really effective antacids should be given four-hourly. This may limit their usefulness.

Gaviscon

- Form:
  - Tablets: alginic acid 500mg, anhydrous aluminium hydroxide 100mg, magnesium trisilicate 25mg, sodium bicarbonate 170mg
  - Liquid: sodium alginate 250mg, sodium bicarbonate 133.5mg, calcium carbonate 80mg in 5mL
  - Dual Infant sachets: sodium alginate 225mg, magnesium alginate 87.5mg with colloidal silical and mannitol per dose (dose = half sachet)
- Dose (oral):
  - Birth–2yrs: 1/2–1 dual infant sachet (do not use other preparations)
  - 2–12yrs: 5–10mL liquid or 1 tablet after meals and at bedtime
  - >12yrs: 10–20mL or 1–2 tablets after meals and at bedtime
- Can cause constipation
- Licence: liquid and tablets licensed for use in children over 2yrs, for children 2–6yrs on medical advice only. Infant sachets licensed for infants and young children but, for children under 1yr, only under medical supervision

Omeprazole

Is the drug of choice for reflux oesophagitis. It is more effective than ranitidine and has a good safety profile. Individuals vary in their response and doses will need titration to achieve effective acid suppression.

- Form:
  - Capsule: 10mg, 20mg, 40mg
  - MUPS dispersible tablets: 10mg, 20mg, 40mg

- Tablets: 10mg, 20mg, 40mg
- Intravenous infusion: 40mg vial
- Intravenous injection: 40mg vial
- Dose (oral):
  - 1 month–12yrs: 700mcg–3mg/kg o.d.—round up to nearest capsule size
  - >12yrs: 20–40mg o.d. or divide dose to give b.d.
- Capsules can be opened and the granules mixed in acidic drink
- Tablets can be dispersed in water or mixed with fruit juice or yoghurt
- Contra-indications and warnings: caution in patients with hepatic impairment
- Interactions: see appropriate text
- Licence: licensed for use in children >2yrs with severe ulcerating reflux oesophagitis

Ranitidine
- Form:
  - Injection: 50mg in 2mL
  - Tablets: 50mg, 300mg. Effervescent tablets 150mg, 300mg
  - Liquid: 15mg in 1mL
- Dose (oral):
  - 6/12 1mg/kg t.d.s.
  - 6/12 2–4mg/kg b.d. (max. 150mg)

Infection

Pneumonia is often the terminal event in children with life-limiting illnesses especially those with neurodegenerative conditions. For this reason, antibiotic treatment may not be appropriate. In some circumstances, however, antibiotics may relieve symptoms and therefore improve the child's quality of life. Antibiotics may also be appropriate early in a life-limiting illness where the child is relatively well. Wherever possible, it is helpful to discuss and record a course of action with the parents, and where appropriate the child, in advance of the terminal phase, making it clear that any decisions can be revised as time goes on. This avoids decisions being made in a crisis and may spare the child from intrusive and futile interventions.

Mouthcare

A painful mouth can cause anorexia, discomfort and difficulties eating. It can also make it difficult for the child to take oral medication. Good mouth care can significantly enhance quality of life for children in the palliative care setting.

A general examination should always include inspection of the mouth as oral problems are readily overlooked but can usually be easily managed.

Consider cause and treat as appropriate

- Oral candidiasis
- Dry mouth
- Ulcers
- Bleeding gums
- Dental caries
- Impacted teeth
- Gum hyperplasia
- Medications e.g. morphine, antidepressants, antihistamines or anticholinergics

Management

General measures

- If using oxygen, try humidifying or using nasal prongs
- Keep mouth clean and moist
- Rinse mouth after vomiting
- If possible, brush teeth, gums and tongue and other mucous membranes two to three times a day with a soft toothbrush
- Clear a coated tongue by gently brushing with a soft tooth brush, or by using effervescent vitamin C
- Sucking pineapple chunks will help maintain a clean mouth
- If the mouth is too painful to brush, regularly clean with pink sponges dipped in water or mouthwash, particularly after eating or drinking
- Avoid preparations containing alcohol
- Try water sprays or atomizers
- Ice chips may be helpful
- Artificial saliva: a number of preparations are available
- Moisten lips with petroleum jelly or lip balm
- Refer to dentist if appropriate

Medication

Oral candidiasis may present as classic white plaques or less commonly as atrophic candidiasis with a red glossy tongue. Remember that candidiasis may extend beyond the line of vision to the oesophagus.

Nystatin

- Form:
  - Pastilles: 100,000 units
  - Oral solution: 100,000 units in 1mL
- Dose (oral):
  - 1 month–18yrs: 1mL or 1 pastille 4–6h
  - For oesophageal candida in the immunocompromised: 5mL 4–6h
- The child should not eat or drink for 20 minutes after taking nystatin
- Continue 48h after clinical cure to prevent relapse
- Licence: licensed for children

Miconazole oral gel
- Form:
  - Oral gel: 24mg in 1mL
- Dose (topical to inside of mouth, then swallow)
  - Birth–1 month: 1–2mL b.d.
  - 1 month–2yrs: 2.5mL b.d.
  - 2–6yrs: 5mL b.d.
  - >6yrs: 5mL q.d.s.

Fluconazole
- Form:
  - Capsules: 50mg, 150mg, 200mg
  - Oral suspension: 50mg in 5mL; 200mg in 5mL
  - (Also available i/v)
- Dose (oral):
  - <2weeks: 3mg/kg every 72h
  - 2 weeks–1 month: 3mg/kg every 48h
  - 1 month–18yrs: 3mg/kg daily for 14 days
- Contra-indications and warnings: reduce dose in renal impairment. Co-administration with terfenadine contra-indicated, interacts with several drugs: see other texts. May cause haematological and biochemical abnormalities particularly in children with HIV or malignancies
- Licence: licensed for use in children

Ulcers/mucositis:
- Often related to neutropaenia resulting from high dose chemotherapy or radiotherapy
- Mouthwash. The type of mouthwash will depend on the severity of the mucositis. Chlorhexidine 0.2 per cent (swished for one minute or swabbed three times daily) is generally adequate for children with mild to moderate mucositis. Hydrogen peroxide mouth rinse (diluted 1 in 8 with water or saline and used two to three times daily) may need to be used in addition to chlorhexidine in children with severe mucositis
- An antifungal agent (see above) should be used. This should be given 20–30 minutes after chlorhexidine
- Mucositis can be extremely painful and analgesia appropriate to the degree of pain should be given. For children with severe mucositis, opioid analgesia may be required

Apthous ulcers
Adcortyl in orabase
- Form:
  - Oral paste
- Dose (topical):
  - All ages: Apply thin layer to affected area b.d.–q.d.s.

Choline salicylate (Bonjela)
- Form:
  - Clear gel
- Dose (topical):
  - >4 months: quarter of an inch of gel up to six times daily; may sting initially

Bleeding gums
📖 See section on Bleeding, p. 486.

Muscle spasm

Muscle spasm may occur in the setting of an upper motor neurone lesion and can cause significant pain and distress. It can be exacerbated by factors such as pain or constipation.

Management

General measures

- Early involvement of a physiotherapist is invaluable for advice on moving, handling, positioning and seating, and is essential to prevent the problem worsening
- Discussion with a paediatric neurologist may be helpful
- Long-standing contractures in a child with a relatively long prognosis can inhibit daily caring and may be managed surgically or with botulinum toxin injection. This should be assessed by an orthopedic surgeon
- While it is generally possible to reduce muscle spasm, it may not be possible to abolish it altogether

Medication:

Analgesia (📖 see section on Pain, p. 520).

Baclofen

- Form:
  - Tablet: 10mg
  - Liquid: 5mg in 5mL
  - Also available as intrathecal injection for specialist use: see below
- Starting dose (oral):
  - >1yr–12yrs: 2.5mg t.d.s.
  - >12yrs: 5mg t.d.s.
  - Increase dose every three days to maintenance dose
- Maintenance dose (oral):
  - 1yr–2yrs: 5–10mg b.d.
  - 2–6yrs: 10–15mg b.d.
  - 6–10yrs: 15–30mg b.d.
  - >12yrs: 10–20mg t.d.s.
- Baclofen can also be used intrathecally as a continuous infusion into the lumbar intrathecal space via an indwelling catheter and subcutaneous pump. The rate of infusion can be altered according to the child's clinical needs at different times of day
- Contra-indications and warnings: May cause drowsiness and increased hypotonia. Avoid rapid withdrawal. Use with caution in epilepsy. See other texts for interactions
- Doses should be reduced in renal impairment
- Licence: licensed for oral use in children >1yr

Diazepam
- Form:
  - Tablets: 2mg, 5mg, 10mg
  - Oral solution: 2mg in 5mL and 5mg in 5mL
  - Suppositories: 10mg; and rectal tubes: 2mg in 1mL: 2.5mg tube, 5mg tube, 10mg tube and 20mg tube; 4mg in 1mL; 10mg tube
- Dose (oral):
  - 1 month–5yrs: 50–100 mcg/kg b.d.–q.d.s.
  - 5–12yrs: 2.5–5mg b.d.–q.d.s.
- May cause sedation
- Licence: tablets and liquid licensed for use in cerebral spasticity and control of muscle spasm in tetany

Dantrolene
- Form:
  - Capsules: 25mg, 100mg
- Dose (oral):
  - Starting dose:
  - 1 month–12yrs: 500mcg/kg o.d.
  - >12yrs: 25mg o.d.
- Titration: Increase dose frequency to t.d.s. then q.d.s. at 7 day intervals. If response unsatisfactory continue increasing dose in increments of 500mcg/kg in children <12yrs, and 25mg in those >12yrs until maximum dose reached
- Maximum dose:
  - 1 month–12yrs: 2mg/kg (or 100mg total) q.d.s.
  - >12yrs: 100mg q.d.s.
- Contra-indications and warnings: Hepatic impairment. Caution with cardiovascular/respiratory disease. Monitor liver function tests
- Licence: not licensed for this indication in children

Nausea and vomiting

Consider cause

- Obstruction: Gastric outflow/bowel
- Constipation
- Uraemia/deranged electrolytes/hypercalcaemia
- Raised intracranial pressure
- Upper gastrointestinal tract irritation
- Anxiety
- Cough
- Pain
- Drugs: opioids, chemotherapy, carbamazepine, NSAIDS
- Intercurrent illness e.g. gastroenteritis, urinary tract infection

Management

General measures

- Treat the underlying cause if possible
- Ensure optimal pain management
- Avoid strong food smells and perfumes which may antagonize nausea
- Keep meals small and remove leftover food quickly

Medication

- Give an appropriate antiemetic according to suspected cause (see below), if this is ineffective or the cause is unclear, a phenothiazine such as levomepromazine will usually be effective. Chlorpromazine is very sedating and is used infrequently
- Levomepromazine is a very effective drug with anticholinergic, antihistaminergic, antidopaminergic and analgesic properties. It is often used in paediatric palliative care
- May need to use parenteral or rectal routes until symptoms are under control then consider oral route
- Review: if treatment is not successful, reconsider cause.

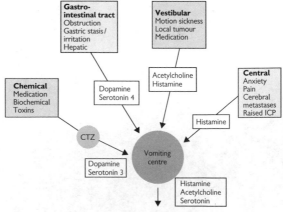

Fig. 7.2 Suspected causes of nausea and vomiting and suggested receptors/neurotransmitters involved

Table 7.1 Receptor site affinities of antiemetics

	D₂ antagonist	H₁ antagonist	ACh antagonist	5-HT₃ antagonist
Metoclopramide	++	0	0	(+)
Ondansetron	0	0	0	+++
Cyclizine	0	++	++	0
Hyoscine hydrobromide	0	0	+++	0
Haloperidol	+++	0	0	0
Prochlorperazine	++	+	0	0
Chlorpromazine	++	++	+	0
Levomepromazine	++	+++	++	0

D_2 =dopamine, H_1 =histamine 1, Ach =muscarinic cholinergic, 5-HT_3 =serotonin group 3

*Adapted from Twycross R, Back I. Nausea and vomiting in advanced cancer. *European J of Pall Care* 1998; **5**: 39–45.

Opioid-induced nausea and vomiting

Opioid-induced nausea is mediated predominantly via dopaminergic pathways. Haloperidol is a dopamine antagonist which acts centrally. It is more potent in this action than metoclopramide. Metoclopramide is a dopamine antagonist and acts on both the CTZ and the gastrointestinal tract (prokinetic action). Like haloperidol, it may cause dystonic side-effects although these can be managed with benztropine. Domperidone is available for oral administration and does not cross the blood brain barrier. This means it is less effective than metoclopramide and haloperidol but is also less likely to cause extrapyramidal side-effects. Dexamethasone may be a useful adjuvant agent. Levomepromazine has antidopaminergic activity in addition to its anticholinergic and antihistamine properties.

Haloperidol
- Form:
  - Tablet: 1.5mg, 5mg, 10mg, 20mg, 500mcg
  - Capsule: 500mcg
  - Oral liquid: 1mg in 1mL, 2mg in 1mL
  - Injection: 5mg in 1mL, 1mL ampoules; 10mg in 1mL, 2mL ampoules
- Dose (oral):
  - 1 month–12yrs: 12.5–50mcg/kg b.d.
  - >12yrs: 500mcg–2mg b.d.–t.d.s.
- Dose (SC):
  - All ages: 25–50mcg/kg over 24h
- Licence: licensed for use in children

Metoclopramide
- Form:
  - Tablet: 5mg, 10mg
  - Syrup/oral solution: 5mg in 5mL
  - Paediatric liquid: 1mg in 1mL
  - Injection: 5mg in 1mL, 2mL ampoule

- Dose (oral/slow i/v /SC):
  - All ages: 100–170mcg/kg t.d.s. Max. 500mcg/kg/24h (max. 10mg)
    Higher doses may be needed but carry an increased risk of
    dystonic side-effects
- Dystonic reactions can occur with any dose although the risk increases
  with dose: reverse with benztropine or procyclidine
- Use with caution if intestinal obstruction suspected: if colic develops,
  reduce dose or stop altogether
- Caution: in moderate renal failure use 75% dose, in severe renal
  impairment use 25–50 per cent dose. Reduce dose in severe liver disease.
- Licence: tablets only licensed in children >15yrs.

Levomepromazine
- Form:
  - Tablet: 25mg
  - Injection: 25mg in 1mL, 1mL ampoule
- Dose (oral):
  - 2–12yrs: 0.1–1mg/kg (max 25mg) o.d.–b.d.
  - >12yrs: 6.25–25mg o.d.–b.d.
- Dose (SC/i/v continuous infusion):
  - all ages: 0.1–0.25mg/kg/24h (max. 25mg/24h)
- Highly sedative in higher doses. (SC dose >1mg/kg/24h)
- May reduce seizure threshold
- Postural hypotension especially if used with opioids
- Little experience in very small children
- Caution: Parkinsonism, postural hypotension, antihypertensive
  medication, epilepsy, hypothyroidism, myasthenia gravis
- Licence: not licensed for use as antiemetic in children

Domperidone
Less effective than metoclopramide but reduced risk of dystonic side-
effects. May be an alternative agent for a patient who has responded well
to metoclopramide but experienced dystonic side-effects.
- Form:
  - Tablet: 10mg
  - Suspension: 5mg in 5mL
  - Suppositories: 30mg
- Dose (oral):
  - 1 month–12yrs: 200–400mcg/kg 4–8 h
  - >12yrs: 10–20mg 4–8 h
- Dose (rectal):
  - 2–12yrs: 15–30mg <25kg: b.d.; 25–35kg: t.d.s.; >35kg: q.d.s.
  - >12yrs: 30–60mg 4–8 h
- Use with caution if intestinal obstruction suspected: if colic develops,
  reduce dose or stop altogether
- Licence: only licensed for use in children in nausea and vomiting
  secondary to radiotherapy/chemotherapy

Chemotherapy/radiotherapy-induced nausea and vomiting

Ondansetron is very effective in relieving nausea and vomiting associated
with chemotherapy. In refractory cases dexamethasone can be combined

with ondansetron. Levomepromazine is recommended as the third line agent. High dose metoclopramide is used in some centres.

Ondansetron
- Form:
  - Tablet: 4mg, 8mg
  - Tablet (melt): 4mg, 8mg
  - Oral solution: 4mg in 5mL
  - Injection: 2mg in 1mL, 2mL and 4mL ampoules
- Dose (i/v over 2–5 minutes):
  - 1 month–12yrs: 5mg/m^2(max. 8mg) b.d.–t.d.s.
  - >12yrs: 8mg b.d.–t.d.s.
- Ondansetron has been used as continuous iv/sc infusion in palliative care
- Dose (oral):
  - 1m.–12yrs: 4mg b.d.
  - >12yrs: 8mg b.d
- Consider co-prescribing laxative (ondansetron is constipating)
- Licence: licensed for post chemotherapy nausea and vomiting.

Dexamethasone
Caution is required when using steroids in children. side-effects including weight gain, and distressing behavioural and emotional changes occur if steroids are used for more than a few days. For this reason it is preferable to prescribe steroids in short courses (3–5 days) and to repeat courses if necessary.
- Form:
  - Tablet: 500mcg; 2mg
  - Oral solution: 2mg in 5mL
  - Injection: 4mg in 1mL can be given orally
- Dose (oral, i/v):
  - <1yr: 250mcg t.d.s.
  - 1–5yrs: 1–2mg t.d.s.
  - 6–12yrs: 2–4mg t.d.s.
  - >12yrs: 4mg t.d.s.
- Co-prescribing: consider antacids and anti-thrush treatment
- Caution: renal disease, cardiac disease or cystic fibrosis. Avoid in cardiac insufficiency
- Licence: not licensed for use as antiemetic in children

Levomepromazine
- Form:
  - Tablet: 25mg
  - Injection: 25mg in 1mL, 1mL ampoule
- Dose (oral):
  - 2–12yrs: 0.1–1mg/kg (max. 25mg)o.d.–b.d.
  - >12yrs: 6.25–25mg o.d.–b.d.
- Dose (SC/i/v continuous infusion):
  - all ages: 0.1–0.25mg/kg/24h (max. 25mg/24h)
- Highly sedative in higher doses. (SC dose >1mg/kg/24h)

- May reduce seizure threshold
- Postural hypotension especially if used with opioids
- No experience in very small children
- Caution: parkinsonism, postural hypotension, antihypertensive medication, epilepsy, hypothyroidism, myasthenia gravis
- Licence: not licensed for use as antiemetic in children

Raised intracranial pressure

Cyclizine

Has anticholinergic and antihistamine activity. Where raised intracranial pressure is a major factor in generating nausea and vomiting, cyclizine is often helpful. Drowsiness is a common side-effect but may be desirable in some circumstances. While it can be given subcutaneously, cyclizine has a propensity to crystallize in syringe drivers and may cause redness at the infusion site.

- Form:
  - Tablets: 50mg
  - Injection: 50mg/mL (1mL)
  - Suppositories: 25mg +12.5mg, 50mg, 100mg ('special')
- Dose (slow i/v bolus):
  - >1m.: 500 mcg–1mg/kg t.d.s. max. single dose
  - <6yrs: 25mg
  - >6yrs: 50mg
- Dose (i/v /SC continuous infusion):
  - <2yrs: 3mg/kg/24h
  - 2–5yrs: 50mg/24h
  - 6–12yrs: 75mg/24h
  - >12yrs: 150mg/24h
- Dose (oral/rectal):
  - <2yrs: 1mg/kg t.d.s.
  - 2–5yrs: 12.5mg t.d.s.
  - 6–12yrs: 25mg t.d.s.
  - >12yrs: 50mg t.d.s.
- Tablets may be crushed
- Caution: hepatic and renal failure, epilepsy, heart failure
- side-effects: dry mouth, drowsiness, blurred vision, headache, urinary retention, restlessness, insomnia, hallucinations
- Cyclizine is compatible with drugs most commonly used subcutaneously including diamorphine
- Incompatible with sodium chloride 0.9 per cent solution
- Licence: Licensed for use in adults and children aged over 6 yrs

Dexamethasone

Caution is required when using steroids in children. side-effects including weight gain, and distressing behavioural and emotional changes can occur if steroids are used for more than a few days. For this reason it is preferable to prescribe steroids in short courses (3–5 days) and to repeat courses if necessary.

- Form:
  - Tablet: 500mcg; 2mg
  - Oral solution: 2mg in 5mL
  - Injection: 4mg in 1mL can be given orally
- Dose (oral/i/v)
  - <1yr: 250–500mcg b.d.
  - 1–5yrs: 1mg b.d.
  - 6–12yrs: 2mg b.d.
  - >12yrs: 4mg b.d.
- Co-prescribing: consider antacids and anti-thrush treatment
- Caution: renal disease, cardiac disease or cystic fibrosis. Avoid in cardiac insufficiency
- Licence: not licensed for use as antiemetic in children

Noisy breathing

Excessive respiratory secretions more often cause distress to parents and carers than to the child. Reassurance may be all that is required. In circumstances where the child is distressed, pharmacological intervention may be warranted. Suction is generally not helpful.

Drug treatment is more effective if started before or immediately after the secretions are evident.

Antisecretory agents may cause drowsiness and anticholinergic side-effects: glycopyrronium has fewer CNS side-effects than hyoscine hydrobromide because it does not cross the blood brain barrier. Sometimes, however, the sedative effect may be helpful.

Management

Medication

Glycopyrronium bromide
- Form:
  - Injection: 200mcg in 1mL, 1mL ampoule
  - Tablets: 1mg, 2mg; named patient basis only
- Dose (i/v /SC):
  - 1 month–18yrs: 4–8mcg/kg (max. 200mcg) t.d.s.–q.d.s.
- Dose (continuous SC infusion):
  - 1 month–18yrs: 10–40mcg/kg/24h (max. adult dose 1200mcg/24h)
- Dose (oral):
  - 1 month–18yrs: 40–100mcg/kg t.d.s.–q.d.s.
- Contra-indications and warnings: see appropriate text
- Compatible with morphine and midazolam
- Licence: not licensed for this indication in children

Hyoscine hydrobromide
- Form:
  - Self-adhesive patch, drug released at rate of 1mg over 72h
  - Injection: 400mcg in 1mL, 1mL ampoule. 600mcg in 1mL, 1mL ampoule
- Dose (topical):
  Caution in children with intracranial malignancy: may cause agitation
  - 2–3yrs: 1/4 patch over three days
  - 3–9yrs: 1/2 patch over three days
  - >10yrs: one patch over three days
- Hyoscine patches can be cut
- Dose (SC, i/v):
  Single dose given over 2–3 minutes:
  - 1–12yrs: 10mcg/kg q.d.s.
  - >12 yrs (>40kg): 400mcg q.d.s.
- Subcutaneous continuous infusion:
  - All ages: 40–60mcg/kg/24h (max. dose 2400mcg/24h)
- Licence: transdermal preparation licensed for use in children >10yrs for motion sickness

Pain

- Adequate pain control can be achieved for the vast majority of children but requires careful attention to recognition, assessment, treatment and review
- Assessment should include a careful history and examination to elucidate the exact nature and likely cause(s) of pain so that the most effective management can be initiated
- Assessment should include discussion with parents/carers and staff as well as the child if possible
- There are a number of pain assessment tools available to aid diagnosis and monitoring of pain and analgesic effect
- Assessment of pain in children, particularly young infants and non-verbal children, may be difficult
- Pain may be under-diagnosed and therefore inadequately treated in children, particularly those unable to communicate readily
- Pain is closely associated with fear and anxiety

Recognizing pain in children with communication difficulties:
- Discuss with family/carers who know the child well
- Look for signs including: crying, becoming withdrawn, increased flexion or extension, hypersensitivity, frowning/grimacing on passive movement, poor sleep, increasing frequency of fits

Management

General measures

- Management should include reducing stress/anxiety as far as possible as well as analgesic measures
- Analgesics should be used in conjunction with non-pharmacological techniques
- Explanations and discussion often help to reduce anxiety
- A calm, quiet environment may help to reduce anxiety.
- Carefully record all information in medical records on a regular basis to enable anyone who consults the records to easily recognize changes

Medication

Choosing an analgesic:
- For mild to moderate pain, it is usual to start by using a non-opioid analgesic on a p.r.n. basis, progressing to regular use
- Some non-opioid analgesics may be used in conjunction with one another or in conjunction with opioids for added analgesic effect (🕮 see below)
- If non-opioid analgesics do not control pain effectively opioid analgesics will usually be helpful
- The oral route is preferred and adequate pain relief can be achieved using this route for most children
- In the palliative care setting where pain is constant, analgesics should be given regularly rather than p.r.n.
- Weak opioids like codeine have a dose limitation. Strong opioids do not, and the dose should be titrated until effective analgesia is achieved or side-effects prevent further escalation. If side-effects are problematic these can be treated with other medication, or the opioid can be changed to a different preparation with a different side-effect profile

- If a patient is having regular analgesia of any kind, it is important to prescribe additional p.r.n. analgesia for breakthrough pain
- Once stable, it may be possible to change to a slow release form of medication
- Discuss the management plan with the family. If opioids are to be used, a careful explanation is required so that families are prepared for drowsiness, understand that laxatives are necessary and are reassured about issues relating to addiction and dependence
- Plan for exacerbations and crises. Make sure appropriate medications and plans for their use are available to the family. This may include parenteral forms of medication for children on oral opioids
- All analgesic regimens should be regularly reviewed, particularly during titration
- Seek advice from appropriately skilled staff if you are unsure or analgesia is not quickly achieved

Non-opioid analgesics for mild/moderate pain
Paracetamol
- Form:
  - Tablet: 500mg; dispersible tablet: 500mg +120mg
  - Oral solution: 120mg in 5mL
  - Oral suspension: 120mg in 5mL; 250mg in 5mL
  - Suppositories: 60mg, 120mg, 125mg, 240mg, 250mg, 500mg, and 30mg as 'special'
- Dose (Oral):
  - Birth–3 months: 20mg/kg t.d.s. 4–6h (max. 60mg/kg/24h)
  - 3 months–1yr: 60–120mg 4–6h (max. 90mg/kg/24h)
  - 1–5yrs: 120–250mg 4–6h (max. 90mg/kg/24h)
  - 6–12yrs: 250–500mg 4–6h (max. 90mg/kg/24h or 4g/24h)
  - >12yrs: 500mg–1g 4–6h (max. 90mg/kg/24h or 4g/24h)
- Dose (rectal):
  - Birth–1 month: 20mg/kg max. t.d.s.
  - 1 month–12yrs: 20mg/kg t.d.s.–q.d.s. (max. 90mg/kg/24h or 4g/24h)
  - >12yrs: 500mg–1g t.d.s.–q.d.s. (max. 90mg/kg/24h or 4g/24h)
- Contra-indications and warnings: dose related toxicity in hepatic failure; in moderate renal failure (creatinine clearance 10–50mL/min/1.73m^2) the minimum interval between doses is six hour. In severe renal failure (creatinine clearance <10mL/min/1.73m^2) the minimum interval is eight hours. Significantly removed by haemodialysis but not by CAPD
- May provide additional analgesia in combination with opioids
- Licence: licensed for analgesic use in children >3months, except 30mg suppository

Non-steroidal anti-inflammatory drugs
- Possess analgesic and antipyretic properties
- Are particularly useful for bone pain
- Individuals may respond better to one agent than another
- Should not be given to children with thrombocytopenia or coagulation disorders

- Can be combined with paracetamol or opioids for additive analgesia
- If gastrointestinal side-effects are likely, it may be useful to prescribe antacids and/or a proton pump inhibitor

Ibuprofen
- Form:
  - Tablet: 200mg, 400mg, 600mg
  - Tablet (slow release): 800mg
  - Capsule (modified release): 300mg
  - Liquid: 100mg/5mL
  - Granules: 600mg/sachet
- Dose (oral):
  - 1 month–12yrs: 5mg/kg t.d.s.–q.d.s. (20mg/kg/24h to a max. 2.4g/24h)
  - >12yrs: 200–600mg t.d.s.–q.d.s. (max. 2.4g/24h)
- Cautions: avoid if peptic ulcer or history of; risk of gastrointestinal bleeding if coagulation defects (ibuprofen considered safer than other NSAIDS); avoid if hypersensitivity to other NSAIDS or aspirin. Caution in renal, cardiac or hepatic impairment and asthma
- Licence: Granules and 800mg slow release tablet not licensed for children. Liquid and immediate release tablets not licensed for children <7kg/<1yr

Diclofenac
- Form:
  - Tablet: (enteric coated) 25mg, 50mg; (dispersible) 50mg; (modified release) 75mg, 100mg
  - Capsules: (modified release) 75mg, 100mg
  - Suppositories: 12.5mg, 25mg, 50mg, 100mg
  - Injection: 25mg in 1mL as 3mL ampoule
- Dose (oral/rectal):
  - 6 months–18yrs: 300mcg–1mg/kg t.d.s. (max. 3mg/kg/24h to max. 150mg/24h)
  - Dose (deep i/m* or i/v– i/v must be further diluted and given over 30–120 minutes)
  - >6 months: 300mcg–1mg/kg o.d.–b.d. (max. 3mg/kg/24h to max. 150mg/24h)
  - *Intramuscular injections not recommended in children. Consider alternative agents/routes
- Cautions and contra-indications: avoid if peptic ulcer or history of; avoid if hypersensitivity to other NSAIDS or aspirin. Caution in renal, cardiac or hepatic impairment and asthma. Avoid suppositories if ulceration of lower bowel/anus. Avoid i/v use if concurrent NSAID or anticoagulant therapy
- Licence: 25mg and 50mg tablets and 12.5mg and 25mg suppositories licensed for chronic arthritis in children >1yr. Other preparations not licensed for use in children

Opioid analgesics for moderate/severe pain
- These are usually commenced when non-opioid analgesics have been tried and have not been fully effective or if pain is severe at presentation
- Always co-prescribe a regular laxative: opioids can be expected to cause constipation and it is better to prevent this from the outset

Other side-effects which should be anticipated and promptly managed are:
- Drowsiness: usually wears off after 3–5 days. Families may need forewarning of this as they may interpret drowsiness as a severe decline in the child's condition
- Nausea and vomiting (□ see section on Nausea and vomiting, p. 512)
- Pruritus: topical measures and antihistamines. Ondansetron may be effective
- Urinary retention: Check that constipation is not a contributory factor. Bethanechol or carbachol may be helpful. Catheterization is required infrequently
- Respiratory depression: this is very unlikely if the dose is titrated appropriately. Naloxone will reverse respiratory depression but this may be at the cost of analgesic effect if not administered carefully
- Euphoria, dysphoria
- Nightmares: a night time dose of haloperidol may be useful
- Physical dependence: opioids should be weaned and not ceased abruptly or a withdrawal reaction may occur
- Tolerance: this is the need for escalating doses to achieve the same therapeutic effect. It is managed by increasing the dose. Families may need to be reassured that tolerance is rare and does not necessarily imply disease progression

Weak opioids
Codeine phosphate
- Form:
  - Tablet: 15mg, 30mg, 60mg
  - Syrup: 25mg in 5mL
  - Linctus: 15mg in 5mL; 3mg in 5mL
  - Injection: 60mg in 1mL (for i/m use, never give i/v), 1mL Amp.
  - Suppositories (specials): 1mg, 2mg, 3mg, 6mg
- Dose (oral/rectal/i/m*):
  - Birth–12yrs: 500mcg–1mg/kg 4–6h (max. 240mg/24h)
  - >12yrs: 30–60mg 4–6h (max. 240mg/24h)
  - *Intramuscular injections not recommended in children. Consider alternative agents/routes
- Constipation common: prescribe laxatives prophylactically
- Cautions and contra-indications and warnings: little experience in young children, avoid in children <3 months. Avoid in renal impairment. Use with caution in hepatic impairment
- Licence: licensed for children >1yr

Dihydrocodeine tartrate
- Form:
  - Tablet: 30mg
  - Liquid: 10mg in 5mL
  - Injection: 50mg in 1mL
- Dose (oral/SC):
  - 1–4yrs: 500mcg/kg 4–6h
  - 4–12yrs: 500mcg–1mg/kg 4–6h
  - >12yr: 30mg 4–6h
- Constipation common: prescribe laxatives prophylactically
- Cautions and contra-indications and warnings: avoid or reduce dose in moderate/severe renal failure, chronic liver disease and

hypothyroidism. Avoid in respiratory depression, cystic fibrosis, head injury and raised intracranial pressure
• Licence: licensed for use in children >4yrs

Strong opioids
Morphine sulphate
• Form:
   • Tablets 10mg, 20mg, 50mg
   • Tablets/capsules (modified release): 5mg, 10mg, 15mg, 20mg, 30mg, 50mg, 60mg, 90mg, 100mg, 120mg, 150mg, 200mg
   • Granules for suspension (modified release): 20mg, 30mg, 60mg, 100mg, 200mg sachets
   • Oral solution: 10mg in 5mL; 100mg in 5mL
   • Injection also available but diamorphine is preferable for this purpose (📖 see below)
   • Suppositories: 10mg, 15mg, 20mg, 30mg. 5mg available as special
• Starting dose (oral/rectal):
   • 1–12yrs: 200–400mcg/kg 4h
   • >12yrs: 10–15mg 4h
• Starting dose (SC/i/v stat):
   • 1–12yrs: 50–100mcg/kg/dose 4 h
   • >12 yrs: 2.5–10mg/dose 4 h
• Starting Dose (continuous infusion):
   • >1yr: 10–15mcg/kg/hr
• NB In children from 6 months–5 years morphine is metabolized more rapidly than in adults, in infants less rapidly
• Prescribing regimen:
   • Always prescribe breakthrough doses (total dose/24h divided by 6)
   • If pain not controlled increase dose by 25–50 per cent
   • Use 4h dosing until pain well controlled, then convert to modified release preparation and prescribe 12h (total dose/24h divided by 2)
   • Slow release preparations normally given b.d. may need to be given t.d.s. in some children
   • Keep required dose under constant review and adjust to give optimum pain control
• Contra-indications and warnings: avoid in paralytic ileus, acute respiratory depression and liver disease. Caution in raised intracranial pressure, head injury, biliary colic, hypothyroidism. Reduce dose in renal failure: use 75 per cent in moderate renal failure (creatinine clearance 10–50mL/min/1.73m^2) and 50 per cent in severe renal failure (creatinine clearance <10mL/min/1.73m^2)
• Licence: Sevredol tablets licensed in children >3yrs. Oramorph SR tablets and Morcap SR capsules are unlicensed for use in children. Oramorph is unlicensed in children <1yr: 5mg suppositories are not licensed

Diamorphine hydrochloride
• Form:
   • Injection: 5mg, 10mg, 30mg, 100mg, 500mg

- Tablets: 10mg but no advantage over morphine sulphate and only one dose available
- Diamorphine is more potent than morphine. Diamorphine is metabolized to morphine but is more water soluble and therefore considered more convenient for SC and i/v injection
- Dose (intravenous):
  - All ages: 12.5–25mcg/kg/h continuous i/v infusion
- Dose (subcutaneous):
  - All ages: 20–100mcg/kg/h continuous SC infusion
- Conversion:
  - The dose of parenteral diamorphine is one third the dose of oral morphine so if converting directly from oral dose: total dose morphine sulphate over 24h divided by three.
- Contra-indications and warnings: paralytic ileus, phaeochromocytoma. Avoid in head injury or raised intracranial pressure. Caution in acute respiratory failure and biliary colic. Reduce dose by 50 per cent in severe renal impairment
- Licence: injection form licensed for children with terminal illness

Fentanyl
Fentanyl is less sedating and less constipating than morphine but it is more difficult to adjust the dose in response to unstable pain when used transdermally. Unless contra-indicated, it is generally better to stabilize the pain using an oral or parenteral opioid before changing to fentanyl patches.
- Form:
  - Patches: for transdermal absorption over 72 h: 25mcg/h, 50mcg/h, 75mcg/h, 100mcg/h
  - Lozenge: for buccal use: 200mcg, 400mcg, 600mcg, 800mcg, 1200mcg, 1600mcg
  - Injection form available but should be used by those with specific experience in paediatric pain medicine
- Dose (transdermal):
  - All ages: To convert from total daily dose of oral morphine sulphate:

Oral morphine (total daily dose) (mg/24h)	<135mg	135–224mg	225–314mg	315–404mg	405–494mg
Fentanyl patch (mcg/hr)	25	50	75	100	125

Converting from oral morphine sulphate:
- Continue oral morphine preparation for up to 12h after first fentanyl patch applied as patch will take 6–12h to reach therapeutic levels
- Wait 24–48h after application before evaluating analgesic effect or changing dose
- Always provide p.r.n. doses of oral morphine for breakthrough pain
- Use new area of skin with each patch change
- Avoid exposure of patch to excessive heat (sun bathing; hot water bottle etc) as heat will increase absorption

- Dose (buccal):
  - Useful for incident and breakthrough pain
  - Dose not related to background analgesic dose, therefore start with 200mcg lozenge and adjust dose according to response
- Although fentanyl may be less constipating than morphine, a laxative should be co-prescribed
- Contra-indications and warnings: see diamorphine. Fentanyl is less problematic in renal failure than diamorphine
- Licence: lozenges and transdermal preparation unlicensed in children

Oxycodone
- Form:
  - Capsules: 5mg, 10mg, 20mg
  - Liquid: 5mg in 5mL; concentrate: 10mg in 1mL
  - Tablets, modified release: 5mg, 10mg, 20mg, 40mg, 80mg
- Dose (oral):
  - **For opioid naïve patients:**
  - 2–12yrs: 0.2mg/kg immediate release preparation 4 h
  - >12 yrs: 5–10mg immediate release preparation 4 h
  - **For children already on opioids:**
  - Conversion ratio from morphine to oxycodone is 2:1 (ie. total daily dose of oxycodone is half the total daily dose of morphine)
  - Alternatively: to determine dose of oxycodone, divide total morphine dose by 12 and give up to 4-h
  - Convert to long-acting preparation when stable
- Contra-indications: acute respiratory depression, paralytic ileus, liver disease, moderate to severe renal failure
- Other opioids such as hydromorphone and methadone are available but their use should be discussed with a paediatric pain or palliative care specialist.

Pain syndromes and adjuvant therapy

Bone pain

Radiotherapy
- Useful for discrete bone metastases
- May be given as a short course or single dose
- Effective treatment with minimal side-effects

Non-steroidal anti-inflammatory drugs
When used in combination with opioids, non-steroidal anti-inflammatory drugs (NSAIDS) may lower the dose of opioid required for effective analgesia. Common choices are:

Ibuprofen
- Form:
  - Tablet: 200mg, 400mg, 600mg
  - Tablet (slow release): 800mg
  - Capsule (modified release): 300mg
  - Liquid: 100mg/5mL
  - Granules: 600mg/sachet
- Dose (oral):
  - 1 month–12yrs: 5mg/kg t.d.s.–q.d.s. (max. 20mg/kg/24h to max. 2.4g/24h)
  - >12yrs: 200–600mg t.d.s.–q.d.s. (max. 2.4g/24h)
- Cautions: avoid if peptic ulcer or history of; risk of gastrointestinal bleeding if coagulation defects (ibuprofen considered safer than other NSAIDS); avoid if hypersensitivity to other NSAIDS or aspirin. Caution in renal, cardiac or hepatic impairment and asthma
- Licence: Granules and 800mg slow release tablet not licensed for children. Liquid and immediate release tablets not licensed for children <7kg/<1yr.

Diclofenac
- Form:
  - Tablet: (enteric coated) 25mg, 50mg; (dispersible) 50mg; (modified release) 75mg, 100mg
  - Capsules: (modified release) 75mg, 100mg
  - Suppositories: 12.5mg, 25mg, 50mg, 100mg
  - Injection: 25mg in 1mL as 3mL ampoule
- Dose (oral/rectal):
  - 6 months–18yrs: 300mcg–1mg/kg t.d.s. (max. 3mg/kg/24h to max. 150mg/24h)
- Dose (deep i/m* or i/v– i/v must be further diluted and given over 30–120 minutes)
  - >6 months: 300mcg–1mg/kg o.d.–b.d. (max. 3mg/kg/24h to max. 150mg/24h)
  *Intramuscular injections not recommended in children: consider alternative agent/route
- Cautions and contra-indications and warnings: avoid if peptic ulcer or history of; avoid if hypersensitivity to other NSAIDS or aspirin. Caution in renal, cardiac or hepatic impairment and asthma. Avoid suppositories if ulceration of lower bowel/anus. Avoid i/v use if concurrent NSAID or anticoagulant therapy

• Licence: 25mg and 50mg tablets and 12.5mg and 25mg suppositories licensed for chronic arthritis in children >1yr. Other preparations not licensed for use in children

Selective COX-2 inhibitors

COX-2 (cyclo-oxygenase 2) inhibitors such as celecoxib are equally analgesic when compared with non-selective NSAIDs. They offer certain advantages in that the risk of gastrointestinal bleeding is reduced, and they have no effect on platelet function.

Bisphosphonates

Bisphosphonates have been shown to reduce bone pain related to malignant and non-malignant causes in adults. They have been used in children. Seek advice before using.

'Resistant' and neuropathic pain

Most pain can be controlled with adequate doses of opioid medication and much of what is regarded as 'resistant' pain can be managed with a dose increase or an alternative route of delivery (e.g. parenteral, spinal). In some instances however, the addition of an adjuvant agent which targets a particular pain mechanism or pathway may be helpful. Neuropathic pain has particular features including a lancinating or burning quality, shock-like features or associated parasthesiae. Antidepressants or antiepileptic medications may be a useful addition to the regimen where these features are present. The choice between the two classes of drug will depend on the child's other symptoms. For example, a child with sleeping difficulties might benefit from a tricyclic antidepressant whereas a child with a coexistent seizure disorder will benefit from an anticonvulsant. If one class of drug is ineffective, a change can be made to another class.

Tricyclic antidepressants

Apart from relieving neuropathic pain, tricyclic antidepressants can enhance opioid-induced analgesia and improve sleep.

Amitriptyline
• Form:
  • Tablets: 10mg, 25mg, 50mg
  • Oral solution: 25mg in 5mL; 50mg in 5mL
• Dose (oral):
  • 1–18yrs: 0.5–1mg/kg nocte
• Starting dose should be at lower end of range, then increase dose by 25 per cent every four days until max. dose (2mg/kg/day) reached or side-effects preclude further titration. Full analgesic effect may not be seen for two weeks
• Contra-indications and warnings: see imipramine
• Licence: not licensed for treatment of neuropathic pain in children

Imipramine
• Form:
  • Tablets: 10mg, 25mg
• Dose (oral):
  • >1 month: 200–400mcg/kg nocte
  • Titrate (50 per cent increase every three days) up to 1–3mg/kg nocte

- Contra-indications and warnings: acute porphyria; hepatic impairment
- Caution with cardiac disease (monitor ECG over 150mg/day)
- Do not use for 3 weeks after discontinuing MAOIs
- Interactions and side-effects: see other texts for full information
- Causes antimuscarinic effects, sedation, cardiac arrhythmias, and lowers seizure threshold
- Licence: not licensed for neuropathic pain in children

Anticonvulsants
Carbamazepine
- Form:
  - Tablets (immediate release): 100mg, 200mg, 400mg; chewable tablets 100mg, 200mg
  - Tablets (modified release): 200mg, 400mg
  - Oral liquid: 100mg in 5mL
  - Suppositories: 125mg, 250mg
- Dose (oral):
  - 1 month–12yrs: start with 2.5mg/kg b.d.
  - Increase by 2.5mg/kg b.d. at weekly intervals to a maximum of 10mg/kg b.d.
  - >12yrs: 200–400mg b.d.–t.d.s.
- The medication should be started at the lower end of the dose range and slowly titrated until therapeutic levels are achieved, symptoms are relieved or side-effects are limiting (e.g. ataxia, drowsiness, nausea.) Titrating slowly minimizes side-effects
- The suspension is absorbed faster than tablets. This might necessitate dividing the total daily dose of suspension into 3–4 doses in order to maintain therapeutic levels
- Contra-indications and warnings: A-V conduction abnormalities, history of bone marrow depression, intermittent porphyria, MAOIs within previous two weeks, sensitivity to tricyclics. Dose reduce in advanced liver disease. Numerous drug interactions
- Licence: licensed for use in children

Gabapentin
- Form:
  - Capsules: 100mg, 300mg, 400mg
- Dose (oral):
  - All ages: start at 10mg/kg once daily for four days then b.d. for four days then t.d.s.
  - Adjust dose according to response. Max. daily dose in adults is 1.8g/24h
  - Capsules can be opened and the contents added to small volumes of fluid or food
- Contra-indications and warnings: avoid abrupt withdrawal. Caution in renal failure: reduce frequency of doses
- Licence: licensed for children >6yrs for epilepsy

Levomepromazine
May be helpful for distressed patients in severe pain unresponsive to other measures.
- Form:
  - Tablets: 25mg
  - Injection: 25mg in 1mL, 1mL ampoule

- Stat Dose (oral, SC):
  - 2–12yrs: 0.5mg/kg o.d–b.d.
  - >12yrs: 6.25–25mg o.d–b.d.
  - Titrate according to response
- Usual maximum daily dose in adults 100mg/day (can be given as a continuous SC infusion) or 200mg/day (p.o.)
- Highly sedative in higher doses. (SC dose >1mg/kg/24h)
- May reduce seizure threshold
- Postural hypotension especially if used with opioids
- Little experience in very small children
- Caution: Parkinsonism, postural hypotension, antihypertensive medication, epilepsy, hypothyroidism, myasthenia gravis
- Licence: not licensed for pain

Ketamine

Ketamine is a useful adjuvant agent for patients with neuropathic pain because of its action on NMDA receptors. It has a tendency to cause agitation and hallucinations in higher doses. Seek advice from a pain management specialist before using.

Nerve blocks/spinal administration/other neuroanaesthetic approaches

May be helpful for children who do not respond to the above measures; consult local anaesthetic team. Spinal infusions can be managed in the community by appropriately trained staff.

Pain associated with tumour-related oedema

Including pain related to intracranial tumours and nerve plexus compression.

Steroids

- Should be used with caution in children
- Short courses (up to five days) can be very effective for this type of pain
- Potential problems include mood and behaviour changes, rapid weight gain and body image changes as well as insomnia and reduced mobility caused by proximal myopathy
- Give entire dose before midday to reduce effect on sleep

Dexamethasone

- Form:
  - Tablets: 500mcg, 2mg
  - Oral solution: 2mg in 5mL
  - Injection: 4mg in 1mL can be given orally
- Dose (oral /SC/i/v):
  - <1yr: 0.25–0.5mg b.d.
  - 1–5yrs: 1mg b.d.
  - 6–11yrs: 2mg b.d.
  - >12yrs: 4mg b.d.
- Higher doses are needed for children with raised intracranial pressure or spinal cord compression
- Contra-indications and warnings: caution if renal disease, cardiac disease or cystic fibrosis. Avoid in cardiac insufficiency
- Licence: licensed for use in children for symptoms associated with brain tumours but not specifically for nerve pain

Painful procedures
- If a procedure is likely to cause discomfort take preventative action!
- Explain all procedures to parents and children as appropriate to reduce anxiety
- Undertake procedures in friendly if not familiar surroundings
- Have parents/carers or the nurse who know the child best present.
- Use anaesthetic creams and distraction techniques appropriate to the age of the child
- Benzodiazepines are often employed in small doses *in conjunction with analgesia* for more difficult procedures e.g. midazolam given buccally, i/v, or intranasally gives light sedation and some amnesia
- Oral
  - 1/12 500mcg/kg max. 15mg
- Buccal/intranasal
  - 200–300mcg/kg dropped into alternate nostrils over 15 seconds. Max. 10mg
- Inhaled nitrous oxide has analgesic and amnesic properties but is non-sedating, so is only useful for co-operative children aged five years or older. Careful supervision is required
- Ketamine is another useful agent but requires careful supervision by trained staff

Psychological issues—anxiety and depression

Management

General measures

- Provide an environment and the opportunity for the child to raise his/her concerns and fears
- Children often find relaxation techniques such as guided imagery very helpful
- Complementary therapies like music therapy may be useful particularly in non-verbal children
- Offer counselling and complementary therapies to parents if possible
- Psychotherapeutic techniques may be necessary

Anxiety

Medication

- Medication should be use in combination with non-pharmacological techniques
- Anxiety may be a manifestation of depression, in which case an antidepressant may be more appropriate
- The choice of benzodiazepine will depend on the circumstance for which it is being prescribed. Children experiencing brief periods of anxiety or panic attacks may benefit from a benzodiazepine with a short half-life, such as midazolam, given buccally or subcutaneously. Sublingual lorazepam is another option for panic attacks or anxiety related to dyspnoea. Children needing a longer duration of action may prefer diazepam

Midazolam

- Form:
  - Injection: 10mg in 2mL; 10mg in 5mL. Injection may be diluted in sodium chloride 0.9 per cent or glucose 5 per cent for buccal and intranasal routes
  - Oral syrup: only available as special
- Single doses:
  - **Intravenous/subcutaneous:**
    - >1month–18yrs: 100mcg/kg
  - **Buccal/sublingual:**
    - >1month–18yrs: 500mcg/kg (max. 10mg)
    - Tastes bitter when given orally but can be mixed with juice or chocolate sauce
  - **Intranasal:**
    - >1month–18yrs: 200–300mcg/kg (max. 10mg)
    - Intranasal route may be unpleasant but has a fast onset of action (5–15 minutes)
  - **Rectal:**
    - >1month–18yrs: 500–750 mcg/kg
    - Continuous intravenous/subcutaneous infusion:
    - >1month–18yrs: 2.5mg/24 h (note: this is not a per kg dose). Titrate to effect

- Contra-indications and warnings: caution with pulmonary disease, hepatic and renal dysfunction (reduce dose), severe fluid/electrolyte imbalance and congestive cardiac failure. Avoid rapid withdrawal after prolonged treatment
- Licence: licensed for sedation in intensive care and for induction of anaesthesia. Other routes and indications not licensed

Clonazepam
- Form:
  - Drops: 2.5mg in 1mL (1 drop = 0.1mg), named patient
  - Tablets: 0.5mg, 2mg
  - Injection: 1mg in 1mL (1mL ampoule)
  - Oral liquid 500mcg in 5mL, 2mg in 5mL 'special'
- Dose (sublingual):
  - All ages: 0.01mg/kg/dose (max. 0.5mg) b.d./t.d.s
  - If necessary, increase by 10–25 per cent every 2–3 days to max. 0.1–0.2mg/kg/day
  - Prescribe as number of drops. Count drops onto spoon before administering
- Irritability and aggression not uncommon in which case drug should be withdrawn. Increased secretions may occur in infants and young children

Lorazepam
- Form:
  - Tablets: 1mg (scored), 2.5mg
  - Suspension: only available as special
  - Injection: 4mg in 1mL, 1mL ampoule
- Dose (sublingual, oral):
  - All ages: 25–50mcg/kg single dose (max. 4mg in adults in 24 h)
  - Most children will not need more than 0.5–1mg for trial dose
- Well absorbed sublingually (good for panic attacks) and child has control
- Injection can also be given sublingually
- Contra-indications and warnings: severe pulmonary disease, sleep apnoea, coma, CNS depression. Caution in hepatic and renal failure
- Licence: tablets licensed as pre-medication in children >5yrs. Injection not licensed in children <12yrs except for treatment of status epilepticus

Diazepam
- Form:
  - Tablets: 2mg, 5mg, 10mg
  - Oral solution: 2mg in 5mL and 5mg in 5mL
  - Injection (solution and emulsion): 5mg in 1mL
  - Suppositories: 10mg
  - Rectal tubes: 2mg in 1mL: 2.5mg tube, 5mg tube, 10mg tube, 20mg tube, 4mg in 1mL: 10mg tube
- Dose (oral):
  - 1 month–12yrs: 50–100mcg/kg b.d.–q.d.s.
  - >12yrs: 2.5–5mg b.d–q.d.s.
- Potential for dependency in prolonged courses
- Licence: rectal preparation is licensed for use in children >1yr with severe anxiety. Tablets and liquid licensed for night terrors and sleep-walking

Levomepromazine and haloperidol are sedatives but are not effective anxiolytics.

Depression

The incidence of depression in terminally ill children (other than adolescents) is unknown, but it is likely that for many it remains unrecognized and untreated.

The clinical picture will depend on the age and developmental stage of the child but the usual features of depressed mood, anhedonia, social withdrawal, and disturbed sleep and appetite may be present. The diagnosis is less dependent on somatic symptomatology because of the coexistence of illness.

Diagnosis may be difficult: trust the instincts of parents and carers and consult a child psychologist at an early stage.

Fluoxetine
- Form:
  - Capsules: 20mg, 60mg
  - Liquid: 20mg in 5mL
- Dose (oral):
  - 6–18yrs: 10mg o.d. increase slowly to 20mg
- Contra-indications and warnings: avoid in hepatic or renal insufficiency. Lowers seizure threshold. Do not use with, or within two weeks of taking MAOIs
- Interactions: see appropriate text
- Licence: not licensed for use in children

Amitriptyline
Although tricyclic antidepressants no longer constitute first line management of depression in children, amitriptyline may be an appropriate choice in circumstances where pain and disturbed sleep are also present.
- Form:
  - Tablets: 10mg, 25mg, 50mg
  - Oral solution: 25mg in 5mL; 50mg in 5mL
- Dose (oral):
  - All ages: 0.5–1mg/kg nocte
  - Start at lower end of dose range and increase by 25 per cent every 2–3 days until maximum dose (2mg/kg/day) reached or side-effects preclude further dose increase. Full effect may not be seen for two weeks

- Contra-indications and warnings: see imipramine
- Licence: not licensed for treatment of neuropathic pain in children

Imipramine
- Form:
  - Tablets: 10mg, 25mg
- Starting dose (oral):
  - 6–7yrs: 25mg nocte
  - 8–11yrs: 25–50mg nocte
  - 12–18yrs: 25mg t.d.s. or 75mg nocte
- Maintenance dose (oral):
  - 12–18yrs only:Increase stepwise to 150–200mg daily in divided doses in first seven days. Continue until definite improvement then gradually reduce dose to long-term maintenance dose of 50–100mg daily
- Contra-indications and warnings: acute porphyria; hepatic impairment. Caution in cardiac disease. Do not use with, or within two weeks of taking MAOIs. Lowers seizure threshold
- Interactions: see appropriate text
- Licence: not licensed for this indication in children

NOTE: The Committee for Safety in Medicines has advised (December 2003) that citalopram, escitalopram, paroxetine, sertraline, venlafaxine, and fluvoxamine are contra-indicated if less than 18 years old.

Sleeplessness

Disturbed sleep has a major impact upon the child and family's quality of life. Adequate sleep may be the difference between a family's ability to cope with the stresses placed upon them or not.

Management:

General measures

- Address the child's fears and concerns
- Consider the sleep pattern: the child may be sleeping a lot in the day and may be reversing the day/night pattern. It may be appropriate to keep the child awake more in the day or to provide extra stimulation during the day—this will depend on the child's stage of illness. The child may not be aware of when he is expected to sleep if intervention is needed around the clock
- Optimize bedtime routine: bath if possible, story, hot drink if appropriate, lights low
- Increase exposure to light in the mornings
- Consider complementary therapies to aid relaxation
- Try and disturb the child as little as possible during the night: this may mean re-scheduling medications

Medication

Temazepam
- Form:
  - Tablets: 10mg, 20mg
  - Oral solution: 10mg in 5mL
- Dose (oral):
  - 1 month–12yrs: 1mg/kg nocte
  - >12yrs: 10–20mg nocte
- Contra-indications and warnings: caution in severe liver disease. Avoid in CNS depression and acute pulmonary insufficiency
- Interactions: see appropriate text
- Licence: not licensed for use in children

Amitriptyline
This is a useful addition in circumstances where pain is also present
- Form:
  - Tablets: 10mg, 25mg, 50mg
  - Oral solution: 25mg in 5mL; 50mg in 5mL
- Dose (oral):
  - 1–18yrs: 0.5–1mg/kg nocte
  - Start at lower end of dose range and increase by 25 per cent every 2–3 days until maximum dose (2mg/kg/day) reached or side-effects preclude further dose increase. Full effect may not be seen for two weeks
- Contra-indications and warnings: see imipramine

Chloral hydrate
- Form:
  - Oral solution: chloral mixture BP: 500mg in 5mL; chloral elixir paediatric BP 200mg in 5mL, extemporaneously prepared
  - Syrup: 500mg in 5mL only available as 'special'
  - Suppositories: 25mg, 50mg, 100mg, 250mg, 750mg only available as 'specials'
  - Tablets: chloral betaine 707mg (= chloral hydrate 414mg)
- Dose (oral/rectal):
  - 1 month–12yrs: 30–50mg/kg (max. 1g) nocte
  - >12yrs: 0.5–1g nocte
- Contra-indications and warnings: avoid in liver disease and severe renal failure. Caution in cardiac disease, respiratory insufficiency, porphyria and gastritis. Avoid prolonged administration and abrupt withdrawal
- Licence: unlicensed in children

Alimemazine tartrate
- Form:
  - Tablets: 10mg
  - Mixture: 1.5mg in 1mL, 6mg in 1mL
  - Syrup: 7.5mg in 5mL
  - Syrup forte: 30mg in 5mL
- Dose (oral):
  - 1m.–12yrs: 1.5–3mg/kg nocte
  - >12yrs: 10mg t.d.s (max 90mg/day)

Promethazine hydrochloride
- Form:
  - Tablets: 10mg, 25mg
  - Elixir: 5mg in 5mL
  - Injection: 25mg in 1mL as 1mL ampoule
- Dose (oral):
  - <1yr: 5–10mg nocte
  - 1–5yrs: 10–20mg nocte
  - 6–12yrs: 20–25mg nocte
  - >12yrs: 25–50mg nocte
- May be useful in mild cases
  - Contra-indications and warnings: Porphyria; CNS depression; hypersensitivity to phenothiazines. Do not use with, or within two weeks of taking MAOIs
- Licence: licensed for use in children >2yrs

Raised intracranial pressure

Consider raised intracranial pressure if the child shows evidence of:
- Confusion
- Personality change
- Drowsiness
- Vomiting
- Headache (especially on waking)
- Focal neurology

Management

General measures

- Investigation should be considered only if it will contribute to management decisions
- Reduction of tumour bulk may improve symptoms e.g. cranial irradiation and chemotherapy. Occasionally a ventricular shunt may be appropriate
- Symptomatic management may include analgesia (see pain section), antiemetics and steroids. The antiemetic of choice is cyclizine

Medication

Dexamethasone

Caution is required when using steroids in children. side-effects including weight gain, and distressing behavioural and emotional changes occur if steroids are used for more than a few days. For this reason it is preferable to prescribe steroids in short courses (3–5 days) and to repeat courses if necessary.
- Form:
  - Tablet: 500mcg; 2mg
  - Oral solution: 2mg in 5mL
  - Injection: 4mg in 1mL can be given orally
- Dose (oral/i/v over 3–5 minutes):
  - <1yr: 0.5–1.0mg b.d.
  - 1–5yrs: 2mg b.d.
  - 6–12yrs: 4mg b.d.
  - >12yrs: 8mg b.d.
  - Do not give after midday as can affect night time sleep
- Dose (SC):
  - Can also be given in equivalent doses SC as single doses or as continuous infusion over 24h
  - If no effect after 3–5 days, stop steroids (no need to tail off)
  - Co-prescribing: consider antacids and anti-thrush treatment
- Contra-indications and warnings: caution if renal disease, cardiac disease or cystic fibrosis. Avoid in cardiac insufficiency
- Licence: licensed for use in children but not as antiemetic

Cyclizine

- Form:
  - Tablets: 50mg
  - Injection: 50mg/mL (1mL)
  - Suppositories: 25mg ('special')

- Dose (i/v stat):
  - 1/12 500mcg/mg/kg t.d.s. Max. single dose <6 yrs: 25mg, >6yrs: 50 mg
- Dose (SC/i/v continuous infusion):
  - 1m.–2yrs: 3mg/kg/24h
  - 2–5yrs: 50mg/24 h
  - 6–12yrs: 75mg/24 h
  - > 12yrs: 150mg/24 h
- Oral/rectal
  - <2yr: 1mg/kg t.d.s.
  - 2–5yrs: 12.5mg t.d.s.
  - 6–12yrs: 25mg t.d.s.
  - >12yrs: 50mg t.d.s.
- Caution: hepatic and renal failure, epilepsy, heart failure
- Side-effects: dry mouth, drowsiness, blurred vision, headache, urinary retention, restlessness, insomnia, hallucinations
- Tablets may be crushed
- Cyclizine is compatible with drugs most commonly used subcutaneously including diamorphine
- Incompatible with sodium chloride 0.9 per cent solution

Skin

Management

General measures

- Like adults, children with terminal illnesses have skin that is susceptible to breakdown with poor healing abilities
- Good nursing care is required to predict and prevent problems, which once established may be difficult to treat
- Frequent and appropriate turning is essential to avoid pressure areas breaking down
- The use of suitable mattresses and mobility aids should be considered
- Consult tissue viability nurse if available

Medication

- At risk areas
  - Protect with Opsite, Tegaderm or Cutifilm
- Broken areas
  - Use Duoderm, Spyrosorb
- Infection
  - Send swab for growth. Use Intrasite gel, Iodosorb paste covered with Opsite or Tegaderm +/- antibiotics
- Cavities
  - Pack with Kaltostat or Sorbsan
- Fungating tumours and odour
  - Use topical metronidazole gel, charcoal dressings or honey and sugar.
- Painful ulcers
  - Consider anaesthetic preparations e.g. lidocaine/prilocaine (EmLa cream) or a topical morphine gel

See also adult section on Skin.

Sweating

Consider cause
- Disease e.g. malignant pyrexia, lymphoma, neuroblastoma
- Drugs e.g. opioids, amitriptyline, chemotherapy
- Infection

Management

General measures
- Disease-modifying treatment may improve sweating if it is part of a malignant syndrome
- Fan, cotton clothing, skin care
- Encourage plenty of fluids to avoid dehydration

Medication
There is no good evidence to support the use of any of the following agents but they may be worth trying

Paracetamol
- Form:
  - Tablets: 500mg; dispersible tablets: 500mg
  - Oral solution: 120mg in 5mL
  - Oral suspension: 120mg in 5mL; 250mg in 5mL
  - Suppositories: 60mg, 120mg, 125mg, 240mg, 250mg, 500mg, and 30mg as 'special'
- Dose (oral):
  - Birth–3 months: 20mg/kg t.d.s. (max. 60mg/kg/24h)
  - 3 months –1yr: 60–120mg 4–6h (max. 90mg/kg/24h)
  - 1–5yrs: 120–250mg 4–6h (max. 90mg/kg/24h)
  - 6–12yrs: 250–500mg 4–6h (max. 90mg/kg/24h or 4g/24h)
  - >12yrs: 500mg–1g 4–6h (max. 90mg/kg/24h or 4g/24h)
- Dose (rectal):
  - Birth–1 month: 20mg/kg max. t.d.s.
  - 1 month–12yrs: 20mg/kg t.d.s.– q.d.s. (max. 90mg/kg/24h or 4g/24h)
  - >12yrs: 500mg–1g t.d.s.– q.d.s. (max. 90mg/kg/24h or 4g/24h)
- Contra-indications and warnings: dose related toxicity in hepatic failure; in moderate renal failure (creatinine clearance 10–50mL/min/1.73m^2) the minimum interval between doses is six h. In severe renal failure (creatinine clearance < 10mL/min/1.73m^2) the minimum interval is eight hours. Significantly removed by haemodialysis but not by CAPD
- Licence: licensed for antipyretic and analgesic use in children >3months, except 30mg suppository

Naproxen
- Form:
  - Tablets: 250mg, 375mg, 500mg
- Dose (oral):
  - >1 month: 5–15mg/kg b.d. (max. 1g/24h)

- Contra-indications and warnings: Contra-indicated in children who have shown hypersensitivity to aspirin or other NSAIDS. Caution in asthma and cardiac, hepatic or renal failure; avoid if creatinine clearance <20mL/min/1.73m². Extreme caution if current or previous history of peptic ulceration
- Licence: not licensed for use in children for this indication

Other

Dantrolene, steroids and H2 receptor antagonists have also been used.

Terminal restlessness

Restlessness and agitation are not uncommon during the terminal phase. Nursing the child in a calm, peaceful and preferably familiar environment is helpful as is having a parent or other trusted adult present. It is important to exclude pain or inadequate positioning as a cause of distress. Hypoxia may also be a factor.

The choice of medication will depend on the clinical circumstances. Midazolam is very effective and can be combined with morphine or diamorphine more commonly in a subcutaneous infusion. Levomepromazine is also compatible with these medications and is an appropriate choice for children who also have pain and nausea.

Medication

Midazolam

- Form:
  - Injection: 10mg in 2mL; 10mg in 5mL
  - Injection may be diluted in Sodium chloride 0.9% or glucose 5% for oral, buccal and intranasal routes
  - Oral syrup: 'special'
- Single doses:
  - Intravenous/subcutaneous:
    - >1month–18yrs: 100mcg/kg
  - Buccal/sublingual:
    - >1month–18yrs: 500mcg/kg (max. 10mg)
    - Tastes bitter when given orally but can be mixed with juice or chocolate sauce
  - Intranasal:
    - >1month–18yrs: 200–300mcg/kg (max. 10mg)
    - Intranasal route may be unpleasant but has a fast onset of action (5–15 minutes). Drop dose into alternate nostrils over 15s
  - Rectal:
    - >1month–18yrs: 500–700mcg/kg
  - Continuous intravenous/subcutaneous infusion:
    - Start at 2.5mg/24 h (note: this is not a per kg dose). Doses of up to 40mg/24 h have been necessary. If high doses required consider changing to a different agent
  - Well absorbed subcutaneously
- Midazolam is compatible in a syringe driver with morphine, diamorphine, cyclizine and other commonly used drugs
- Contra-indications and warnings: caution with pulmonary disease, hepatic and renal dysfunction (reduce dose), severe fluid /electrolyte imbalance and congestive cardiac failure. Avoid rapid withdrawal after prolonged treatment
- Midazolam raises seizure threshold making it a good choice for children likely to fit
- Licence: licensed for sedation in intensive care and for induction of anaesthesia in children >7yrs. Other routes and indications not licensed

Clonazepam
- Form:
  - Drops: 2.5mg/mL(1 drop = 0.1mg), named patient basis
  - Tablet: 0.5mg, 2mg
  - Injection: 1mg in 1mL (1mL ampoule)
  - Oral liquid: 500mcg in 5mL, 2mg in 5mL 'specials'
- Dose (sublingual):
  - All ages: 0.01mg/kg/dose (max. 0.5mg) b.d./t.d.s.
  - If necessary, increase by 10–25 per cent every 2–3 days to max. 0.1–0.2mg/kg/day
  - Prescribe as number of drops. Count drops onto spoon before administering
- Irritability and aggression not uncommon in which case drug should be withdrawn. Increased secretions may occur in infants and young children
- Licence: not licensed for this indication

Levomepromazine
- Form:
  - Tablets: 25mg
  - Injection: 25mg in mL, 1mL ampoule
- Dose (continuous SC/i/v infusion):
  - All ages: 0.5–1mg/kg/24h. Titrate to effect. (max. adult dose 300mg/24h)
- Also acts as antiemetic
- May lower seizure threshold
- Can be used in conjunction with midazolam
- Highly sedative in higher doses (SC dose > 1mg/kg/24h)
- Postural hypotension especially if used with opioids
- Little experience in very small children
- Caution: Parkinsonism, postural hypotension, antihypertensive medication, epilepsy, hypothyroidism, myasthenia gravis
- Licence: not licensed for use as an antiemetic in children

Emergency drugs summary

The following information is given as a rough guide for quick reference only.

Many of the following drugs, doses or indications are unlicensed in children.

Table 7.1 Analgesics

Drug	Route	1month–1yr	2–12 yrs	12–18 yrs	Notes
Morphine	p.o./PR	100mcg/kg	200–400mcg/kg	10–15mg	4-h starting doses
Diamorphine	CSCI	20–100mcg/kg/24h	20–100mcg/kg/24h	20–100mcg/kg/24h	24h starting dose
	SC/i/v stat	5–15mcg/kg	5–15mcg/kg	2.5–5mg	4-h as needed
Ibuprofen	PPO	5mg/kg	5mg/kg	200–600mg	t.d.s–q.d.s Maximum 2.4g/day

Table 7.2 Antiemetics

Drug	Route	1 month–2yr	2–12 yrs	12–18 yrs	Notes
Cyclizine	p.o./PR	1mg/kg t.d.s.	2–5yrs: 12.5mg t.d.s.	25–50mg t.d.s	
Cyclizine	SC i/v continuous infusion	3mg/kg/24h	2–5yrs: 50mg/24h 6–12yrs: 75mg/24h	150mg/24h (max.)	
Cyclizine	i/v stat	>1month 500mcg–1mg/kg t.d.s. (max. 25mg)	2–5yrs: 20mg (max. 25mg) 6–12yrs: 25mg (max. 50mg)	>12yrs: 50mg (max.)	Give slowly over 3–5 minutes
Haloperidol	p.o.	12.5–50mcg/kg b.d.	12.5–50mcg/kg b.d.	0.5–2mg b.d.–t.d.s.	Increased risk of extrapyramidal side-effects in children.
Ondansteron	i/v	5mg/m² b.d.–t.d.s. (max. 8mg)	5mg/m² b.d.–t.d.s. (max. 8mg)	8mg b.d.–t.d.s	Give over 3–5 minutes Can be given as continuous infusion
Ondansteron	p.o.	1mg b.d.–t.d.s	2–4mg b.d.–t.d.s 4–12yrs 4mg b.d.–t.d.s	8mg b.d.–t.d.s	
Metoclopramide	p.o./i/m /slow i/v/SC	100–170mcg/kg t.d.s.	100–170mcg/kg t.d.s.	100–170mcg/kg t.d.s.	Increased risk of extrapyramidal side-effects in children
Levomepromazine	p.o.		0.1–1mg/kg o.d.–b.d.	6.25–25mg o.d.–b.d.	Very sedating in doses over 1mg/kg/24 h
Levomepromazine	SC i/v continuous infusion	0.1–0.25mg/kg (max. 25mg/24h)	0.1–0.25mg/kg (max. 25mg/24h)	0.1–0.25mg/kg (max. 25mg/24h)	

Table 7.3 Sedatives

Drug	Route	<1yr	1–12 yrs	12–18 yrs	Notes
Diazepam	p.o./PR	50–100mcg/kg/dose	50–100mcg/kg/dose	2.5–5mg b.d.	Repeated as needed
Lorazepam	p.o./sublingual	25–50 mcg/kg/dose	25–50mcg/kg/dose	25–50mcg/kg/dose	Max 4mg in 24 h
Midazolam	CSCI	>1 month–18yrs: 2.5mg/24h			
	SC/i/v stat	>1month–18yrs: 100mcg/kg			
	Buccal stat	1 month–18yrs: 500mcg/kg (max 10mg)			

Table 7.4 Antisialogogue (for death rattle)

Drug	Route	2–18 yrs	Notes
Hyoscine hydrobromide	SC stat	1–12yrs: 10mcg/kg <12yrs (>40kg): 400mcg	Repeat every 4h as needed Sedating
Hyoscine hydrobromide	CSCI	40–60mcg/kg/24h	Max dose 2400mcg/24h
Glycopyrronium	SC/i/v stat	1month–18yrs: 4–8mcg/kg	Repeat every 6–8h as needed Doses for drooling much lower, max. 200mcg/dose
Glycopyrronium	CSCI	1month–18yrs: 10–40mcg/kg/24hr	Max adult dose 1200mcg/24h

Table 7.5 Average weights for healthy children

Age	Mean weight Kg	% Adult dose
Newborn	3.5	12.5
6 months	8	22
1 yr	10	25
3 yrs	15	33
5 yrs	20	40
7 yrs	25	50
12 yrs	40	75
Adult male	70	100
Adult female	60	100

NB Wt. in stones × 6 ≈ wt. in Kg.

The percentage adult dose should only be used as a rough guide when paediatric doses in mg/kg are not available.

Further reading

Books and articles

Bluebond-Langner M. (1978) *The Private Worlds of Dying Children*. Princeton: Princeton University Press.

Goldman A. (1994) *Care of the dying child*. Oxford: Oxford University Press.

Herbert, M. (1996) *Supporting bereaved and dying children and their parents*. Leicester: BPS Books.

Jassah SS. (2002) *Basic symptom control in paediatric palliative care: The Rainbow Children's Hospice Guidelines*. 4th edn. Loughborough: Rainbow Children's Hospice.

Leikin S. (1989) A proposal concerning decisions to forgo life-sustaining treatment for young people. *J Pediatrics* **115**: 17–22.

Lidstone V. et al. (2003) *Paediatric Palliative Care Guidelines*. London: The South West London and the Surrey, West Sussex and Hampshire Cancer Networks.

Orloff S., Huff S. (2004) *Homecare for Seriously Ill Children: A Manual for Parents*. Alexandria: CHI.

Royal Children's Hospital, Brisbane. (1999) *A Practical Guide to Paediatric Oncology Palliative Care*. Brisbane: Royal Children's Hospital.

Royal College of Paediatrics and Child Health (2003) *Medicines for Children*. 2nd edn. London: RCPCH.

Royal College of Paediatrics and Child Health (1997). *Withholding or Withdrawing Life-saving Treatment in Children*. London: RCPCH.

Waechter EH. (1971) Children's awareness of fatal illness. *Am J Nurs.* **7**: 1168–72.

Palliative care in non-malignant disease

The majority of patients in the UK (over 90 per cent) receiving specialist palliative care services have cancer. There is increasing recognition of the unmet need in patients with other progressive, incurable, non-malignant diagnoses which has been highlighted by recent publications. The Department of Health in the UK is striving to redress this balance, dictating that all patients with end-stage illness should have access to the services offered by multidisciplinary palliative care teams.

Specialist palliative care teams have traditionally been wary about taking responsibility for patients in whom the prognosis is uncertain, with the fear that precious resources would become overburdened by patients with longer term chronic illness. Studies in motor neurone disease (MND), however, showed that patients did not 'block' specialist beds any more than any other patients and most hospices now accept patients with MND into their programmes. It was perhaps the emergence of AIDS in the mid 1980s that made all specialist units take notice of a group of dying patients for whom they felt obliged to take some responsibility.

Patients with end-stage non-malignant disease suffer from as many distressing symptoms as those with cancer. Despite this there remains a lack of confidence in looking after patients with less familiar illnesses. This may partly stem from the fact that the dying phase is often different from that seen in cancer. Patients dying from cancer tend to deteriorate gradually over time, and usually it becomes obvious when the terminal phase is entered and when treatment and interventions can be aimed more at comfort. Patients dying from chronic heart or lung disease, on the other hand, are often deteriorating over a somewhat longer period of time, interspersed by acute episodes that may be better managed within a hospital environment, where acute care management is both appropriate and readily available. This may highlight educational and training issues, but does not mean that the palliative care team should take over the rôle of other specialist teams. Rather they should work alongside specialists in the other fields, ensuring that the principles of palliative care are upheld and that patients and families receive optimal treatment.

The percentage of the population over 65 years has increased and will continue to do so. The main causes of mortality are heart disease, cerebrovascular disorder, chronic respiratory disease and cancer. Palliative care teams will need to find a way to deliver appropriate care to all patients regardless of diagnosis. To this end, there is a higher percentage of patients with non-malignant disease in the hospice movement in the USA (20–30 per cent) and there is evidence that this trend is increasing in the UK, particularly within hospital specialist palliative care services.

With increasing dialogue, partnership, research and funding, the vision of providing services where they are needed should be a realistic aim.

AIDS in adults

Introduction

AIDS is a cluster of clinical conditions that inevitably occur in a person infected by the Human Immuno-deficiency Virus (HIV). As this virus attacks and weakens the cellular immune system the infected person develops an increasing number of infections, often from weak but oppor-tunistic micro-organisms. The virus also directly attacks various body tissues, resulting in chronic diarrhoea, severe weight loss, painful peripheral neu-ropathy, progressive dementia or profound pancytopenia. In the advanced stages of HIV infection, there is also an increasing incidence of malignancies such as Kaposi's sarcoma and cerebral lymphoma, that were previously extremely uncommon.

HIV affects principally the T-lymphocytes, resulting in impaired cell-mediated immunity. Certain lymphocytes (T4 cells) have a surface protein (CD$_4$) which has a high affinity for HIV. The CD$_4$ count declines with advancing disease and increasing immunodeficiency. Counts below 200/microlitre are associated with a high risk of developing opportunistic infection. The viral load is high following the initial infection and then declines as the immune system partially recovers after about 12 weeks. It remains at a low level for a variable period of time and then increases again with the collapse of the immune system.

Historical background

There has been much heated debate about the origins of AIDS. It was initially recognized in the gay community in the USA in the early 1980s and since then has gradually spread to the wider world community. Transmission is through contact with blood or other body fluids infected with HIV. Those most vulnerable to HIV infection are thus persons with multiple sexual partners, intravenous drug users, babies of infected mothers, persons receiving blood transfusions and health professionals who sustain needle-stick injuries.

Complexity

The course of the illness is unpredictable, the presentation is variable and, even with anti-retroviral drugs (ARVs), death from AIDS is inevitable. Added to this complex clinical picture is the emotional, social and economic impact that this pandemic is having, especially in sub-Saharan Africa. Fear, stigma, rejection, repeated bereavement and conflicting messages accompany this disease. With the rising death rate, declining life expectancy, prolonged suffering and economic disruption that is occurring as a direct result of AIDS, this condition is the single greatest health challenge to our world in the twenty-first century.

Statistics

The confusing and sometimes conflicting statistics that are presented tend to muddle rather than help, at a time when we need clear reasoning and constructive planning for the future. What is certain is that this pandemic is very large and is growing rapidly. Despite all the recent preventive strategies and medical advances, it is showing no signs of abating. By 2000, the WHO estimated that 40 million people worldwide were infected. The vast majority of these live in Sub-Saharan Africa where it is estimated that 1 in 5 adults is infected.

Even in the UK, where more than 50,000 people had been infected with HIV by 2000, the number of infections has continued to rise despite the introduction of ARVs. AIDS is also spreading rapidly in Asia and South America.

Clinical features

AIDS has replaced syphilis and tuberculosis as the great mimic. It may present in such a myriad of ways that it should be considered as a possibility in any patient of any age with almost any complaint anywhere in the world. There are, however, a number of clinical presentations that are typical and even some that are diagnostic of AIDS. Loss of weight of more than 10 per cent, diarrhoea or fevers lasting more than a month, generalized lymphadenopathy especially including the submental and epitrochlear nodes, are very suggestive. Herpes zoster in a young adult, dry itchy skin and small darkly pigmented itchy bumps would also raise the suspicions of any health worker in an endemic area. Kaposi's sarcoma, cryptococcal meningitis and cerebral lymphoma are pathognomonic.

The classification devised by the WHO is a useful way of staging the illness clinically, especially when CD$_4$ counts and viral loads are not available (see Table 8a.1).

Table 8a.1 WHO clinical staging of HIV/AIDS (modified)

	Clinical stage			
	Sero-conversion (1)	Early (2)	Intermediate (3)	Late (4)
Feature				
Activity	Normal	Rests occasionally	Rests for <50% of day	Rests for >50% of day
Weight loss	No	< 10%	> 10%	Wasted/ cachectic
Fever	Mild in 50%	Occasional	> 1/12	> 1/12
Diarrhoea		Occasional	> 1/12	> 1/12
Respiratory infections		URTIs Pneumonia Pleural effusion	Recurrent pneumonia Chronic otitis media	Pneumocystis carinii pneumonia (PCP)
Pulmonary TB			Miliary Lower lobes Mediastinal nodes	Extensive bilateral Resistant
Other TB				Pericardial Peritoneum Spine/bone Meningitis
Skin		Shingles H. simplex Dry Itchy papules Tinea corporis	Severe shingles Pellagra Stevens–Johnson syndrome Vaginal thrush	Persistent genital ulcers

Table 8a.1 (Continued)

	Clinical stage			
	Sero-conversion (1)	Early (2)	Intermediate (3)	Late (4)
Mouth		Aphthous ulcers Reiter's syndrome Gingivitis	Oral thrush Progressive gingivitis	Oesophageal thrush
CNS		Bell's Palsy Guillain–Barré syndrome		Painful feet Paraplegia 25% dementia Cryptococcal meningitis Toxoplasmosis
Cancer				Kaposi's sarcoma Invasive cancer of cervix Lymphoma
Lymph nodes	Generalized	Generalized	Generalized	Generalized or absent

Natural history

Following infection by HIV, the natural progression of this illness is very variable. For many there are few symptoms initially and it is only after several years of relatively normal health that the typical clinical features of AIDS become apparent. In others, the initial sero-conversion may be more pronounced with fever, body pains, headache, ulceration of the mucosa of the mouth and genitalia, a maculo-papular rash, hepatosplenomegaly and generalized lymphadenopathy. These symptoms usually resolve spontaneously over a few weeks. During this phase the person may, however, develop Bell's palsy or the Guillain–Barré syndrome, indicating early neurological involvement.

After about 12 weeks the body reaches a steady state with partial recovery of the immune system and a decline in the number of circulating viral particles. Now follows a phase of clinical latency where the only clinical signs may be generalized lymphadenopathy and occasional episodes of sweating, especially at night.

While a small proportion of infected people may progress rapidly to full-blown AIDS within one or two years, in the majority AIDS takes eight to ten years to develop. A few individuals progress very slowly and may be still alive after 20 years, even without ARVs.

As the immune system begins to become exhausted, the person becomes susceptible to a wide range of infections including recurrent upper respiratory tract infections, pneumonia, tuberculosis, a wide variety of intestinal micro-organisms, cryptococcal meningitis, herpes zoster and monilial infections of the mouth, vagina and oesophagus.

The variability of the resilience of the immune system and the potentially fatal nature of some of the infections, make it difficult to estimate the prognosis of an individual.

The effects and limitations of highly active anti-retroviral therapy (HAART)

The advent of Highly Active Anti-Retroviral Therapy (HAART) has radically changed the prospects for many people with AIDS. An emaciated person who appears to be beyond all help may start rapidly improving on ARVs. This has been nicknamed the 'Lazarus Syndrome'. In Europe and North America, numerous hospices and hospital wards dedicated to caring for dying AIDS patients have been able to empty their beds and concentrate on other forms of care.

ARVs are the best form of palliation for AIDS that is available at present. The decision of when to start ARVs and which combination to use may at first seem complex. The key to success is for the affected person and the doctor to negotiate the most suitable timing of the start of ARVs and the most suitable combination.

Good stories are a very effective way of explaining the use of ARVs and getting the right message across to less well developed educated communities e.g.

> Imagine you are hiking through the bushveld and enjoying the birdlife and the game. But, in the distance, you see a lion stalking you. You aren't too worried because you have a gun. But there are only two bullets in the gun, so you need to be quite sure about the best time to shoot. If you shoot too soon there is a good chance that you will miss the lion, and that the explosion will chase away all the wildlife. If you leave it too late the lion may be on top of you before you can take aim.
>
> The lion represents AIDS and the distance between you and the lion shows how strong your immune system is—the closer the lion the weaker your immune system. The gun with the two bullets is your anti-retroviral therapy, which you need to learn how to use properly so that you don't hurt yourself. The sound of the gun being fired represents the potential side-effects of the antiretroviral therapy—a real nuisance if the lion is far away, but the last thing you'd worry about when the lion is getting close!

The decision to start ARVs must not be hurried. Anti-retrovirals (ARVs) need to be used responsibly.[1] Time needs to be taken to help the person understand as fully as possible the various options and the need for strict adherence.
- Treatment needs to be taken for life
- It is very important to choose the first treatment regimen carefully as it is the one most likely to have the best results
- Once the virus has been exposed to ARVs, subsequent regimens are less likely to give good results
- The start of ARVs should be delayed until the CD_4 count is below 200/microlitre, or the symptoms of the infection are very troublesome
- Social and psychological problems, especially depression, need to be resolved where possible before starting ARVs as these will make adherence difficult
- The choice of drugs is growing rapidly. The inexperienced clinician should ask for advice from someone experienced with using ARVs

- In an effort to make the decision as simple as possible, the WHO is recommending fixed combinations in a similar way to the TB regimens. See www.who.int/hiv/pub/prev_care/draft/en/
- Efavirenz or nevirapine (NNRTIs) should be used in combination with zidovudine and lamivudine or stavudine and lamivudine (NRTIs from different categories) (see Table 8a.2).

Table 8a.2 Classification of anti-retroviral drugs*

Category I (NRTIs)	Category II (NRTIs)	Category III (NRTI)	Category IV (NNRTIs)	Category V (PIs)
Stavudine (d4T)	Didanosine (ddI)	Abacavir (ABC)	Nevirapine (NVP)	Nelfinavir (NFV)
Zidovudine (AZT)	Lamivudine (3TC)		Efavirenz† (EFV)	Indinavir/RTV (IDV)
	Zalcitabine (ddC)			Saquinavir/RTV (soft gel) (SQV)
				Lopinavir/RTV (combination)
				Ritonavir (RTV)‡

NRTI = nucleoside reverse transcriptase inhibitor

NNRTI = non-nucleoside reverse transcriptase inhibitor

PI = protease inhibitor

*For initiation of therapy in an ARV-naïve patient use 2 NRTIs (one from category I and one from category II) together with one NNRTI (category IV).

† EFV is teratogenic.

‡ RTV is most often used in combination with another PI at a low dose of 100 mg twice daily. Here it is used as a $_p$450 inhibitor to boost the levels of the combined PI. It is not a useful anti-retroviral agent at this low dose. In adults it is rarely used as an anti-retroviral in its own right (600mg twice daily) due to increased adverse events (e.g. diarrhoea).

- The immune-compromised person who develops TB presents the clinician with an additional dilemma, as ARVs do not combine well with the standard anti-TB drugs. Where possible, the TB should be treated first
- The initial euphoria about ARVs is now abating somewhat as the problem of viral resistance to many of the drugs becomes apparent. Already 10 per cent of new infections in Europe are resistant to at least one drug. Strict adherence (>97 per cent) to complex drug regimens is needed to suppress the replication of the virus. Poor compliance leads to resistant strains developing rapidly with resultant treatment failure and disease progression. Although minor side-effects such as rashes are common, usually soon after initiating treatment, these can be managed symptomatically. Serious side-effects, such as lactic acidosis, may occur on d4T, ddI or AZT and may be fatal if not detected early

1 Brechtl JR., Breitbart W., Galietta M. et al. (2001) The use of highly active anti-retroviral therapy (HAART) in patients with advanced HIV infection: impact on medical, palliative care, and quality of life outcomes. Journal of Pain & Symptom Management. **21**: 41–51.

Initial small, well-controlled trials of ARVs have been shown to be very effective in some African countries. Patients adhere to their drugs as well as patients in Europe and America. The distribution of ARVs on a large scale, however, is likely to overwhelm the already over-extended primary health services in countries such as South Africa unless there is a massive injection of funds into the health system. The cost of the drugs needed to cope with this pandemic is large, but even more will be needed to build up the infrastructure and improve the capacity of the hospitals and health centres to provide the treatment and monitor patients. The vast distances and poor public transport services in rural areas will limit access to ARVs for many patients.

A number of companies, especially the large mining companies in South Africa, have made ARVs available to their staff at no cost. They have realized that it is better to keep their skilled staff healthy rather than constantly to recruit and retrain new workers.

The 'brain drain' of skilled doctors and nurses from developing countries to places such as Canada, Australia, the UK and the Middle East is compounding the difficulties. The Melbourne Manifesto on the recruitment of health professionals, adopted at the World Rural Health Conference in May 2002, needs to be taken seriously.

See http://www.globalfamilydoctor.com/aboutwonca/working-groups/rural_training/melbourne_manifesto.htm

The rôle of palliative care

As mentioned, current ARVs do not cure AIDS, but merely delay its natural progress. For many years to come the vast majority of infected people in the world will not have access to such drugs, some who are able to obtain them will not respond well or will be unable to adhere to the strict regimens required to suppress the virus. In the forseeable future we will still be faced with millions of people, dying slowly of AIDS, who will need effective palliative care. Such care should have the same focus as palliative care in other situations, namely promoting quality of life, excellent symptom control, effective communication and appropriate support for both patient and family.

Pain

Pain is common and is often undertreated. Surveys have shown that up to 98 per cent of advanced AIDs sufferers will have significant pain.

- Headache is a frequent symptom and cryptococcal meningitis (CM) and tuberculous meningitis (TBM) need to be excluded as these are treatable if diagnosed early. CM may be associated with raised intracranial pressure and the resulting severe headache can be relieved by daily serial lumbar punctures (LPs), draining off 15–20 mL of cerebrospinal fluid (CSF) with great care. Focal signs may indicate a space-occupying lesion. If possible a scan should be done to confirm the diagnosis. In Africa toxoplasmosis is the commonest cause
- Severe sensory neuropathies are present in 30 per cent of patients. Most are due to direct damage to peripheral nerves by the virus, but some may occur from the toxic effects of anti-TB treatment or ARVs (ddC, d4T and ddI)

- Herpes zoster may occur early in the course of the illness and may be severe with persisting post-herpetic neuralgia
- Persisting mouth and genital ulcerations are common and very debilitating. Once again, treatable conditions such as candida and sexually transmitted infections (STIs) should be sought. Chronic ulceration due to persisting herpes simplex can be very frustrating, but some good results are reported from resource poor areas in Africa where aciclovir tablets are crushed and applied topically
- Painful swallowing (odynophagia) may be due to oesophageal candidiasis, acid reflux and TB, which are treatable, or due to infection by cytomegalovirus (CMV) or Kaposi's sarcoma (KS), which often respond poorly to treatment
- Abdominal pain occurs in 20 per cent of patients and may be due to many different causes. Patients with abdominal pain should be approached like all other patients. Surgical emergencies should be referred appropriately, rule out lactic acidosis or pancreatitis due to ARVs (ddI, ddC, and d4T), treat infections such as salmonella, shigella or tuberculosis and provide effective analgesia for all
- Muscle and joint pains are also common. The same approach applies. Identify treatable infections and conditions and provide effective analgesia for all. Pyrazinamide used to treat TB commonly causes severe arthralgia

Follow the principles of pain management: 'By mouth', 'By the ladder', 'By the clock' with careful follow-up and review. (📖 See Chapter 6a.)

The biggest challenge in poorly resourced areas is making morphine and other effective drugs available and accessible. Great progress has been made in Uganda with the introduction of appropriate legislation allowing the distribution of morphine at clinic level. In Zimbabwe, trained palliative care nurses are able to prescribe morphine. Other developing countries need to follow their example.

Diarrhoea

Recurrent and persisting diarrhoea may be present in more than 50 per cent of patients with advanced AIDS. In places with poor sanitation, good hygiene has been shown to reduce this percentage significantly. Half of the patients with chronic diarrhoea will have an identifiable infection. The presence of fever or blood in the stool should be investigated for a treatable cause. In resource-poor areas, a short empirical trial of metronidazole and co-trimoxazole may be tried. Loperamide or morphine should be titrated up to an effective dose to reduce the frequency of diarrhoea to manageable levels. Trying to cope with profuse diarrhoea without proper sanitation or easily accessible running water is a reality for most affected families in many areas in third world countries. This places an extra burden and risk on already overwhelmed families. Chronic diarrhoea needs to be taken just as seriously as pain.

Fever

Sweating and fever are frequent throughout the course of AIDS. It may be part of the immune response or it may indicate the onset of yet another opportunistic infection. Careful assessment for possible treatable causes such as pneumonia or TB needs to be made. Extra fluids and antipyretics can be given until any possible treatable cause is identified.

Neurological

See p. 622.

Skin problems

Almost all patients with AIDS will have some kind of skin problem.

- Dry skin and itching is frequent. Discourage excessive bathing, especially in warm water, and apply aqueous cream twice a day to the whole body. The judicious use of appropriate steroid creams and oral antihistamines (especially H_1 blockers) may bring relief of itching
- Itching may also be caused by 'Itchy bump disease' (pruritic papular eruption). This is very common in Africa and is a group of conditions causing inflamed, very itchy, papules that leave small darkly pigmented bumps on the limbs and trunk
- Seborrhoeic dermatitis and psoriasis are common and should be treated appropriately
- Scabies should be considered in any patient with itching. It may present in the usual form of red itchy papules with burrows in the web spaces of the fingers and around the ano-genital area. Occasionally scabies may present in a scaly, less itchy form (hyperkeratotic scabies) on the scalp, hands and trunk. Large thick crusts on the body with cracking may also be due to scabies
- Multiple purple-brown nodules of varying size scattered all over the body especially, on the face and in the mouth, are characteristic of Kaposi's sarcoma. It may occur at any stage of the illness and although it is often slowly progressive at first, it may spread to involve internal organs and be rapidly fatal. Pain and dyspnoea are then often present and may be controlled with morphine. Palliative radiotherapy, intralesional chemotherapy and topical cryotherapy can be tried especially if the patient is still reasonably well ($CD_4 < 200$/microlitre)

Emotional and mental symptoms

The diagnosis of being HIV positive presents the infected person not only with the prospect of a fatal illness but also the stigma associated with AIDS. Many strong emotions crowd the mind including:

- fear of rejection by others
- fear of infecting others
- anger and sense of betrayal
- sense of shame for having contracted the disease
- sorrow in anticipation of the loss of everything
- worry about how to cope and how one's children will survive

It is little wonder that anxiety and depression are common throughout the course of illness, especially shortly after the diagnosis and again as the symptoms of advanced AIDS become apparent. Family and community support, however, can help the infected person come to terms with the situation. Without support, the HIV positive person may lose hope. Suicide then becomes a strong possibility.

Support groups for people living with AIDS have proved very effective in Africa in countering the despair and hardship that so often accompanies this illness. Many HIV positive people have become involved in caring for those that are sick at home, looking after the infants left behind and comforting the grieving. Some have been brave enough to speak out in public and have been very effective in breaking down stigma and prejudice. This has never been easy and at times it has been dangerous, kindling the wrath of an already outraged community.

Being a neurotropic virus, over 80 per cent of people with AIDS will show some cognitive impairment while 25 per cent will go on to develop HIV-associated dementia or psychosis. Most are apathetic and withdrawn while a few may become delirious and agitated, requiring sedation.

Nutrition

While good nutrition is essential to maintain an adequate immune system, great care needs to be taken to ensure that the rôle of particular diets, such as the use of garlic, lemon juice and olive oil, is not seen as an alternative to effective medical care. The sick have always been vulnerable to exploitation by quacks and 'snake oil' salesmen. While vitamins and other micronutrients have their place, 'a round pill' should not replace 'a square meal'.

In the underprivileged areas of developing countries, vegetable gardening and small-scale subsistence farming needs to be encouraged both as a means of survival and for the sense of well-being that it encourages.

Social issues

The young adult is the main age group affected by the AIDS pandemic. Young adults may be the main 'bread-winners' and the parents of small children. Their deaths have a devastating effect on the community. In developing countries, the loss of income, the multiple bereavements, the growing orphan population, the child-headed households or children having to leave school to care for dying parents and siblings are all causing great economic and emotional suffering.

Impact on Africa

In a survey of affected households in South Africa in 2002, it was found that 45% had an income of less than $150 a month, 57% had no running water inside their homes and 25% had no toilet. The plight of children is desperate. It was found that 22% of children under 15 years had lost at least one parent and 50% of children often went to bed hungry. The sick family members required care for extended periods, often as long as 12 months. Twenty per cent were too weak to wash and 16% were incontinent. The average life expectancy in South Africa has dropped by 10 years. (SA Health Review 2002)[2]

Despite some countries having child support grants and disability pensions, multiple administrative obstacles may prevent access to these funds. The capacity of the health and social welfare services to cope in most sub-Saharan countries is being stretched to the limits.

2 http://www.hst.org.za/publications/527

Spiritual issues

Fear, discrimination, stigma, rejection and isolation have added to the burden of those affected and infected by HIV/AIDS. While community organizations and religious groups are playing a rôle in helping those in need, the perception that AIDS sufferers have 'only themselves to blame' is still prevalent and will take much wisdom and compassion to overcome.

Health professionals need to be aware of the way different communities perceive illness and misfortune. In Africa there is a common perception that some conditions are 'natural' while others are not. Unfamiliar illnesses or conditions that are not easily cured may be attributed to evil influences of 'sorcerers' or the jealousy of neighbours. In addition to seeking help from health professionals at a hospital or clinic for the symptoms of the disease, the affected person will consult a traditional healer to discover the person responsible for the misfortune. The 'victim' will also expect to be given some means of protection from this evil.

An example of this is the common interpretation for the persistently painful feet of the peripheral neuropathy that so often accompanies AIDS. This will be interpreted as being caused by an enemy who has sprinkled 'poison' just outside the front gate of the home of the affected person. Unless the poison can be neutralized there will be no lasting cure.

Great care is needed in dealing with spiritual issues, especially if there are cultural and language differences between the ill person and the healthcare worker. A helpful approach is for the health professional to admit his/her ignorance of the beliefs and customs of the community and to ask the ill person or the family for help in understanding their needs.

Medico-legal issues

AIDS is a minefield of medico-legal issues. The right to confidentiality, the concerns of the public and the fears of the health professionals have caused many heated debates and even several court cases. The way information is entered into medical records and on death certificates has needed to be revised and improved. Disclosure even to another health worker must be on a legitimate 'need to know' basis and only after proper informed consent.

Laws relating to employment, dismissal and benefits need to be reviewed. When others are at risk, especially within a family, the infected individual needs to be helped and encouraged to disclose their HIV status.

Communities also need to deal with the issues of HIV positive children attending community schools. Proper education and the introduction of universal precautions have helped to allay the fears of parents in most cases.

Care during the dying phase

The transition from fighting against a terminal illness to preparing for death is never easy, especially when the person is young. In addition, the opportunistic infections are often treatable. Thus both doctor and patient may remain focused on cure. Families find it equally difficult to let go. However, a time comes sooner or later when despite all efforts, recovery does not take place. The same approach is needed to care for patients dying from AIDS as for those dying with cancer. The medication regimen should be simplified to only those drugs needed for good symptom control. This may include stopping ARVs and even anti-TB treatment. As long as the person is no longer sputum positive for TB, there is little risk to others. It may be prudent to continue antifungals and agents for herpes simplex.

Treatment and ongoing prophylaxis for CMV retinitis may also be important, especially if retinal lesions are near the optic nerve or fovea. Fifty per cent of patients develop progressive sight deterioration within 2–3 weeks of stopping treatment.

Home-based care in developing countries has become a practical alternative to overcrowded public hospitals. With the support of established hospices, community groups have taken on the task of supporting affected families.

Bereavement and AIDS

Loss and grief are difficult to deal with at the best of times. Friends, neighbours and family members usually rally round and help to bear the burden of coping without the lost loved one. In developing countries, the multiple deaths of the AIDS epidemic are leaving the survivors with little support. It is not uncommon for an elderly widow who has been struggling to survive on her small pension, to find herself having to care for six or seven grandchildren whose parents have died one by one in a short space of time. In this state of 'distracted grief' there is little time for anything other than survival. The stigma of AIDS creates further barriers within the wider community.

Frustrations, fears and compassion fatigue

Despite the warnings and predictions of the scale and complexity of the AIDS epidemic in the late 1980s, most health services in developing countries were ill prepared for the numbers of sick and dying patients that began to crowd hospitals and clinics in the 1990s. In South Africa, this dramatic rise began in 1997. Wards in public hospitals became overcrowded with emaciated men and women with chronic diarrhoea and persisting cough. More than 50 per cent of deaths in the adult wards could be directly attributed to AIDS while in the paediatric wards the figure was closer to 85 per cent.

Advances

The identification of the causative organism, accurate diagnostic testing, HAART and the initial development of vaccines against this virus are some of the advances that have taken place. Although there is a long way to go yet before we can even begin to consider that AIDS is under control, the future looks a lot brighter than it did ten years ago.

The challenge

> AIDS is no longer just a disease, it is a human rights issue.
>
> Nelson Mandela, November 2003.

The WHO is leading the challenge with its new '3 x 5' campaign. It hopes to have three million people on ARVs by 2005. It rightly acknowledges that to achieve that will require more than the money for the drugs: the entire infrastructure of health services in developing countries will need supporting.

Resources

The following are a small selection of internet sites with information on AIDS:

Africa Alive—a forum for sharing ideas and strategies.
Web site: http://www.africalive.org
AIDS Education Global Information System—a wide range of HIV/AIDS related topics.
Web site: http://www.aegis.com
Aidsmap—The British HIV Association
Web site: http://www.aidsmap.com/
JAMA HIV/AIDS Information Centre—recent developments and treatment guidelines.
Web site http://www.ama-assn.org/special/hiv/hivhome.htm
Medscape—a web site of educational activities
Web site: http://hiv.medscape.com/

Further reading

Books

O'Neill J., Selwyn P. and Schietinger H. (eds) (2003) *A Clinical Guide to Supportive and Palliative Care for HIV/AIDS*. Washington: US Dept of Health and Human Services. (The guide is available as a free download from www.hab.hrsa.gov.)

Wilson D., Naidoo S., Bekker L.-G., Cotton M. and Maartens G. (eds) (2003) *Handbook of HIV Medicine*. Oxford: Oxford University Press.

Articles

Cameron D. (2002) Saving the history of the defeated and the lost—ethical dilemmas in the midst of the AIDS epidemic. *SA Fam Pract*, **25, 4**: 15–18.

Fassin D. and Schneider H. (2003) The politics of AIDS in South Africa: beyond the controversies. *BMJ*, **326**: 495–7.

Orrell C. and Wilson D. (2003) The art of HAART: a practical approach to antiretroviral therapy. *CME*, **21, 6**: 306–12.

Palliative care in non-malignant respiratory disease

Introduction

- The course of chronic respiratory disease is often marked by slow, inexorable decline with prolonged periods of disabling dyspnoea, reducing exercise tolerance, recurrent hospital admissions and premature death
- This is associated with loss of dignity, social isolation and psychological problems for the individual and pressure on family and carers. There is much potential gain with the application of a holistic approach to care
- Recent studies have recognized the similarity in symptoms between patients dying with malignant and non-malignant disease, and it is accepted that, regardless of diagnosis, the needs of the dying patient should be met by palliative care services

A difficulty with this is determining when chronic disease becomes terminal, as most end-stage respiratory disease progresses with periods of stability interrupted by major life-threatening exacerbations.

The potential requirement for palliative care in end-stage pulmonary disease

Respiratory disease accounted for 153,168 of 632,062 (24.2 per cent) deaths in the United Kingdom in 1999:

Condition	Deaths (%)
All respiratory disease	deaths 153,16 cases (100)
Pneumonia and TB	67,591 cases (44.1)
Cancer	35,879 cases (23.4)
Progressive non-malignant causes	39,939 cases (25.1)
COPD + asthma	(21.0)
Pulmonary circulatory disease	(4.1)
Pneumoconiosis	(0.8)
Cystic fibrosis	(0.1)
Sarcoidosis	(0.07)
Others (congenital, foreign body, etc.)	9,759 cases (6.4)

Research into symptomatology, survival, appropriate care and utilization of services is needed if the needs of this population are to be met.

Terminal symptoms, quality of life, and survival of patients with end-stage pulmonary disease

Symptoms presenting in the final weeks and months of life include dyspnoea, cough, fever, haemoptysis, stridor and chest wall pain—a similar picture to symptoms experienced by lung cancer patients.

The inability to predict disease trajectory in patients with non-malignant terminal disease makes end-of-life decisions difficult. Studies indicate that quality of life is at least as poor as those suffering from malignant lung disease.

Symptom pathophysiology and assessment

Less than 5% of patients with non-malignant disease die in hospices compared to at least 20% of lung cancer patients. More palliative care services are available to cancer patients.

Dyspnoea

Dyspnoea can be defined as difficult, uncomfortable or laboured breathing or when an individual feels the need for more air. It is the most frequently experienced symptom in those with end-stage respiratory disease and is multifactorial in origin.

Not clearly understood, the mechanism of dyspnoea has been described as a mismatch between central motor activity and incoming afferent information from chemo- and mechanoreceptors. A person's emotional state, personality and cognitive function also influence its perception.

A good history and examination is invaluable. (📖 See Chapter 6e.)

Recurrent aspiration

This is often a feature in the development of respiratory failure. There may be a bulbar cause e.g. MND, CVA or there may be repeated micro-aspiration leading to bronchiectasis.

The right main bronchus is the most direct path to the lungs leading more commonly to right lower lobe infections. Diagnosis can be made clinically, on CXR or on barium swallow.

Treatment includes:
- Nursing in semi-recumbent position
- Speech and language therapy assessment
- Thickened foods
- Nasogastric tube
- Treatment of the associated pneumonia with antibiotics and physiotherapy

Management of end-stage respiratory disease

The end-stage is not easy to recognize but usually comprises:
- Persistent dyspnoea despite maximal therapy
- Poor mobility
- Increased frequency of hospital admission
- Decreased improvements with repeated admission
- Expressions of fear, anxiety
- Panic attacks
- Concerns expressed about dying

Drugs For dyspnoea

Anxiolytics
Anxiety can exacerbate breathlessness. Clinical experience suggests that low dose anxiolytics (diazepam) can result in improvements despite a lack of evidence.

Antidepressants
TCAs and serotonin selective re-uptake inhibitors have been shown to be beneficial

Oral opioids
- Site of action may be central (brain stem) or peripheral lung receptors or help by decreasing anxiety. Opioids can cause serious side-effects such as CO_2 retention, nausea, drowsiness and respiratory depression, so care is needed
- A trial of opioid in COPD patients without CO_2 retention is appropriate with close monitoring
- Low doses and small increments should be used e.g. 2.5mg morphine elixir 4-h
- Subcutaneous diamorphine can be used in patients not able to swallow
- In the terminal phase, opioid therapy is justified for treatment of dyspnoea even in the presence of CO_2 retention

Nebulised opioids
Currently no good evidence to support use. 'As effective as nebulised saline.'

Mucolytics
N-acetylcysteine can be used, as can steam inhalers and nebulised saline.

Palliative oxygen therapy
A significant proportion of patients will have resting hypoxia, although its degree does not correlate with the level of dyspnoea. Symptoms may be improved by oxygen. Even in the absence of hypoxia, oxygen may relieve dyspnoea in COPD patients.

Non-pharmacological measures

General
- Vaccinations—influenza and pneumococcal
- General nursing care—fan, open windows, regular repositioning, relief of constipation
- Good nutrition
- Physiotherapy—forced expiratory technique, controlled coughing, chest percussion

- Psychological support—help patient cope, provide strategies to relieve symptoms, maximize quality of life etc.
- Pulmonary rehabilitation—centres around exercise conditioning by general exercise and specific muscle training
- Controlled breathing techniques—pursed lip/slow expiration etc.
- Non-invasive mechanical ventilation—shown to decrease need for intubation
- Lung reduction surgery—initial benefit in FEV_1 lasts only 3–4 years
- Lung transplantation—emphysema is most common indication

COPD

Pharmacological treatments

Bronchodilators

- beta-2 agonists, e.g. Salbutamol
- anticholinergic agents (may aggravate prostatism or glaucoma) e.g. ipratropium bromide
- Inhaled bronchodilators +/– spacers should be used where possible as nebulizers deliver medication less efficiently

Inhaled/oral steroids

These benefit 15–20 per cent of stable COPD patients and as such a trial with steroids is indicated, where at least a 20 per cent increase in FEV_1 should indicate continued use.

Theophylline

The pharmacokinetics are unstable and there is a narrow therapeutic range, but if used judiciously they have a place in COPD management.

Oxygen

- Has a definite place in the management of selected hypoxic patients
- Usually employed overnight, followed by intermittent daytime use through to continuous use
- Care needs to be taken where headaches, drowsiness or confusion appear indicating potential carbon dioxide retention

Long-term oxygen therapy (LTOT)

This can extend life expectancy if administered for 12–15 h per day, although there is a lack of evidence to support increased quality of life.

> **Indications for LTOT:**
> - PaO_2 < 7.3 kPa when breathing air
> - $PaCO_2$ may be normal or > 6.0 kPa
> - Two measurements separated by 4 weeks when clinically stable
> - Clinical stability = no exacerbations or peripheral oedema for four weeks
> - FEV_1 < 1.5l and FVC < 2.0l
> - Non-smokers
> - PaO_2 between 7.3 and 8.0 kPa together with secondary polycythaemia, peripheral oedema or pulmonary hypertension
> - Nocturnal hypoxia (SaO_2 below 90 per cent for > 30 per cent of the night)
> - Interstitial lung disease or pulmonary hypertension where PaO_2 < 8 kPa
> - Palliation of terminal disease

Interstitial/fibrotic lung disease

These include:
- Idiopathic fibrotic disorders, e.g. idiopathic pulmonary fibrosis, autoimmune pulmonary fibrosis
- Connective tissue disorders, e.g. SLE, rheumatoid arthritis, scleroderma etc.
- Drug-induced diseases, e.g. nitrofurantoin, amiodarone, gold, radiation etc.
- Occupational, e.g. silicosis, asbestosis, farmer's lung etc.
- Primary unclassified, e.g. sacoidosis, amyloidosis, AIDs, adult respiratory distress syndrome (ARDS) etc.

These conditions are, however, rare.

Treatment includes immunosuppressants such as steroids, cyclophosphamide, azathioprine, and penicillamine with variable success.

Neuromuscular, restrictive and chest wall disease

These cause respiratory muscle weakness or loss of compliance in the respiratory cage. Muscular function can be affected at various sites from the spinal cord to the muscles themselves.

Features that characterize some of these conditions include:
- Increased ventilatory drive with inadequate ventilatory response
- Sleep disorders
- Unbalanced weakness of spinal and thoracic muscles leading to kyphoscoliosis
- Bulbar incoordination
- Diaphragmatic paralysis
- Pulmonary embolism

Supportive treatments:
- Oxygen
- Antibiotics
- Physiotherapy
- Techniques to clear secretions
- Inspiratory muscle training
- Beta-2 agonists

Ventilatory support can include:
- Rocking beds
- Abdominal pneumatic belts
- Negative pressure body ventilators
- Non-invasive positive pressure ventilation
- Nasal continuous positive airways pressure
- There have been many advances in this field, but many patients still choose to refuse such invasive treatments

Bronchiectasis

Survival of patients has improved markedly with the advent of antibiotic therapy. Conditions associated with bronchiectasis include:
- Cystic fibrosis
- HIV infection
- Rheumatoid arthritis
- Infection, inflammation
- Bronchopulmonary sequestration

- Allergic bronchopulmonary aspergillosis
- Alpha1-antitrypsin deficiency
- Congenital cartilage deficiency
- Immunodeficiency
- Yellow nail syndrome
- Bronchial obstruction
- Unilateral hyperlucent lung

Diagnosis is usually made by high resolution CT scanning.
Treatment involves:
- Antimicrobial drugs—directed by sputum microbiology, usually treated for longer periods
- Bronchodilator therapy
- Chest physiotherapy
- Nebulised recombinant human deoxyribonuclease
- Anti-inflammatory treatment
- Supplemental oxygen
- Immunoglobulin administration/enzyme replacement
- Surgery
- Management of haemoptysis
- Management of halitosise—e.g. broad-spectrum antibiotics, mouth and gum care

Cystic fibrosis
- Affects 1 in 2,500 newborns
- Marked by alteration in ion and water transport across epithelial cells resulting in recurrent pulmonary infection, bronchiectasis, lung fibrosis and pancreatic insufficiency
- Most care takes place in specialized units with home support teams trained in the principles of palliative care

HIV-associated
Pulmonary complications:
- bacterial e.g. Strep. pneumoniae, Pseudomonas aeruginosa
- mycobacterium e.g. M. tuberculosis, M. avian complex
- fungi e.g. Pneumocystis carinii, Cryptococcus neoformans
- viruses e.g. Cytomegalovirus
- parasites e.g. Toxoplasma gondii
- Malignancies e.g. Kaposi's sarcoma, non-Hodgkin's lymphoma
- Interstitial pneumonitis e.g. lymphocytic pneumonitis
- Other e.g. COPD, pulmonary hypertension

Tuberculosis
Recurrent reactivation results in severe pulmonary scarring, cavitation and secondary aspergillosis infection and, if left unchecked, respiratory failure, recurrent bacterial infection and massive haemoptysis.

Chronic bronchitis and emphysema

These conditions cause 80 per cent of pulmonary hypertension. Treatment usually involves:
- Oxygen
- Non-invasive ventilation
- Beta-2 agonists
- Diuretics in the management of fluid retention in acute phase of cor pulmonale
- The use of pulmonary vasodilators is of doubtful significance

Obstructive pulmonary hypertension
- This is often caused by repetitive, silent pulmonary embolism. Other causes include vasculitis, sickle cell anaemia and infective endocarditis
- Treatment can involve anticoagulation, and occasionally pulmonary thromboendarterectomy or the insertion of inferior vena caval filter

Primary pulmonary hypertension
- Of unknown aetiology
- Symptoms can include progressive dyspnoea, decreased exercise tolerance, central chest pain and syncope
- Occasionally it is associated with haemoptysis, fluid accumulation and sudden death
- Treatment involves oxygen, anticoagulation and vasodilators such as hydralazine and nifedipine

Pulmonary embolism (📖 see Chapter 6l)

There is an increased incidence of thromboembolism in dependent, hospitalized patients.
- The triad of venous stasis, alteration in coagulation and vascular injury are fundamental in the pathogenesis
- A clinical suspicion is possible with dyspnoea, pleuritic pain and haemoptysis being classical symptoms
- Forty per cent of high-risk patients with proximal DVT's are asymptomatic when pulmonary embolism occurs

Investigation includes:
- Arterial blood gas (Not commonly available in in-patient palliative care units.)
- ECG
- CXR
- Doppler ultrasonography/contrast venography
- V/Q scan
- Angiography
- Enhanced spiral CT scan

Prevention involves adequate hydration, promotion of mobility, the avoidance of venous obstruction, compression stockings and low molecular weight heparin (LMWH).

Treatment usually involves heparinization with LMWH and consideration of warfarinization, or vena-caval filters.

For patients with metastatic malignancy there is increasing evidence
that warfarin is not as effective as LMWH. (📖 See Chapter 6l.)

Pneumothorax and pleural disease

Pathogenesis includes spontaneous and iatrogenic causes. Treatment usually involves intercostal tube drainage if appropriate, or oxygen, analgesia and opiates in the terminally ill.

- Causes of pleural effusion are multiple but include infection, cardiac failure, hypoalbuminaemia and renal impairment
- Treatment may consist of intermittent aspiration +/− chemical pleurodesis
- Localized pleural pain may be secondary to rib fracture, infection or pneumothorax and may respond to normal analgesia, or may require a local anaesthetic intercostal nerve block

Respiratory terminal care and palliative sedation

In terminal phase, simple measures are important:

- constant draught from fan or open window
- regular sips of water
- sitting upright

In the terminal stages, the emphasis changes from active interventions to supportive and symptomatic measures.

- Non-invasive ventilatory support and active physiotherapy may be withdrawn
- Drugs for palliating symptoms are often unavoidable
- The oral route should be used where possible, but failing this, drugs may be given by the subcutaneous route

The 'rattle' associated with loose respiratory secretions, although probably not distressing to the patient, may be addressed by re-positioning, or by the use of hyoscine hydrobromide or glycopyrronium bromide.

- As many patients approaching death with end-stage respiratory disease will have uncontrolled dyspnoea, sedation and opioid use should not be withheld because of an inappropriate fear of respiratory depression
- Options include benzodiazepines or opioids. The risks and benefits must be carefully considered and the justification for sedation clearly defined. Such decisions are often made by teams rather than individuals and it is appropriate that patients and families are fully involved in the decision making process

Further reading

Books

Ahmedzai S. (1998) Palliation of Respiratory Symptoms. In D. Doyle, G. Hanks, N. MacDonald: *Oxford Textbook of Palliative Medicine*. 2nd edn. Oxford: Oxford University Press.

Back, I. (2001) *Palliative Medicine Handbook*. 3rd edn. Cardiff: BPM Books.

Davis C. L. (1998) Breathlessness, Cough and Other Respiratory Problems. In M. Fallon, B. O'Neill (eds.) *ABC of palliative care*. London: BMJ Books.

Doyle D., Hanks G., Cherny N. and Calman K. (2004) *Oxford Textbook of Palliative Medicine.* 3rd edn. Oxford: Oxford University Press.

Fallon M. (ed.) *ABC of Palliative Care.* London: BMJ Books.

Watson M. and Lucas, C. (2003) *Adult Palliative Care Guidelines.* London: The South West London and the Surrey, West Sussex and Hampshire Cancer Networks.

Wilcock A. (1997) *Dyspnoea.* In P. Kaye (ed.) *Tutorials in palliative medicine,* pp. 227–49. Northampton: EPL Publications.

Palliative care in heart failure

Definition

Chronic heart failure is a progressive, fatal disease and is the final common pathway of many cardiovascular diseases. Heart failure is defined by the European Society of Cardiology as the presence of symptoms of heart failure at rest or during exercise, and objective evidence of cardiac dysfunction (usually on echocardiography).

Incidence

Heart failure is the only major cardiovascular disease with increasing incidence. It is predominantly a disease of old age (mean 75 years). There are 63,000 new cases per annum in the UK.[1] A diagnosis of heart failure has huge cost implications: patients with heart failure occupy up to 2 per cent of all inpatient bed days and account for up to 2 per cent of NHS costs (most of which are hospital not community).

Prognosis

An estimated 5 per cent of all deaths in the UK (24,000 per annum) are from heart failure. (Death certification explicitly discourages doctors from recording heart failure as a cause of death—the true number is probably much higher). Forty per cent of patients die within one year of diagnosis. Fifty per cent of patients with heart failure die suddenly and 25 per cent without worsening of their heart failure symptoms. This can occur at any stage of the disease. There are no reliable prognostic models either for poor overall prognosis or sudden death.

Relevant pathology and physiology

Coronary artery disease and hypertension are the commonest causes of heart failure. The direct insult is of mechanical pump failure, but this initiates an ongoing, complex cascade of haemodynamic, metabolic, neuroendocrine and renal dysfunction that is the syndrome of chronic heart failure.

Clinical features

Breathlessness and fatigue are the classic symptoms of heart failure. Orthopnoea is a sensitive 'measure' of fluid overload.

Fluid retention causes not only breathlessness, cough and dependent oedema, but also anorexia, nausea, abdominal bloating and pain.

Other common symptoms which are poorly recognized and therefore frequently not treated include:

• Pain (common, severe, prolonged and distressing). Probably due to a combination of angina, liver capsule distension, lower limb swelling and co-morbid disease, e.g. arthritis

1 Petersen S., Rayner M., Wolstenholme J. (2002) Coronary heart disease statistics: heart failure supplement 2002 edition.

- Anxiety and depression (severe in a third of hospitalized patients). Depression adversely affects mortality and hospital readmission[2]
- Disordered sleep
- Memory loss and confusion
- Anorexia, nausea, vomiting and constipation
- Weight loss (usually mild, but severe cachexia is a poor prognostic sign)
- Loss of libido

Poor information, communication and understanding for patients are widespread and contribute to psychological morbidity.

Significant functional impairment in activities of daily living and social isolation are common, long before the end-of-life. Despite this there is poor access to social and therapy services. The pattern of functional decline is slow, compared to the classic patient with cancer who exhibits a precipitous decline approximately five months before death.[3]

Disease burden

The burden of chronic heart failure has physical, psychological and social dimensions. These needs have been demonstrated to be prevalent, severe, prolonged and usually unrecognized and unrelieved.

The disparity in symptom control and support offered to those dying from heart failure compared to cancer is described tellingly by those who have lost a parent to each disease.

Table 8c.1 New York Heart Association (NYHA) functional classification (summary)

Class	Symptoms
I	Heart disease present, but no undue dyspnoea.
II	Comfortable at rest; dyspnoea on ordinary activities.
III	Less than ordinary activity causes dyspnoea, which is limiting.
IV	Dyspnoea present at rest; all activity causes discomfort.

Management

Disease-specific management

Education of patients and carers including diet (salt intake, alcohol, weight), smoking and exercise advice.

The cornerstones of drug treatment are angiotensin-converting enzyme (ACE) inhibitors and beta blockers. They both improve symptoms and slow disease progression. Diuretics are used to control fluid overload. Angiotensin-II antagonists, spironolactone and digoxin are used where appropriate.

Symptom management

1 Ensure specific heart failure treatments are optimal. This is the first step in achieving good symptom control. Diuretics may need quite frequent dose changes to control fluid overload. Avoid over-diuresis which may cause dizziness, nausea, poor sleep and fatigue.

2 Avoid where possible drugs which may worsen cardiac function. These include some drugs commonly prescribed in cancer palliative care practice. (See Table 8c.2.)

3 Actively seek out and manage other likely symptoms. Bear in mind the likely causes of symptoms in a patient with heart failure and the renal function.
   • Pain: follow the WHO ladder. Avoid NSAIDs and alter opioid dosing schedules as per renal function
   • Nausea: try haloperidol for a biochemical cause and metoclopramide for gastric stasis
   • Anxiety and depression: treat conventionally (with or without drugs). Newer classes of antidepressant such as sertraline (a selective serotonin re-uptake inhibitor) and mirtazepine are safer than tricyclics. They are less likely to affect cardiac conduction, cause postural hypotension or interact with other drugs
   • Breathlessness management: this may include correction of anaemia, low dose opioids and the non-pharmacological approaches used in respiratory rehabilitation and lung cancer management
   • Adopt a palliative approach to psychological, social, spiritual, information and communication needs, actively pursuing and managing identified needs. Patients and carers may need help to manage the uncertainty of a future with a high chance of sudden death

End-of-life care

Diagnosing dying in heart failure is extremely difficult. The disease trajectory is of a steady decline punctuated by unexpected sudden death.

Features suggested as characterizing a subgroup of patients with a poor prognosis are:[4]
• Previous admissions with worsening heart failure
• No identifiable reversible precipitant
• Optimum tolerated conventional drugs
• Deteriorating renal function
• Failure to respond soon after admission to changes in vasodilators or diuretics

In these patients, invasive treatments and monitoring should be reviewed and emphasis on palliation should predominate. Discontinuation of cardiac drugs may be appropriate. When a patient is clearly dying, use of a guideline such as the Liverpool care pathway for the dying patient[5] is recommended.

Models of care

Although chronic heart failure is increasingly being managed across the community/hospital interface by multiprofessional heart failure teams, most

2 Jiang W., Alexander J., Christopher E., Kuchibhatla M., Gaulden L. H., Cuffe M. S. *et al.* (2001) Relationship of depression to increased risk of mortality and rehospitalization in patients with congestive heart failure. *Arch Intern Med,* **161, 15**: 1849–56.

3 Teno J. M., Weitzen S., Fennell M. L., Mor V. (2001) Dying trajectory in the last year of life: does cancer trajectory fit other diseases? *J Palliat Med,* **4, 4**: 457–464.

4 Ellershaw J. and Ward C. (2003) Care of the dying patients: the last hours or days of life. *BMJ,* **326**: 30–4.

5 http://www.lcp-mariecurie.org.uk

patients currently never see a heart failure specialist. These teams should aim to address the disease management and supportive and palliative care needs of the majority of patients with heart failure. The minority of patients with extraordinary palliative needs may need direct involvement from specialist palliative care services, often in concert with active heart failure team management. Mutual support and education, plus joint management by heart failure and specialist palliative care teams should be objectives for the future.

Table 8c.2 Key drugs to avoid in heart failure patients

Drugs	Reason for avoidance
Non-steroidal anti-inflammatory (NSAID)	Salt and water retention and worsen renal function
Tricyclic antidepressants	Cardiotoxic
Lithium	Salt and water retention
Cyclizine	Probably cardiotoxic
Steroids	Water retention
Progestogens	Water retention
Flecainide/mexiletine	Depress myocardial function

Diuretics

Furosemide is less effective when given orally rather than parenterally in heart failure, cirrhosis and probably any hypoalbuminaemic state. It is more affected by food intake than bumetanide which may be better absorbed orally than furosemide. Continuous infusion of furosemide may be given i/v and has been given by CSCI. Spironolactone is used for ascites particularly if associated with liver metastases, steroid-induced fluid retention and possibly heart failure. Metolazone is a weak thiazide diuretic which can be used alone but is also synergistic with furosemide.

Further reading

Articles

Gibbs J. S. R., McCoy A. S., Gibbs L. M., Rogers A. E., Addington-Hall J. M. (2002) Living with and dying from heart failure: the rôle of palliative care. *Heart*, **88** (Suppl. 2): ii36–ii39.

Remme W., Swedberg K. (2001) Task Force for the Diagnosis and Treatment of Chronic Heart Failure. *European Heart Journal*, **22**, **17**: 1527–60.

Ward C. (2002) The need for palliative care in the management of heart failure. *Heart*, **87**, **3**: 294–8.

Palliative care in non-malignant neurological disease

Multiple sclerosis (MS)

There are an estimated 80,000 to 90,000 people with multiple sclerosis in the UK. In the majority (70–80 per cent), the course of the disease is relapsing and remitting in nature at the onset. Half of these patients will enter a progressive phase within 10 years (secondary progressive MS). In a smaller group of patients the disease is progressive from the onset (~15 per cent). In a population of patients with MS approximately 20–30 per cent have marked paraparesis, hemiparesis or paraplegia, 15 per cent are wheelchair-bound and 5 per cent have severe cognitive impairment. It is estimated that only about 25 per cent of patients who are severely disabled are alive at 10 years.

Death is commonly due to secondary complications of MS (e.g. aspiration pneumonia, pulmonary embolus). If sudden neurological deterioration occurs, precipitating factors such as infection should be looked for. If there is no resolution of symptoms, a course of steroids is usually given which has a high chance of improving symptoms for a further year or so.

Symptom management

Immobility

Walking is usually affected if the disease is progressive, through a combination of weakness, spasticity, fatigue, disuse, pain, cerebellar ataxia and sensory loss particularly proprioception. Immobility inevitably becomes difficult towards the end-of-life, leading to many problems, which need to be addressed by the majority of members of the multidisciplinary team.

Pain

Chronic pain may be present in 60 per cent and some studies have shown inadequate control in 40 per cent of patients, with significant adverse effects on quality of life. Neuropathic pain, which may present as a persistent burning discomfort often affecting the lower limbs, is usually treated with standard agents for neuropathic pain such as the tricyclic antidepressants.

Trigeminal neuralgia is a common paroxysmal pain and is classically treated with carbamazepine. Gabapentin has also been used. Neurosurgical procedures such as percutaneous denervation may be considered, although this may leave the patient with paraesthesiae.

Lhermitte's sign is a syndrome of intermittent burning sensations or 'electric shocks' occurring on neck flexion. It is probably due to demyelination in the posterior columns of the spinal cord and can occur in up to two-thirds of patients at some time during the course of the disease. It is often self-limiting but, if persistent, a cervical collar and carbamazepine may be needed.

Musculoskeletal pain is common, particularly back pain, and results from prolonged immobility, poor posture and gait abnormalities. It is probably caused by a combination of spasticity leading to muscular pain and abnormal stresses resulting in mechanical pain. Osteoporosis should also be considered and treated as appropriate. Simple analgesics or NSAIDs can be prescribed. Physiotherapy is needed to improve poor posture and to ensure that correct seating and wheelchair adaptations are provided. Passive and active exercises, TENS, massage and acupuncture may also be helpful.

Spasticity

Increased muscle tone occurs in the majority of patients with MS. It may cause difficulty with function of the affected limb, painful muscle spasms and, when severe, difficulty in nursing care. Neurophysiotherapists teach patients and their carers stretching techniques for shortened spastic muscles and passive joint exercises to maintain movement which should be carried out regularly. Splints may be used and TENS may alleviate the frequency of painful muscle spasms and improve sleep. Aggravating factors such as urinary tract infections, pressure sores and constipation should be avoided and/or treated.

Baclofen can be built up slowly by 5mg every few days starting from 5mg t.d.s. up to a maximum of 80mg daily. Transient neuropsychiatric and gastrointestinal symptoms may occur. Reduction of baclofen should be gradual to avoid fits or hallucinations. Intrathecal baclofen can be used for severe spasticity and muscle spasms if they are affecting quality of life and have proved unresponsive to other therapies.

Benzodiazepines such as diazepam can be given at night if painful spasms disturb sleep.

Dantrolene is less sedating than other muscle relaxants but can further weaken muscles and is therefore often reserved for those patients who are wheelchair-bound. Liver function should be monitored.

Tizanidine, an alternative to baclofen, is associated with less muscle weakness than baclofen or diazepam. The starting dose is 2mg increased every 3–4 days in 2mg increments up to 24mg daily in divided doses. It can cause sedation and dry mouth and liver function should be monitored for the first four months. Gabapentin is an alternative.

Intramuscular botulinum toxin can be effective for focal spasticity that interferes with hygiene or nursing care. It is generally only used when maintenance of function is less important. It should always be accompanied by a physiotherapy regime of passive stretching.

Tenotomies (surgical release of tendons) or other nerve blocks most commonly obturator, perineal, adductor, or pudendal may be needed.

Ataxia and tremor

Feeding, correct seating and head control can be very difficult. The rôle of the occupational therapist is crucial. There is some evidence, although minimal, for the benefits of propranolol and clonazepam. Severe tremor can be treated with stereotactic thalamotomy but with initial benefit only. Other techniques of deep brain stimulation may be promising.

Urinary system

Assessment and treatment is important in order to improve symptoms and to minimize complications such as pressure atrophy of the kidneys, urinary tract infections and skin breakdown secondary to incontinence. Incontinence can lead to profound embarrassment and social breakdown. Adequate fluid intake, bladder emptying (particularly if residual volume is more than 100ml) and treatment of infection are the principle priorities.

Hyperreflexia of the bladder is associated with a low volume capacity bladder and possible symptoms of mild urgency, frequency and incontinence. Treatment is usually with anticholinergic drugs such as oxybutinin or tolterodine. Incomplete bladder emptying, induced by these drugs, may require intermittent self-catheterization. Nocturnal incontinence may be relieved with desmopressin nasal spray 10–40 mcg at night. If the overactive bladder is resistant to conventional management, transvesical phenol capsaicin may provide some benefit.

Bladder hypotonia and sphincter dyssynergia (sphincter contracts when voiding) results in incomplete emptying, of which the patient may be unaware. Catheterization will be needed. Intermittent catheterization is associated with less risk of UTI than a permanent indwelling catheter. However, the latter may be needed if all other methods fail to fully empty the bladder frequently enough to avoid problems. Even with a permanent catheter, an anticholinergic may still be needed for bladder spasm and urinary bypassing. If all else fails a urinary diversion may be the only viable option.

Constipation

Constipation is common due in large degree to delayed gut transit time, immobility and anticholinergic medication. Adequate dietary fibre and fluid intake are important and regular oral laxatives or suppositories/enemas are frequently needed.

Fatigue

Fatigue is severe and disabling in the majority of patients, reflecting muscle weakness and sleep interruption (e.g. from nocturia or spasms). It presents as overwhelming tiredness which is not relieved by exercise or rest. It does not necessarily directly correlate with mood disturbance or the severity of the MS.

Precipitants such as exposure to hot baths and hot weather should be avoided. Amantadine and modafinil offer modest benefit. Explanation, reassurance, and advice on modification in lifestyle such as pacing activities, taking rest periods and gentle exercise are essential.

Mood/cognitive disturbance

Clinical depression is common in MS. The estimated lifetime risk of developing depression is 50 per cent and the risk of suicide is 7.5 times that of the healthy population. Depression is contributed to by many factors including the breakdown in family relationships, public embarrassment, social isolation and other losses of work, money, sexual abilities and confidence. Antidepressants should be selected according to their side-effect profile; for example, a tricyclic antidepressant might be used if an overactive bladder and additional neuropathic pain are a problem. Conversely, an SSRI which is less sedating than a tricyclic would be preferable if the patient feels fatigued.

There is some degree of cognitive impairment in 50–60 per cent of patients. The most common deficits relate to short-term memory, attention and speed of processing information and impaired learning. Personality and behaviour may change. Moderate to severe dementia is seen in 10 per cent of patients with long-standing MS. Pathological laughing and crying is a problem in 10 per cent, for which amitriptyline may be tried.

Multiple sclerosis is usually only managed in late advanced-stage disease by specialist palliative care teams, although they may have an earlier rôle in providing respite. The principles of palliative care apply through the illness trajectory and should aim to provide the best and most acceptable quality of life for the individual. Good symptom control and support for families are paramount.

Further reading

Articles

Cornish C. J. et al. (2000) Symptom management in advanced multiple sclerosis. *CME Bulletin Palliative Medicine*, **2, 1**: 11–16.

Gibson J., Frank A.O. (2003) Supporting individuals with disabling multiple sclerosis. *Journal of the Royal Society of Medicine*, **96, 5**: 256–7.

Parkinson's disease

Parkinson's Disease (PD) is the commonest neurodegenerative disease, after Alzheimer's disease, with an estimated incidence of 2/1000. It affects just under 1 per cent of people over the age of 65 years. PD is probably not one disease but several with common clinical features.

Criteria for the diagnosis of Parkinson's Disease

Bradykinesia (slowness and progressive decrease of amplitude of movement) plus at least one of the following:
- Tremor (frequently 'pill rolling')
- Rigidity (often cogwheeling in nature) or
- Disorders of posture (flexion of neck and trunk)
- Disorders of balance (loss of righting reflexes)
- Disorders of gait (short steps, shuffling, festination and freezing)

Classical pathological lesions seen in PD include loss of dopaminergic neurones in the substantia nigra and locus coerulus with formation of Lewy bodies in the cytoplasm. Degeneration of the nigrostriatal pathway leads to depletion of the neurotransmitter dopamine.

The aetiology is unknown, although neurotoxins such as 1-methyl-4-phenyl-1,2,3,6-tetrahydropyridine (MPTP), pesticides and herbicides have been linked to causation. There is a two- to threefold risk of developing PD in first-degree relatives.

Management

Research is underway into transplantation of human and animal foetal cells or allogenic stem cells, and therapy with nerve growth factors.

Surgical options such as subthalamic nucleus (STN) lesions may be effective for disabling dyskinesias (abnormal, involuntary movements), relieving rigidity and tremor. Alternatively, deep brain stimulation using implantable electrodes and a pacemaker-like generator may be used, allowing flexibility to modify the response and reduce side-effects.

The mainstay of management is the control of symptoms with medication with the aim of achieving optimal quality of life. Patients with PD should be monitored by doctors and teams specializing in PD, who should be alerted if there are any changes to the basic clinical pattern; reversible factors adversely affecting the PD should be pursued and subtle changes in medication advised, where appropriate.

Motor symptoms

Levodopa preparations

Dopamine does not cross the blood–brain barrier (BBB). To circumvent this problem, levodopa, which is able to cross the BBB, is used. Levodopa is converted to dopamine by the enzyme aromatic-L-amino-acid decarboxylase. The striatum is thus provided with the essential dopamine. However, the presence of too much dopamine outside the blood–brain barrier causes side-effects such as nausea. To circumvent this problem, inhibitors of the converting enzyme, which do not cross the BBB, are given to reduce peripheral dopamine. Carbidopa and benserazide are used in this way and combined with levodopa as the preparations sinemet and madopar respectively.

These compounds are available as modified release and immediate release preparations. They are also available in the dispersible form to aid administration with an oral syringe or through a nasogastric or gastrostomy tube where necessary. The timing of medication and dose are individualized, some patients benefitting from a 'kick start' dose in the mornings and others by avoiding late night medication which may interfere with sleep. Others benefit from long-acting medication at night to reduce painful stiffness. Any changes in dose should be undertaken slowly, allowing several weeks for the change in regimen to stabilize. The drugs should never be withdrawn unless severe side-effects develop, since patients may become unable to move, swallow and adequately protect the airway.

Unfortunately, the efficacy of levodopa is marred by unwanted actions that become progressively more prominent with advancing disease. These patients may develop severe drug-induced dyskinesia, often alternating with sudden unpredictable loss of mobility (freezing and hesitancy).

Dopamine agonists
These act directly on dopamine receptors and include bromocriptine, pergolide, ropinerole, pramipexole and cabergoline. Lisuride is rarely used in the UK. They are more likely than levodopa to cause dopaminergic side-effects such as nausea, vomiting, drowsiness, hallucinations and confusion and should be titrated up slowly; domperidone cover may be needed to treat the nausea.

Apomorphine is usually administered subcutaneously either as boluses or as a continuous infusion using a portable minipump. Its rapid onset of action can 'rescue' patients from sudden 'off' periods. It is most commonly reserved for patients experiencing severe and frequent motor fluctuations despite adequate trials with other oral medications. Domperidone is needed for three days prior to starting treatment to prevent nausea. Painful nodules which ulcerate may develop and sites of injection should be changed daily. Apomorphine treatment should be guided by a specialist in PD.

Drugs that delay the breakdown of levodopa
Entacapone achieves this by inhibiting the enzyme catechol-0-methyl transferase (COMT). It usually relieves motor fluctuations and allows dose reduction of levodopa-containing drugs.

Anticholinergics
These are sometimes effective for tremor but not bradykinesia and rigidity. Dry mouth, urinary retention, drowsiness and confusion often limit their usefulness.

Glutamate inhibitors (e.g. amantadine)
Amantadine may help rigidity and bradykinesia. It can be useful as adjunctive therapy and may be beneficial in reducing levodopa-induced dyskinesias. Common side-effects include peripheral oedema, livedo reticularis and hallucinations.

Monoamine oxidase type B selective inhibitor (e.g. selegeline)
This boosts the dopamine available in the brain by reducing the metabolism, and may be useful symptomatically. It is controversial as to whether or not selegeline has a neuroprotective rôle. Selegeline is now available as both an oral and a buccal melt preparation.

Other general measures for management of motor symptoms include input from members of the multidisciplinary team, particularly the physiotherapist, occupational therapist, speech therapist and dietician.

Nausea and vomiting

This may be due to drug treatment for PD or for another unrelated reason. Neuroleptics should not be used, in particular haloperidol, metoclopramide and prochlorperazine. (Most phenothiazines should be avoided since they may aggravate PD, except for clozapine and quetiapine which do not have extrapyramidal side-effects.) The safest drug to use is domperidone which can be given orally or rectally. A 5-HT$_3$ inhibitor such as ondansetron may also be tolerated.

Depression

This may occur in 40 per cent of patients with PD. It is not known whether it is an inherent feature of PD or secondary to a reaction to the disability caused by PD. Drugs such as the tricyclic antidepressants may aggravate postural hypotension and cause dry mouth. The selective serotonin reuptake inhibitors (SSRIs) may be helpful although they may worsen symptoms of PD and can cause postural hypotension. Mirtazepine has proved helpful in relieving depression and anxiety and reducing tremor.

Constipation

This may be caused by a lack of adequate neurotransmitter in the myenteric plexus. Advice on diet, adequate fluids and exercise should be given. Aperients are usually needed.

Swallowing difficulties

The ability to take food, chew and swallow may vary during the day, especially in more advanced disease. The speech and language therapist may be able to analyse the cause of the difficulty and to provide useful advice. Also the dietician may be required to advise on diet. The occupational therapist can help by providing appropriate feeding implements. Special seating and head and neck supports may be required.

Patients often lose a significant amount of weight in late stage PD, since the severe dyskinesias use up a significant amount of calorific energy. Feeding difficulties are often associated with periods of motor disability. Patients may choose to use their good functional moments to attend to activities of daily living or to pursue what they want to do, rather than wasting these precious moments on eating. They should be advised to eat little and often to make efficient use of time and energy intake. A deterioration of PD can be triggered by minimal dehydration and patients should be encouraged to drink adequately, especially during hot weather. High calorific drinks and other nutritional additives are useful to supplement an often inadequate diet.

Urinary urgency and nocturia

Urinary urgency may be helped with drugs such as tolterodine, oxybutynin and trospium. Severe distressing nocturia may be helped by a nocturnal dose of desmopressin, but care should be given to ensure that hyponatraemia and congestive cardiac failure are not induced by this treatment.

Postural hypotension

Patients should be given general advice on rising carefully from a lying or sitting position. It may be helpful to raise the head of the bed and some patients may tolerate compression stockings. If symptoms are severe, fludrocortisone may be needed. If dizziness is experienced, encourage the patient to take a full glass of water with medication, especially with the first dose of the day.

Sleep

Sleep disorders occur in 70–80 per cent of patients with PD and are distressing for patients and carers alike. The patient may be awoken by motor fluctuations; they may wake up and be unable to move and any effort to turn may cause painful muscle spasms; painful neck extension and leg cramp may occur. Attempts should be made to maintain nocturnal levels of levodopa, including avoiding high protein meals in the late evening (amino acids compete with dopamine for receptor sites) and by giving domperidone in the evenings (if needed) to avoid a delay in gastric emptying. Restless leg syndrome (RLS), characterized by an urge to move the legs, with painful cramps, paraesthesiae and a burning sensation in the calves may be relieved by standard levodopa therapy and dopamine agonists.

Amantidine and selegeline are stimulant and should be avoided if possible in the evenings. If PD is associated with dementia a reversal of the sleep-wake cycle may occur. Short-acting hypnotics can be used if necessary. Hallucinations and panic attacks may also keep patients awake at night and may be due to dopamine agonists and other antiparkinsonian medication therapy. (📖 See the section on confusion/hallucinations below).

Communication

Difficulties in communication can be very distressing, especially if the patient is cognitively intact but has unpredictable episodes of being unable to communicate adequately. As with other symptoms in PD, it may worsen in stressful situations. Impaired emotional expression (mask-like facies), so characteristic of PD, impairs the very important non-verbal aspects of communication and should be recognized. Speech therapists can be helpful in improving symptoms.

Dementia

May occur in up to 40 per cent of patients.

Confusion/hallucinations

This may occur as part of the PD itself or as a result of medication. Nocturnal hallucinations are a particular problem and may improve if medication is avoided just prior to sleep. Patients will sometimes tolerate a degree of hallucinosis provided that the other features of the disease, such as motor disability, are reasonably well controlled. The newer antipsychotic agents such as clozapine (beware agranulocytosis), risperidone or olanzepine may help, although should be avoided if there is cerebrovascular disease. Quetiapine is also a very useful medication in this regard but for some is too sedating. Antimuscarinics should be avoided if possible. All medication may have to be reduced if symptoms persist. The anti-dementia drugs such as donepezil, rivastigmine, galantamine and memantine are proving very effective in suppressing drug-induced hallucinations and confusion.

Pain

Pain is a feature of PD and may be relieved by treating the stiffness with levodopa or dopamine agonists. Pain of a sensory nature often occurs in PD and should be treated appropriately. It is important to remember that patients, if demented, may not be able to communicate the presence of pain.

Anxiety

This occurs in 40 per cent of patients but in over 90 per cent of depressed patients with PD. Symptoms of PD such as tremor and dyskinesia often worsen in situations induced by anxiety or emotional excitement (even watching a television programme). A benzodiazepine may help, although it may result in muscle weakness and falls due to loss of muscle tone. Very small doses such as diazepam 1mg b.d. can be effective, therefore this dosage should be carefully titrated from this low start dose.

The terminal phase

PD may worsen with infection, dehydration or other illnesses. Any reversible factors should be corrected where appropriate alongside the management of the PD itself, preferably in a specialist centre. Care and consideration needs to be given to continuing on the antiparkinsonian drugs for as long as possible in order to keep patients as comfortable as possible and able to communicate and swallow. However, if the patient is developing distressing side-effects from the medication, withdrawal of therapy may be in the patient's best interests.

All patients should be encouraged, with help from the family and professionals, to discuss their attitudes and wishes for the management of acute life-threatening medical problems that may occur, such as pneumonia. An Advanced Directive may be helpful in ascertaining patients' wishes for interventions.

Multiple system atrophy (MSA)

Progressive supranuclear palsy (PSP)

Multiple system atrophy (MSA)

MSA is a progressive neuro-degenerative disorder that results in autonomic dysfunction in addition to parkinsonian and at times cerebellar features. It is not hereditary and affects adults usually in the fourth or fifth decade. Post-mortem studies of patients diagnosed with PD indicate that between 10–25 per cent had MSA. It is poorly responsive to levodopa. The mean survival is nine years. As with PD, a multidisciplinary approach is essential.

Progressive supranuclear palsy (PSP)

PSP is the most common cause of an atypical Parkinsonian syndrome with dementia. It occurs more commonly in men than women, with a peak incidence in the early 60s. It comprises postural instability associated with parkinsonism, vertical opthalmoplegia and progressive subcortical dementia. Patients are limited in their ability to move their eyes downwards on request, although the eyes are able to move downwards reflexly, such as when a patient is asked to stare at a stationary object and the head is gently rotated backwards.

Limited upwards eye movement is also common in PSP, but is not diagnostic. Within one year of diagnosis the majority of patients have frequent falls, are slow in performing activities of daily living and have speech difficulties. Twenty-five per cent are confined to a wheelchair by one year following diagnosis increasing to 70 per cent by four years. The mean duration of the illness is four–six years, though this is often shorter in older patients.

Further reading

Bhatia K. et al. (2001) Updated guidelines for the management of Parkinson's disease. *Hospital Medicine* (London) 62, **8**: 456–70.

Global Parkinson's Disease Survey (GPDS) Steering Committee (2002) Factors impacting on quality of life in Parkinson's disease: results from an international survey. *Movement Disorders*, 17, **1**: 60–7.

O'Sullivan J. (2000) What PD therapies to use and when. *Health and Ageing*, January: 16–18.

Olanow CW. (2001) An algorithm (decision tree) for the management of Parkinson's Disease: treatment guidelines. *Neurology*, **56** (11 Suppl 5): S1–S88.

Rascol O. et al. (2002) Treatment interventions for Parkinson's Disease: an evidence-based assessment. *Lancet*, **359**: **9317**: 1589–98.

Schapira AHV (1999) Science, medicine and the future: Parkinson's disease. *British Medical Journal*, **318**: 311–314

Scott S. (2002) *Swallowing Problems and Parkinson's*. PDS Information Sheet 52. London: PDS.

Motor neurone disease

> When I wake each morning I decide ...
> This can be a good day or a bad day—my choice.
> I can be happy or sad—my choice.
> I can complain or I can cope—my choice.
> Life can be a chore or a challenge—my choice.
> I can take from life or give to life—my choice.
> If all things are possible,
> How I deal with those possibilities is—my choice.
>
> Steve Shackel, diagnosed with MND, (alternatively referred to as amyotrophic lateral sclerosis (ALS))[1]

Motor neurone disease (MND) is a disease of unknown aetiology in which there is progressive degeneration of both upper and lower motor neurones, leading to wasting of muscles and weakness. The average survival is 40 per cent at five years although older patients presenting predominantly with bulbar signs may have a worse prognosis and conversely, younger patients with largely lower motor neurone involvement may have a better than average prognosis. The mean age of onset is 56 years.

UPPER MOTOR NEURONE involvement leads to generalised spasticity, hyper-reflexia and often emotional lability.

LOWER MOTOR NEURONE involvement leads to flaccidity, muscle wasting and fasciculation.

Involvement of BULBAR innervated muscles leads to dysarthria and dysphagia. Interestingly the third, fourth and sixth cranial nerves and those of the lower segments of the spinal cord are usually spared such that eye movements, bladder, bowel and sexual function are generally unaffected. Furthermore intellect, memory, sight and hearing are also usually preserved.

Symptoms in MND are often similar to patients with cancer and include:
- weakness (100 per cent)
- constipation (65 per cent)
- pain (50–60 per cent)
- cough (50–60 per cent)
- insomnia (40–50 per cent)
- breathlessness (40–50 per cent)
- dribbling (30–40 per cent)
- anxiety and depression

In addition problems related to mobility, communication and psychosocial issues, both for the patient and their families, must be addressed necessitating a fully multidisciplinary approach.

1 http://home.goulburn.net.au/~shack

Symptoms

Weakness

Attention to individual needs for maximum comfort is crucial in order to prevent pain and other problems such as skin trauma, contractures and joint dislocation. The rôle of the physiotherapist is important, not only for the patient but also to educate and advise relatives. Although it is important to maintain muscle function and to keep joints mobile, over-enthusiastic physiotherapy may tire the patient and be counterproductive.

Insomnia

It is important to ascertain as far as possible the cause of insomnia, which may range from pain and depression to the overwhelming anxieties of choking and the fear of dying. There is a general reluctance to prescribe night sedatives to patients with MND for fear of respiratory depression. In practice this rarely happens and is insignificant in relation to the morbidity associated with chronic fatigue.

Pain

Management of cause of pain
- Stiff joints—careful positioning/physiotherapy
- Inflammation—NSAID
- Joint pains—Intra-articular steroid injections
- Muscle cramp—quinine sulphate
- Muscle spasm diazepam/baclofen
- Skin pressure—regular turning/turning beds, analgesic ladder

Neuropathic pain is not a feature of MND per se, however patients may complain of pain associated with sensory disturbance and tricyclic antide-pressants may help.

The use of opioids in MND

There has been a reluctance to prescribe opioids for fear of respiratory depression in patients whose lung function may already be compromised. However, one study showed that over 80 per cent of patients had been treated with morphine without detriment.

Dysphagia

The speech therapist will help in analysing the exact cause of dysphagia in order to recommend specific techniques to aid swallowing. A common cause is spasticity of the tongue causing difficulty in propelling a food bolus to the pharynx.

Ice packs applied to the neck or chips of ice placed in the mouth may result in relaxation of the tongue and ease swallowing.

The subject of artificial feeding via a gastrostomy tube should be discussed with the patient and the advantages and disadvantages outlined. In the end-stages of the disease, tube feeding may not necessarily prolong life. However, earlier in the disease, particularly if the patient is ambulant, gastrostomy feeding may slow the inevitable weight loss and its associated weakness and depression.

The dietician will advise on food consistency and general nutritional requirements, and the speech therapist on the timing of endoscopic percutaneous gastrostomy tube insertion.

Dysarthria

The speech therapist should be involved early to teach the patient various techniques relevant to his/her own special needs. Various aids are available and include Lightwriters with or without synthesized voice function. Other computerized systems are available from specialized centres including electronic equipment, telephone devices and communication boards which may be adapted to the physical abilities of the individual patient. It is essential to plan ahead since motor function may deteriorate rapidly.

Breathlessness

This is due to diaphragmatic and respiratory muscle weakness. The physiotherapist may suggest breathing techniques and help with chest drainage if appropriate. Antibiotics may be useful in controlling symptoms but if the patient is in a terminal stage they may be inappropriate, serving only to prolong dying.

Nocturnal hypoventilation is characterized by poor sleep and nightmares, early morning headaches and daytime tiredness with subsequent impaired concentration. At an early stage in the disease, it may be appropriate to consider some form of limited ventilatory assistance, such as non-invasive positive pressure ventilation to aid respiration at night time. As breathing becomes weaker, this form of ventilation may continue during the day time.

Patients must be fully informed of the pros and cons of assisted ventilation. More invasive ventilation through a tracheostomy is generally not used in the UK. The wishes of patients for respiratory support should be discussed well in advance of acute problems arising. Patients with MND may die suddenly and unexpectedly with respiratory failure.

Choking

The normal reflexes which protect the airway are impaired so that swallowing food or saliva may result in choking. Although it is a common fear, patients rarely, if ever, die as a result of choking. Speech therapists may help by advising different techniques for protecting the airway such as chewing carefully and slowly, breathing in, swallowing and then deliberately coughing. This technique serves to clear the larynx and to minimize the possibility of choking.

Some patients find suction to the upper airways useful. For others it is avoided since it not only causes trauma, fright and discomfort but may also be very distressing for the relatives to witness.

The Motor Neurone Disease Association (MNDA) supplies a box known as a Breathing Space Kit which provides support for patients and carers. It is a small box with two drawers which contain drugs prescribed by the GP. One side may contain rectal diazepam for the family to administer in an emergency and the other side, drugs such as diamorphine, hyoscine and diazepam, for the doctor or nurse to give.

The multidisciplinary team

All members of the team will have been involved in the care of a patient with MND at some time. These include the neurologist, physiotherapist, occupational therapist, speech therapist, dietician, case manager, GP, district nurse, social worker, palliative physician and palliative home care team.

The MNDA provides an invaluable service not only in terms of liaising, supporting and educating patients and carers but also in facilitating the loan of equipment and helping financially.

Further reading

Borasio G., Voltz R. (1997) Palliative care in amyotrophic lateral sclerosis. *Journal of Neurology*, **244**(Suppl. 4): S11–S17.

Borasio G. D. *et al.* (2001) Clinical characteristics and management of ALS. *Seminars in Neurology*, **21**: 155–66.

Carter H. *et al.* (1998) Health professionals' responses to multiple sclerosis and motor neurone disease. *Palliative Medicine*, **12, 5**: 383–94.

Dawson S., Kristjanson L. (2003) Mapping the journey: family carer's perceptions of issues related to end stage care of individuals with Muscular Dystrophy or Motor Neurone Disease. *Journal of Palliative Care*, **19, 1**: 36–42.

Leigh N. *et al.* (2001) Motor neurone disease. *European Journal of Palliative Care*, **8**, 1: 10–12.

Oliver D. (1998) Opioid medication in the palliative care of motor neurone disease. *Palliative Medicine*, **12, 2**: 113–15.

Oliver D. *et al.* (eds) (2000) *Palliative Care in Amyotrophic Lateral Sclerosis (Motor neurone disease)*. Oxford: Oxford University Press.

Polkey M. I. *et al.* (1999) Ethical and clinical issues in the use of home non-invasive mechanical ventilation for the palliation of breathlessness in motor neurone disease. *Thorax*, **54, 4**: 367–71.

Neurological complications of AIDS

Prevalence: up to 65 per cent.

AIDS dementia complex

- A syndrome of progressive cognitive loss with motor and behavioural dysfunction in HIV- infected patients
- Clinical features: apathy, social withdrawal, impaired concentration, slowing of speech and movement, unsteady gait, can progress to being bedridden with paraparesis, urinary incontinence and faecal incontinence
- Investigations:
  - Need to exclude opportunistic infection with toxoplasmosis or CMV
  - CT scan—cerebral atrophy and ventricular enlargement
  - MRI scan—white matter abnormality
- Management: anti-retroviral drugs may improve symptoms and prolong survival

Vacuolar myelopathy

- Aetiology: unclear but vacuolization of the white matter in spinal cord is seen at post-mortem
- Clinical features: progressive weakness, spasticity and ataxia, urinary incontinence, faecal incontinence
- Management: no current treatment

Peripheral neuropathy

- Distal symmetrical polyneuropathy is the most common feature and may occur in 10–30 per cent. It is characterized by a symmetrical distal painful sensory loss which is associated with weight loss and dementia
- Management: trial of amitriptyline
- Inflammatory demyelinating neuropathy is characterized by progressive weakness and loss of tendon reflexes. It is usually mild
- Inflammatory polyradiculopathy can be due to CMV infection and is characterized by a progressive distal weakness, sensory problems and incontinence
- Management: no treatment available
- Cranial nerve neuropathy, can involve the facial nerve

HIV-associated myopathy

Symptoms are progressive with symmetrical painless weakness of the proximal limbs and facial muscles.

- Investigations: electromyography (EMG), muscle biopsy
- Management: consider corticosteroids and plasmapheresis

Opportunistic infections of the CNS

- Common organisms: Toxoplasmosis gondii, cryptococcus neoformans, JC virus, CMV
- Clinical features: headache, confusion, fever, seizures, focal signs
- Investigations: CT scan, MRI scan, lumbar puncture—CSF analysis
- Management:
  - Cerebral toxoplasmosis—pyrimethamine and sulphadiazine
  - Cryptococcal meningitis—amphotericin B

- Progressive multifocal leucoencephalopathy (JC virus)—no effective treatment
- CMV infection—ganciclovir

Further reading

Article

Janssen R. S. *et al.* (1989) Human immunodeficiency virus (HIV) infection and the nervous system: report from the American Academy of Neurology AIDS Task Force. *Neurology*, **39, 1**: 119–22.

Creutzfeldt-Jakob disease (CJD)

CJD is a rare degenerative disorder of the central nervous system. Prion proteins occur naturally but it is the abnormal development and accumulation of rogue prion proteins in brain cells that leads to the development of CJD.

The most common form of the disease, accounting for 80 per cent of all cases, is '**sporadic**', presenting as a rapidly progressive multi-focal dementia with poor memory and cognition, impaired balance and mobility, myoclonic jerks, slurred speech and visual problems. The incidence of sporadic CJD is 0.5–1 new case/million population per year.

'**Inherited**' prion disease, accounting for around 10 per cent of cases, is due to autosomal dominant inheritance of a genetically-mutated prion protein. The clinical course of inherited forms is usually more protracted than other forms.

'**Acquired**' prion disease occurs when rogue proteins have inadvertently been introduced into the individual (e.g. secondary to treatment with human derived growth hormone, following transplant of infected organs such as corneas, or the inadvertent use of contaminated neurosurgical instruments).

'**Variant**' (vCJD) was first described in 1996 and has been linked to the UK Bovine Spongiform Encephalopathy (BSE) epidemic of the 1980s. The median age at onset is younger than for patients with sporadic disease, at 26 years. Common early features are dysphoria, withdrawal, anxiety and hallucinations, with subsequent neurological decline. The time course is longer than for sporadic disease (14.5 months mean duration compared with four months).

Unpublished research into the palliative care of patients with CJD has shown that many patients are being cared for by specialist palliative care services, and that the key issues in their care include managing agitation and movement disorders, impaired communication and the dilemmas associated with end-of-life decisions. There is frequently a high level of distress amongst those emotionally close to the patient, in keeping with the younger age of patients, the distressing nature of the illness and its high media profile.

Following the death of a patient, the case should be discussed with the coroner, who may require a *post-mortem*. As with any coroner's case, a *post-mortem* can be carried out without permission from the next of kin which may cause great distress, particularly with some cultural/religious groups who will need a great deal of support at this time. All *post-mortems* for CJD are usually carried out in designated neuropathology institutions. Following removal of the brain and spinal cord, families are able to view the body again if they wish. There is usually no visual evidence that the body has been tampered with. The brain and spinal tissue are then sent to the CJD Surveillance Unit where a formal tissue diagnosis may take months. The Unit has information for relatives and handles the situation sensitively, organizing the return of body parts to the family's funeral director for cremation or burial when the tests are completed.

Further reading

Articles

Carter H., McKenna C. *et al.* (1998). Health professionals' responses to multiple sclerosis and motor neurone disease. *Palliat Med*, **12, 5**: 383–94.

Oliver D. (1998) Opioid medication in the palliative care of motor neurone disease. *Palliat Med*, **12, 2**: 113–5.

Bailey B., Aranda S., Quinn K., Kean, H. (2000) Creuzfeldt-Jakob disease: extending palliative care nursing knowledge. *Int J Palliat Nurs*, **6**: 131–9.

Brown P. (2001) Bovine Spongiform Ecephalopathy and variant CJD. *British Medical Journal*, **322**: 841–4.

Spencer M., Knight R., Will R. (2002) First hundred cases of variant CJD: retrospective case note review of early psychiatric and neurological features. *BMJ*, **324**: 1479–82.

Meek J. (1998) A case study: team support for a patient with CJD. *Community Nurse*, **4**: 27–28.

Useful contacts

Multiple Sclerosis Resource Centre
7 Peartree Business Centre
Peartree Road
Stanway
Colchester
Essex CO3 5JN
Tel: 01206 505444
Freephone: 0800 783 0518
E-mail: themsrc@yahoo.com
Web Site: http://www.msrc.co.uk
Also provide a 24 hour MS telephone counselling service on 0800 783 0518

Multiple Sclerosis Society
MS National Centre
372 Edgware Road
London NW2 6ND
Tel: 020 8438 0700
MS Helpline: Freephone 0808 800 8000, 9am–9pm
E-mail: info@mssociety.org.uk
Web Site: http://www.mssociety.org.uk
Provides information, support and practical help to anyone affected by MS
and to those working with them. Also provide respite care centres and
holiday homes.

Motor Neurone Disease Association
PO Box 246
Northampton NN1 2PR
Tel: 01604 250505
Fax: 01604 638289/624726
Helpline: 08457 626262
E-mail: enquiries@mndassociation.org
Web Site: http://www.mndassociation.org
Links to other sites and documents can be accessed through this site.
Telephone: 0131 537 2128
National Prion Clinic: www.st-marys.nhs.uk/specialist/prion/clinicinfo.htm

The National C-JD Surveillance Unit
Western General Hospital
Crewe Road
Edinburgh EH4 2XU
Web Site: http://www.cjd.ed.ac.uk

NHS National Prion Clinic
Box 98
National Hospital for Neurology and Neurosurgery
Queen Square
London WCIN 3BG
Tel: 020 7405 0755
E-mail: help.prion@st-marys.nhs.uk
Web Site: http://www.st-marys.nhs.uk/specialist/prion/clinicinfo.htm

Palliation in the care of the elderly[1]

Old age is associated with disease, it does not cause it.

The large majority of the population over the age of 85 years live at home; 20 per cent live in nursing homes. Elderly patients with palliative care needs often have a constellation of complex and chronic requirements including:
- Appropriate therapeutic interventions that can preserve function and independence and help patients maintain quality of life
- Clear communication on the usual course of illness so that they and their family members can make appropriate arrangements
- Recognition and management of caregiver stress
- Management of physical and psychological symptoms of both acute and chronic illnesses

Elderly people in the UK may receive palliative care in a number of settings, including;
- At home with the care of a GP and community nursing team
- In a residential or nursing home with the care of a GP and local nursing staff
- In a Community Hospital
- On a care of the elderly unit/facility
- In an acute hospital following an acute admission

Background
- While a child born in 1900 could expect to live fewer than 50 years, life expectancy for a child born in 2010 is expected to increase to 86 years for a girl and 79 years for a boy.[2] The implication for increasing input from supportive and palliative care is clear
- In developed nations, the overwhelming majority of deaths occur in elderly patients suffering from multiple coexisting and progressive chronic illnesses
- Some studies suggest that elderly patients are excluded from life-prolonging interventions even if they might be appropriate. This difference may be due to de facto rationing based on age rather than emphasis on individualizing the goals of care. Specialists in care of the elderly are skilled at devising goals of care which are appropriate for the individual's particular needs
- Data suggests that elderly patients receive less pain medication than younger persons for both chronic and acute pain. Chronic pain syndromes such as arthritis, and other musculoskeletal problems affect 25–50 per cent of the community-dwelling elderly and are also typically undertreated

1 Meier D. and Monias A. (2004) In D. Doyle, G. Hanks, N. Cherny and K. C. Calman *Oxford Textbook of Palliative Medicine*. 3rd edn. pp. 935–44. Oxford: Oxford University Press.

2 Field M. J. and Cassel C. K. (1997) Approaching death: Improving care at the end of life. In Institute of Medicine, ed. Washington, DC: National Academies Press.

Caregiver burden

- The tremendous growth in numbers of people over 65 years with chronic health problems has challenged both national and personal resources
- In the UK, the duration of caring for an elderly relative may exceed ten years
- Fifty per cent of caregivers have financial difficulties
- Caregiving in general is not valued in western societies, where sometimes those involved in full time caring can be made to feel that life is passing them by

Risks to the carer include:
- Physical risks
  - Development of musculoskeletal diseases through lifting and handling
  - Increased mortality—Many of the carers are themselves elderly and vulnerable
- Emotional risks
  - Major depression, and associated comorbidities
- Social risks
  - Isolation and loss of contact with friends and social circle. Close to 90 per cent of caregivers say they need more help in caring for their loved ones in one or more categories including
  - Personal care
  - Nursing
  - Transportation
  - Loss of income
  - Loss of status within society

How can we address the needs of an elderly, frail and depressed woman who is shortly to be bereaved, and who through the course of caring for her demented husband over many years has lost contact with any support network of friends or family?

Medical goal-setting in care of the elderly with chronic illness

Table 8e.1 A checklist for palliative care throughout the course of chronic illness in the elderly

Early	Middle	Late
Discuss diagnosis, prognosis, and course of disease	Assess efficacy of disease-modifying therapy	Discuss goals of care with patient and family
Discuss disease-modifying therapies	Review course of disease	Confirm previous advance directives
Discuss goals of care, hopes, and expectations	Reassess goals of care and expectations	Actively manage symptoms
Discuss advance care planning	Confirm advance directives and ensure a health care proxy is appointed	Review financial resources and needs

Table 8e.1 (Continued)

Early	Middle	Late
Manage comorbidities Advise financial planning/consultation with a social worker for future needs including long-term care	Recommend physio/ occupational therapies to preserve function and promote socialization Behavioural and pharmacological symptom control	Review long-term care needs and discuss options
Inform patient and family about support groups Inquire about desire for spiritual support	Treat mood disorders Suggest support groups for patient and caregiver	Consider if palliative care needs are being well met in current care setting
Behavioural and pharmacological symptom control	Offer social and emotional support to caregivers	Referral/planning to ensure peaceful death
Treat mood disorders	Review long-term care options and resource needs	Assess spiritual needs Offer respite care

Reproduced from *Oxford Textbook of Palliative Medicine*.[3]

Early in illness

Health care professionals should discuss goals of care with their patients. These goals may change as the disease progresses but may include:
- Prolonging life
- Preserving autonomy and independence
- Maintaining social activities
- Forming a plan for advanced stages of disease
- Staying at home.

Mid-disease

The middle disease period is characterized by:
- Increased medical needs
- Declining function
- Loss of independence, and increased dependence on caregivers for assistance in basic activities of daily living, e.g. patients with dementia require increased supervision while patients with Parkinson's disease, heart failure, or rheumatological diseases may need more assistance with ambulation.

Needs during mid-disease period include:

Patient needs
- Treating physical symptoms of chronic disease such as pain, dyspnoea, anorexia, nausea, vomiting, changes in bowel habit and insomnia which may become prominent during this phase of disease. These symptoms should be effectively treated as outlined in other chapters

3 Meier D. and Monias A. (2004) In D. Doyle, G. Hanks, N. Cherny and K. C. Calman *Oxford Textbook of Palliative Medicine*. 3rd edn. pp. 935–44. Oxford: Oxford University Press.

Caregiver needs
- Help in supervision of the patient, the lack of which results in great caregiver stress, leading to unnecessary consideration of nursing home placement
- Information for carers about local resources for adult day care, respite care, home care services, and support groups
- Helping the caregiver to maintain physical, financial, and emotional strength for the multi-year tasks ahead by providing opportunities to discuss and address their particular difficulties
- Where appropriate encourage a regular rotating schedule of respite support from family and friends

Ageism and the care of the Elderly

Ageist attitudes can inhibit the quality of palliative care available to elderly patients. Such attitudes may be displayed overtly or covertly by:
- Society at large— 'a disproportionate percentage of patients who are left waiting on trolleys for hospital admission in the UK are elderly'
- Doctors and Nurses—'He is too old to benefit from a hip replacement'
- Relatives—'Granny wouldn't want to be told about her disease'
- The elderly themselves—'Why should anyone bother with me? I've had my day'

Home needs
- Home evaluation for adaptive devices such as raised toilet seats, shower seats, and grab bars

Late in disease of chronic illness

In later stages of disease, goals may shift to providing maximum comfort and security.

Patient needs
- Careful attention to symptom control as, particularly in the last few months of life, patients may lose the ability to complain of pain and other symptoms. (e.g. Pain is often undertreated in end-stage dementia.)
- To be treated as an individual, and as a person with particular characteristics and needs
- Ensuring that patients' wishes, fears, and concerns as far as possible are discussed and addressed
- Enjoyment in the modalities of life where joy is possible, e.g. food which the patient enjoys
- At this stage of disease, mortality is 50 per cent at six months, and the goals of care shift to minimise suffering and maximize quality of life, according to the values and expressed wishes of the patient
- Physicians should discuss the merits, or otherwise, of continuing painful routine procedures with the patient and carers

Carer needs
- Patients in the end-stage of a chronic disease may be bed or chair-bound. They can become completely dependent on caregivers for feeding,

toileting, bathing, and dressing and are often incontinent, which can be
extremely distressing both for the patient and the carer
- As patients deteriorate carers can enter a chronic state of loss as they
witness their relative's physical and mental deterioration. Recognition
of the loneliness and pain of such a state can bring important comfort
and help
- Due to increased care demands and exhaustion of family caregivers,
patients' families may benefit from respite admissions in order to allow
the patient's choice to stay at home long term to be achieved

Placement needs
- It is important that efforts are made to find out where a patient
would prefer to die, and where possible to ensure that this decision
is respected
- Patients who reside in a nursing home and want to remain in the
comfort and security of familiar surroundings may not want to be
transferred routinely to the hospital for intercurrent illness or for
symptoms that can be managed in the nursing home. 'Do not transfer'
instructions should be discussed with patient, family, and staff where
possible, and if appropriate, to prevent an emergency move to an acute
setting when the patient's condition deteriorates
- No one place is the ideal setting for terminal care for every person, as
physical, emotional and social resources will all need to be balanced in
the selection of place of care

Common issues in palliative care of the elderly

Physical issues

Infection

- The late stages of many terminal illnesses are commonly complicated by life-threatening infections
- Immobility, malnutrition, incontinence, lung aspiration, and decreased immunity increase the risk of pneumonia, cellulitis, decubitus ulcers, urinary tract infections, and sepsis
- Decreased ability to express oneself and atypical presentation may lead to delayed recognition of infections
- Palliative care should focus on reducing risk factors for infection in providing patients with good skin care, ambulation training, and aspiration precautions
- As with all other treatments, the risks and benefits of antibiotic therapy need to be weighed

Pressure ulcers

- Many patients who are bedbound, incontinent, and poorly nourished do not develop decubitus ulcers in large measure due to the excellence of care provided
- Importantly those who do develop ulcers often do so in spite of excellent care—the appearance of the ulcer being a marker of deteriorating physical condition rather than deteriorating medical or nursing care
- Use of pressure relieving mattresses and cushions prior to the development of skin problems, and quality nursing care are the mainstays in preventing ulcers developing
- In the terminal phase, care should focus on relieving pain and limiting odour, not on aiming for ulcer cure
  - Analgesia should be provided prior to all dressing changes
  - Odour can be controlled with topical metronidazole gel, silver sulfadiazine, or charcoal dressings
- Although the development of decubitus ulcers is not an independent risk factor for death, the presence of a pressure wound is a marker of advanced stage of disease and poor prognosis

Pain

Treatment of pain in the elderly generally follows the same guidelines as in younger adults. Studies on clinical pain perception indicate that pain from headache and visceral pain decrease in the elderly, but musculoskeletal, leg, and foot pain increase with aging. Pain is undertreated in the elderly.

Concomitant diseases likely to cause chronic pain have a higher prevalence in the elderly and often exist alongside the prime pain causing problem, i.e. the development of bowel cancer will not prevent a patient from continuing to suffer the pain of rheumatoid arthritis.

Such chronic illnesses include:

- Arthritis
- Polymyalgia rheumatica

- Atherosclerotic disease
- Cancer
- Herpes zoster

Such diseases cannot be ignored if holistic quality symptom control is to take place.

Nausea and vomiting
Common causes of nausea and vomiting in the elderly include:
- Drug reactions, including opioids
- Gastroparesis due to autonomic system dysfunction (especially caused by diabetes)
- Constipation

Management for nausea and vomiting in the elderly is the same as for younger patients, with particular attention being paid to the possible side-effects from antiemetic medication. ('Start low, go slow.')

Constipation
Constipation is a nearly universal complaint of elderly patients. Over half of the community-dwelling elderly report constipation.
  Risk factors include:
- female gender
- medication
- depression
- immobility
- chronic diseases—Parkinson's disease, hypothyroidism, diabetes mellitus, diverticular disease, irritable bowel syndrome, and haemorrhoids
- Common medication includes opioids, calcium, iron, calcium channel blockers, antihistamines, tricyclic antidepressants, and diuretics

Management
A patient who presents with a history of constipation should always be examined rectally to exclude faecal impaction. If impaction is present, the patient should be manually disimpacted, with some sedation to minimise distress, and treated with suppositories and/or enemas prior to receiving oral laxatives. (☐ See Chapter 6b.)

Diarrhoea
If patients are bedbound this symptom can be particularly exhausting and demeaning to patients and caregivers.
  Common causes of diarrhoea in the elderly include:
- Overflow incontinence
- Antibiotics
- Clostridium *difficile* enterocolitis
- Malabsorption
- Enterocolitis
- Stress

Note: The onset of diarrhoea can also herald the onset of a gastrointestinal haemorrhage.

Management
- Exclude reversible causes
- Consider bulking agents if patient mobile and able to drink enough fluid

- Loperamide, co-phenotrope or codeine may help
- Octreotide is effective to reduce intestinal secretions and leaking fistulae in special circumstances

Cough

Non-malignant causes of chronic cough in the elderly include oesophageal reflux disease, COPD, heart failure, and post-nasal drip. Cough can also be a result of medications such as ACE inhibitors.

Dizziness

- Dizziness is a common symptom in elderly patients with chronic disease. Prevalence ranges from 13–38 per cent
- It is multifactorial in origin and can be due to decreased proprioception secondary to diabetic neuropathy, vascular disease, vestibular disorders, and cardiac arrhythmias. Postural hypotension may also result in dizziness, as can certain medications
- Dizziness has been identified as a syndrome of the elderly because of its prevalence and the frequency with which no single cause is isolated

Drug management includes treating any obviously reversible pathology and appropriate consideration of antihistamines, such as betahistine, or occasionally anxiolytics. Secondary prevention is also important, reducing the risks of falls through education, and risk assessment of the patient's home.

Oral symptoms

Elderly patients can present with mouth pain, dryness, and halitosis.

- The differential diagnosis of mouth pain includes aphthous ulcers, mucositis from chemotherapy, fungal infection secondary to decreased immunity or antibiotics, dental caries, periodontal disease, and poorly fitting dentures
- Infection should be treated appropriately and patients and caregivers instructed on oral hygiene
- Medications are the most common cause of dry mouth in elderly patients and should be kept under constant review
- When symptoms are not relieved with sips of water or ice, artificial saliva or commercial preparations containing mucin may provide relief
- Some patients experience mouth pain despite a normal oropharyngeal examination. These patients often benefit from viscous lidocaine

Ethical issues

Artificial nutrition and hydration (📖 See Chapter 1)

General issues

- Patients suffering from end-stage dementia and other chronic neurological illnesses may develop dysphagia, which predisposes them to aspiration pneumonia
- In the late stages of dementia, patients frequently refuse food, clamp their mouths shut, or hold food without swallowing
- Feeding may become a frustrating battle between the patient and caregiver, who may feel that the patient is deliberately being difficult. Carers will need support and information to understand that this may be involuntary and due to the dementia

Possible management options
- Changing the texture of the diet to purée, or liquids thickened with cornstarch or potato starch, may support safe swallowing
- Improving the taste of food may provide increased enjoyment of the process of eating
- Caregivers should be trained to feed the patient in an upright position, with the head forward, using small spoonfuls

Artificial nutrition and hydration is an emotionally charged issue for many caregivers.

They may believe that their loved one would suffer hunger without artificial nutrition and hydration.

Family members should understand that loss of appetite is an integral part of the dying process

📖 For a fuller discussion of these issues see Chapter 1.

Prescribing in the elderly
This is a huge issue, and many patients are admitted to hospital each year due to the effects of injudicious prescribing, particularly in the elderly population.

Particular concerns include the following:
- Decreased renal function and liver metabolism places elderly patients at higher risk of drugs accumulating to toxic levels
- Multiple complex physical and psychological conditions can lead to a wide range of medication being prescribed for different complaints, with increasing likelihood of drug interactions causing dangerous side-effects
- Complexity of prescribing schedules and lack of support networks can lead to irregular medicine ingestion with higher risks in a population where memory, eyesight and dexterity may not be as good
- It is easier to increase medication than it is to reduce or stop drugs which have been started by another specialist team
- Elderly patients may be particularly sensitive to the confusional side-effects of medication, and in situations where patients suddenly develop confusion it is important to exclude iatrogenic cause
- Medication which a patient has taken faithfully for many years to help with a symptom due to e.g. high blood pressure may no longer be strictly necessary, but the patient or family may have a belief in that particular tablet, which makes stopping it even in the last days of illness very difficult
- Routes of administration can become an important issue in prescribing if an elderly patient loses the ability to swallow

General rules
- As few medications as possible
- Start medication at low doses and slowly increase
- Regular review of medication and reduce any unnecessary tablets
- Use of pre-filled drug administration boxes or other devices may help with compliance
- Age should not exclude patients from either effective, expensive, or innovative drug therapy where it is appropriate and prescribed with care and consultation

Emotional issues

Dementia: 'a syndrome consisting of progressive impairment in two or more areas of cognition sufficient to interfere with work, social function or relationships in the absence of delirium or major non-organic psychiatric disorders.'

Some 5–8% of all people over the age of 65 suffer from moderate to severe dementia, with the prevalence doubling every 5 years reaching over 20% in 80 year olds

Agitation in the chronically confused

- Seventy per cent of patients with dementia may have insomnia or 'sun-downing', a syndrome of increasing confusion during the evening
- Daytime exercises, a consistent bedtime routine, and minimizing daytime napping can help improve sleep patterns
- Encouraging patients to participate in their own grooming and bathing may decrease agitation
- Sponge baths and adjusting water temperature may make bathing less threatening
- Familiar music and frequent social activities may also exert a calming influence
- Early in the disease, behavioural abnormalities in patients with dementia can be helped by disease-specific cholinesterase inhibition with drugs such as donepezil, galantamine, or rivastigmine. (Often such improvement does not last more than a few months.)
- Low doses of neuroleptics can ameliorate confusion, hallucinations, and delusions
- Second-generation antipsychotic medication (risperidone, and olanzapine) causes less extrapyramidal toxicity than first-generation antipsychotics; however, patients still need to be monitored for parkinsonism, and doses should always be started as low as possible to minimise side-effects
- Successful management of agitation can prevent hospital admissions and nursing home placement

Anxiety

Being elderly and ill can often provoke considerable anxiety. Such anxieties may relate to:

- Concern about the process of dying. Such patients may have had experiences of illness and dying which lead them to believe it will inevitably be pain-filled and difficult
- Concerns about leaving dependent relatives, or family, particularly if there are unresolved conflicts or issues within the family
- Concerns about financial or housing matters

Such anxieties will usually be helped by open discussion and isolation of the particular points of concern. General, non-specific, 'don't worry' advice tends to increase rather than decrease anxiety levels, as patients need a plan as to what they can do to address their concerns.

Common sources of suffering and discomfort in the elderly

- Patients may suffer even when they are free of pain or other symptoms
- Health care professionals need to ask about suffering as well as pain
- Questions should be open-ended in order to help make the patient comfortable with discussing fear, anxiety, and other non-physical symptoms. 'How are you feeling inside yourself?'
- A sample question to family members is, 'are you concerned that your family member may be suffering or uncomfortable?'

As in younger patients, relief of pain goes hand in hand with treatment of the emotional and spiritual components that contribute to it.

Care of the caregiver

Caregivers of elderly patients in the end-stage of chronic disease often need as much or more attention from the medical team as the patient. While family caregivers may take enormous satisfaction from their ability to provide safe and loving care for their loved one, most also feel varying degrees of exhaustion, guilt, and frustration.

- Listening to and trying to help address the concerns of caregivers, the medical team conveys the fact that the caregiver is not alone and that the concerns are legitimate and important
- Caregiver stress does not end after placement of the patient in a nursing home
- Caregivers continue to worry about the patient as well as suffer guilt over the necessity of nursing home placement
- Caregivers universally face difficult medical (and goals of care) decisions when the question of tube feeding, hospitalization for predictable infection, and use of antibiotics arise

Hospice Care and the Elderly Population

Concern exists within the palliative services of being overwhelmed by elderly patients with chronic long term care needs

- Although hospice care may be appropriate for certain patients with end-stage dementia and other chronic illnesses, hospice is accessed less frequently for these patients than for those with cancer
  This may be because: It is more difficult to accurately identify a limited prognosis among such patients
- The needs of elderly patents suffering from long term illnesses in the last year of life may far exceed the needs of patients with malignancy, yet the services available to meet those needs are often much less
- Quality palliative care does not require admission to a hospice but does require access to a healthcare team committed to providing holistic, individualised, planned and communicated care in whatever setting is appropriate for the particular patient

Conclusions

Growing old is a natural process which often changes our bodies, minds and what we regard as being important. A life which has been well lived can provide an elderly person with great comfort and satisfaction as they contemplate their pending death.

Having the opportunity to 'sort things out' and to 'tidy up loose ends' can provide ease of mind to someone who is coming to the end of their life, and is a process that should be facilitated and not regarded as 'morbid'.

The essence of palliative care is providing holistic care tailored to the particular needs of individual patients. The same can be said of care of the elderly.

Remaining open to all the possibilities of old age and the dying journey will prevent our care of the elderly in this very important part of their lives becoming stereotyped or sentimental and help carers face the realities of their own mortality.

Further reading

Books

Meier D. and Monias A. (2004) *Oxford Textbook of Palliative Medicine.* 3rd edn. pp. 935–44. D. Doyle, G. Hanks, N. Cherny and K. C. Calman. Oxford: Oxford University Press.

Articles

Bernabei R., Gambassi G. *et al.* (1998) Management of pain in elderly patients with cancer. SAGE Study Group. Systematic Assessment of Geriatric Drug Use via Epidemiology. *JAMA,* **279, 23**: 1877–82.

Feldt, K. S. and Gunderson J. (2002) Treatment of pain for older hip fracture patients across settings. *Orthop Nurs,* **21, 5**: 63–4, 66–71.

Krulewitch H., London M. R. *et al.* (2000) Assessment of pain in cognitively impaired older adults: a comparison of pain assessment tools and their use by nonprofessional caregivers. *J Am Geriatr Soc,* **48, 12**: 1607–11.

Lawlor P. G., Fainsinger R. L. *et al.* (2000) Delirium at the end of life: critical issues in clinical practice and research. *JAMA,* **284, 19**: 2427–9.

Spiritual care

The awareness and appreciation of a patient's individual spiritual orientation (spiritual issues, spiritual needs, spiritual pain, spiritual care, spiritual practices and nurturing) is essential to holistic care.

Holistic care in human life is governed by social, psychological, physical and spiritual influences. A dying person is more than a failing physiological system.

The doctor most often credited with founding the modern hospice movement, Dame Cicely Saunders, approached palliative care from the rather unique perspective of multiprofessional training. Her insights into the dying journey were enhanced by her social work background—listening and recording the experiences and feelings of patients, her nursing experience—dealing in practical terms with the physical needs of patients and her medical training—scientifically and systematically diagnosing and treating the cause of distressing symptoms.

The concept of holistic care was not discovered in St Christopher's Hospice, but the search to improve care for patients who appeared to have been sidelined by modernist over-confidence in scientific and medical advances resonated with a deeply felt need throughout the world.

Spiritual care is inseparable from holistic care, despite the difficulties which it brings with it in secular, multi-faith societies and to communities divided by religious and ethnic conflicts. Spirituality remains a challenging and vital presence at the heart of palliative care provision.

- The concept of spiritual care is inherent in the practice of holistic palliative care
- Spiritual matters are often referred to as those things that give life meaning and value
- In order to carry out holistic care, we must attend to the three indivisible facets of the human condition—the mind, body and spirit of humankind.[1]

In one study, 93 per cent of patients with cancer said that religion helped sustain their hopes.[2]

1 Hopper A. (2000) Meeting the spiritual needs of patients through holistic practice. *European Journal of Palliative Care*, **7, 2**: 60–3.

2 Roberts J. A. *et al.* (1997) Factors influencing views of patients with gynecologic cancer about end-of-life decisions. *American Journal of Obstetrics and Gynecology*, **176**: 166–72.

Definitions

Central to the problematic nature of 'spiritual care' is how 'spirituality' is defined.

- A definition which *includes* religious elements may cause a sense of exclusion among those who hold to a different belief system
- A definition which *excludes* all religious elements may exclude those within society who subscribe to a particular belief

The term 'spirituality' has strong religious connotations in the monotheistic religions of Christianity, Judaism and Islam, and it has been used in the religious context for hundreds of years to refer to particular practices and theological meanings.

In the context of eastern religions, with growing influences in the West both directly and through new age movements, spirituality has a less defined but no less central significance.

To disentangle completely 'spirituality' from such religious associations which have interpreted and developed understandings and insights into 'spirituality' over hundreds of years in the context of faith communities seems disingenuous.

However, paradoxically 'spirituality' is also used, in the context of patient care, as a term to refer to a particular characteristic of an individual which can exist without reference to any particular body of beliefs.[3]

Thus no single definition of 'spirituality' can capture its full meaning.

O'Brien defines spirituality very broadly as: That which inspires one to transcend the realm of the material.[4]

> Spirituality can be defined as what we do with our pain. We can either transform it or transmit it.
>
> R. Roar

... the word 'spiritual' has become a portmanteau into which we tend to stuff what is left over when we have removed what we can identify with and describe in terms of the body or the mind. Theologically, this runs the risk of leaving only the gaps in our understanding to God. Philosophically, it is perhaps an extension of Descartes' reductionist emphasis on the division of mind and body, adding a third dimension—the spirit.[5]

Spirituality is therefore not simply an intellectual proposition but consists of cognitive, emotional, and behavioural components that contribute to defining a person and to the way life is experienced.[6]

> The essence of what it means to be human, spiritual issues are the issues of the soul and concern our deepest values and meaning.
>
> M. Kearney

> And almost everyone when age,
> Disease, or sorrows strike him,
> Inclines to think there is a God,
> Or something very like him
>
> From 'There is no God', Arthur Hugh Clough 1819–61

- The concept of spirituality, which may seem abstract and ethereal to a scientifically trained doctor or nurse, is ignored at the peril of providing substandard care

- Spirituality forms the context in which patients respond to care, choose their treatment options, deal with relationship matters and face death
- The type of care shown to the patient will inevitably impact on the patient's own sense of meaning, worth and hence 'spirituality'
- The expression of spirituality is shaped by the accepted practices and beliefs of a particular culture, as well as by other influences such as institutionalized religion, or reaction to institutionalized religion
- How people live and understand their life can provide a framework for helping them face their own mortality and death
- Being forced to face imminent mortality can challenge belief systems profoundly, and sometimes beliefs cannot withstand such challenge without changing. A disintegration of beliefs evidenced by doubts, conflict and confusion can cause severe distress to the individual and family involved
- Conversely, spiritual beliefs which have long lain dormant can sometimes become central when a person experiences the suffering associated with a serious life-threatening illness
- It is important to realize just how dynamic the concept of spirituality is, especially in the palliative care setting
- Those involved in looking after patients need to be aware of the spiritual impact that their interaction with the patients can have
- Spiritual beliefs have been shown to affect the ways in which a patient deals with illness. Holland studied patients with malignant melanoma and discovered that those who rated religious and spiritual beliefs as highly important often used successfully active—cognitive means of successful coping. She felt that such coping strategies provided a sense of connection, involvement and meaning which helped patients accept their illness.[8]
- Others have claimed that those with strong religious beliefs, including atheistic convictions, are better able to deal with mortality issues, than those who have lukewarm beliefs which can contribute to increased anxiety and fear as death approaches

Spirituality and religion

'Religious practices have been developed to impose sense and order on the inherent mysteries of spiritual things, and sacraments have evolved to express the seemingly inexpressible.'[5]

The tension between the religious elements of 'spirituality' and the non-religious elements cannot be ignored. To ignore one aspect will lead to a distorted concept of spirituality that is either so culturally rooted to a particular set of beliefs as to manifest itself as tribalism, or to be so unrelated

3 Cobb M. (2003) Spiritual care. In M Lloyd-Williams (ed.) *Psychosocial Issues in Palliative Care*, pp. 135–47. Oxford: Oxford University Press.

4 O'Brien M. E. (1978) The need for spiritual integrity. In H. Yura and M. B. Walsh (eds) *Human Needs and the Nursing Process.* Norwalk, Connecticut: Appleton-Century-Crofts.

5 Hopper A. (2000) Meeting the spiritual needs of patients through holistic practice. *European Journal of Palliative Care*, **7, 2**: 60–3.

6 Argyle M. (2000) *Psychology and Religion*. London: Routledge.

7 Murray R. B., Zentner J. P. (1989) *Nursing Concepts for Health Promotion*. London: Prentice Hall.

8 Holland J. (1999) The rôle of religious and spiritual beliefs in coping with malignant melanoma. *Psycho-oncology*, **8, 1**: 14–26.

to human existence, as experienced by the vast majority of the population in their day-to-day existence, as to be irrelevant.

Experiencing the tension of such a paradox can be uncomfortable for those unused to paradoxical thinking, though less so for those whose philosophical or religious upbringing has provided insight into paradox.

Various understandings in the nature of the relationship between spirituality and religion have been explored.

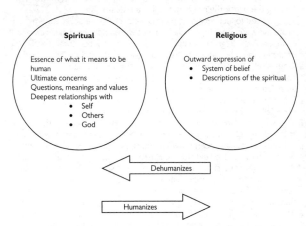

Fig. 9.1 The relationship between spirituality and religion. Leonard Lunn/Margaret, 1990.

When Rajendra was admitted to the Hospice it was clear that his prognosis was very limited. His district nurse had asked that he be admitted to a side room because his family, who were devoutly Hindu, wanted to be able to fulfil their familial and spiritual responsibilities to him without upsetting other patients. The family were extremely attentive to his personal physical care and also to his religious requests.

Through the reading of the Hindu scriptures and the burning of incense Rajendra seemed to derive great comfort.

The Hospice was a Christian foundation, with strong links to the local churches and an active chaplaincy department who visited Rajendra regularly at his request.

Several members of staff found the overt Hindu practices very distressing as they were concerned about demonic influences. A decision was taken that such members of staff would be assigned to different patients.

Several weeks after his death the family returned to say how much they had valued their last days together with Rajendra in the Hospice. They had been nervous when admission had been suggested because they had been aware of the Christian ethos of the Hospice.

They also shared how Rajendra's greatest spiritual comfort and solace in his last days had come from the sense of love, care, and acceptance he had received from hospice staff, particularly because in his business life as a shop owner, he had had to put up with a great deal of racial and religious harassment.

Faith practices

Compare spirituality with nutrition; neither is a subject that healthcare providers can take for granted. Inadequate nutrition is costly. If people are not fed properly, resistance weakens and wounds do not heal. Evidence is growing in volume and quality that this holds for spiritual sustenance too. [9]

For many people spirituality is not just an idea but has daily practical, social and material meaning. In short 'spirituality' has form as well as content.
These forms may include:
- **Rituals:** such as prayer, meditation, pilgrimage, and sacraments
- **Social group values**: beliefs, dietary restrictions, and morals
- **Material manifestations**: buildings, icons, prayer beads, symbols etc
- Patients may have practices and rituals which they would wish to maintain because of their beliefs
- These practices may be disrupted because of illness
- Illness and treatment may affect energy levels and therefore interfere with the routines of normal life and the opportunities for contact from other members of the faith community
- Those from minority faith traditions may find particular difficulty in accessing religious support

Faith practices can be very helpful particularly in times of stress and change. In the context of illness and the inevitable medicalisation inherent in modern treatment pathways, faith practices can help to maintain an identity separate from that of 'patient'.

For the carers of such patients it is *dangerous to make assumptions* about faith practices.
- Those with no identifiable religious affiliation may wish to be involved with, and derive obvious comfort from, faith rituals or prayer and meditation
- Conversely those with identifiable religious affiliations may find the expected practice of their faith rituals unhelpful and burdensome

Faith practices have a particular importance around the period of death which underscore the transition from life to death and help patients and relatives make sense of their loss, to be supported through hurt and to provide a framework for dealing with the process of letting go.

9 Koening H. K. et al. (2001) *Handbook of Religion and Health.* Oxford: Oxford University Press; Quoted by Culliford L. (2002) Spirituality and clinical care. *BMJ,* **325**: 1434–5.

Suffering

> The realization that life is likely to end soon may well give rise to feelings of the unfairness of what is happening, and at much of what has gone before, and, above all, a desolate feeling of meaninglessness. Here lies, I believe, the essence of spiritual pain.[10]
>
> Dame Cicely Saunders

This is echoed by Frankl's dictum that: 'Man is not destroyed by suffering, he is destroyed by suffering without meaning.'[11]

Suffering involves more than the activation of nerve pathways and the experience of physical pain. Suffering involves the experience which a person undergoes when their personhood is threatened or damaged.

In the palliative care context this threat often relates to that posed by a serious illness which not only threatens the individual's physical health, but also their emotional well-being, social standing and identity.

Suffering affects people in very personal ways which are particular to the individual involved. How people respond to such suffering will vary greatly. Some will find a resilience to transcending their suffering, others may feel completely overwhelmed by it. In part, the different responses are nurtured by previous encounters with suffering and what methods people have used in the past to deal with it.

Some will focus on accepting their suffering, others will talk in terms of 'fighting it'. Some will try to play their suffering within a larger landscape, in which all of their life experience can be incorporated and in which they seek to find wholeness through incorporating the many differing experiences of being human.

The religious traditions of the world have different interpretations of suffering and have practices and theologies which help people to transcend their immediate suffering through prayer, meditation or other religious ritual.

For others, suffering may so completely overwhelm them that they may describe themselves as 'living in hell'—isolated, hopeless and abandoned. Such patients may need psychiatric assessment to exclude a major depressive episode. For those providing spiritual care, such suffering provides a severe challenge in which words offered in an attempt to bring comfort can sound platitudinous and trite.

Remaining in contact with such patients can be exhausting, as their alienation and aloneness can quickly drain those carers who feel they have a responsibility to find an answer to the suffering.

Maintaining a regular presence and offering the chance of connectedness is more sustainable if carers recognize that not all suffering can be 'cured'.

Less suffering	More suffering
• Identified cause of pain	• Life threatening cause of pain
• Pain can be dealt with	• Intractable
• Short lived	• Reflects hopeless prognosis

Twycross 1994

'When I was diagnosed with lung cancer, in the space of a few days everything changed. I had to stop working. I went onto chemotherapy which made me tired, and at home suddenly instead of being the person who provided for my wife and children, they were having to look after me. I felt myself to be nothing more than a burden, no longer fit to be a husband, or father. I just felt that I might as well be dead'

Spiritual pain

- Spiritual pain can be defined as an individual's perception of hurt or suffering associated with seeking to transcend the realm of the material
- It is manifested by a deep sense of hurt stemming from feelings of loss or separation from one's God or deity, a sense of personal inadequacy before God and man, or a lasting condition of loneliness of spirit
- Spiritual pain has been defined as: 'a disruption in the life principle that pervades a person's entire being and that integrates and transcends one's biological and psychosocial nature'

Given that spirit is experienced, not proven, it may be suggested that the spirit manifests itself through the expression of its needs (Mount 1993)
- Need to find meaning, purpose in life, suffering, death. 'The person who has a 'why' to life can bear with it almost any how,' (Victor Frankl 1971)
- Need for hope and creativity
- Need for a belief and love in self, others and a power beyond the self
- Need to find forgiveness and acceptance
- Need to be listened to with respect
- Need for a source of hope and strength
- Need for trust
- Need for expression of personal beliefs and values
- Need for spiritual practices

Some Elements of Spiritual Pain

Experience of:-
- Disconnection
- Disharmony

- Lack of meaning (why me?)
- Hopelessness
- Feeling of emptiness
- Despair
- Feelings of injustice
- Pointlessness
- Powerlessness
- Feelings of being abandoned
- Spiritual guilt
- Anxiety/fear of God (What will happen after death? Heaven, hell, annihilation)

10 Saunders C. (1998) Spiritual pain. *Journal of Palliative Care,* **4**: 29–32.

11 Frankl V. (c. 1962) *Man's Search for Meaning.* London: Hodder & Stoughton.

Assessment

Spiritual needs can be broadly categorized as the need for meaning and purpose in life, the need for love and harmonious relationships with humans, living entities and God, the need for forgiveness, the need for a source of hope and strength, the need for trust, the need for expression of personal beliefs and values, and the need for spiritual practices.[12] The point of assessing a patient's spirituality is so that an appropriate response can be initiated to meet such needs.

An assessment provides information for the whole palliative care team which allows decisions to be made in the context of the patient's beliefs and spirituality. Conversely the assessment process can illustrate clearly to the patient how important the individual's beliefs are to the professionals caring for them. Assessment continues beyond the initial interview, as a patient's spirituality may change during the course of an admission.

Information gained from the initial and the subsequent assessments must be recorded in the patient's notes along with other physical and psychosocial assessment information.

- Spiritual assessment for its own sake, without any potential benefit to the patient, is of dubious ethical status
- Spiritual assessment needs to be carried out using a methodology which acknowledges each person's 'right to their own values and beliefs and to respect their right to remain silent about them'.[13]
- The initial assessment needs to address the importance of spirituality to the patient
- If the patient has indicated that spirituality is a meaningful aspect of their life and that they are willing to talk about it, then questions clarifying the nature of the patient's spirituality are appropriate
- Finally the patient should be offered the opportunity to speak further about their spirituality

Examples of helpful questions in an initial assessment

(Cobb, M. Spiritual care. In: Lloyd-Williams M, editor. (2003). *Psychosocial Issues in Palliative Care*. Oxford: Oxford University Press: 135–147.)

'I see from your notes that you describe your religion as Jewish, can you tell me about this?'
Or
'Do you have any spiritual or religious beliefs?'/'Can you tell me about them?'
'Is your faith/spirituality/religion helpful to you?'
'Are there ways in which we can support you in your faith/spirituality/religion?'
'Are there things we need to know about your faith/spirituality/religion that would help us in caring for you?'
'Would you like to talk to someone about these matters?'
'We have a chaplain who is part of our team, would you like to see him/her?'
'Would you like us to arrange a member of your faith community to come and see you?'

Providing spiritual care

'Having no solution is not the same as having no response'.

Leonard Lunn

Before initiating effective spiritual care, professionals must know and understand their own level of spiritual awareness, which involves an examination of personal beliefs and values, combined with a positive attitude towards spiritual health.

An awareness of one's own prejudices and biases will ensure that clients are dealt with sensitively, and that one's own values and beliefs are not imposed on others, especially spiritual doctrines. Self-awareness helps to prevent forming judgements or attempting to convert another to one's own beliefs or cultural understanding.[12]

In a much-quoted paper about spiritual pain, Cicely Saunders wrote that although work is pressing, patients are very ill and there may be no available opportunity to talk about matters of the spirit, but 'we can always persevere with the practical'. She seems to suggest that while spiritual care on one level is related explicitly to what we say, it is in practice implicit in the detail of care. It rests not just in what is said, but rather in what is to be done. The very word 'palliative' conveys some sense of this. That which is palliative is not 'what one can do when nothing else can be done', but rather 'what there is to do'.[14]

It is instructive to distinguish cure of symptoms from healing of people.[15,16] The words 'heal' and 'whole' have common roots. Healing entails restoration of psychobiological integrity, with the implication of personal growth and a sense of renewal.[17]

12 Dom H. (1999) Spiritual care, need and pain—recognition and response. *European Journal of Palliative Care*, **6, 3**: 87–90.

13 Stoll R. (1979) Guidelines for spiritual assessment. *American Journal of Nursing*, **79**: 1574–7.

14 Leone S. (1997) Pain as an ethical and religious problem. *European Journal of Palliative Care*, **4, 2**: 54–7.

Some Principles of Spiritual Care

Presence: To be maximally useful to patients and their experiences, we must be fully aware of our own biases and distortions

Listening: Listening attentively with genuineness and acceptance.

Facilitate exploration: Meaning cannot be given by another, it must be found by the person him/herself.

Allow for mystery: Some issues will always defy explanation.

Allow for paradox: Conflicting priorities in the care of patients may mean that some questions are difficult to answer. The emotional pain of this needs to be recognised and supported.

Foster *realistic* hope: To give unrealistic hope that life will be prolonged is unethical but there is always something more that can be done to bolster hope in a realistic way.

Create 'space' for patients: Patients need to feel that they still have some choice and control.

Combination: Professionalism with compassion.

Remain in touch with your own spiritual needs: To maintain spiritual equilibrium.

Skills needed to provide spiritual care

The spirituality of those who care for the dying must be the spirituality of the companion, of the friend who walks alongside, helping, sharing and sometimes just sitting, empty handed, when one would rather run away. It is a spirituality of presence, of being alongside, watchful, available, of being there.[18]

- Spiritual care is relevant in all aspects of a patient's care and may include giving good support during treatment such as radiotherapy, providing tasty food and privacy and the opportunity for prayer, or laughter etc. according to wishes. Spiritual need is best addressed by offering practical care in a way that responds to the patient as a unified individual experiencing life and dying in every facet of their being
- Excellent communication skills
- Empathetic and active listening, where the patient is unconditionally accepted
- Being able to detach from your own orthodoxies and concentrate on your orthopraxies (from beliefs to practices)
- Helping a patient to deal with:
  - Past issues
  - Present issues
  - Future issues

15 Swinton J. (2001) *Spirituality and Mental Healthcare: Rediscovering a Forgotten Dimension*. London: Jessica Kingsley.

16 Culliford L. D. (2002) Spiritual care and psychiatric treatment—an introduction. *Advances in Psychiatric Treatment*, **8**: 249–58.

17 Culliford L. (2002) Editorial: Spirituality and clinical care. *BMJ*, **325**: 1434–5.

18 Cassidy S. (1998) *Sharing the Darkness*. London: Darton, Longman & Todd.

- Ability to foster hope and provide strategies to support or restore hope in some way
- A broad perspective

'Compassion is about being with others in their suffering. It is about entering into that pain in such a way that one is no longer an observer but an integral participant.

Compassion does not mean 'feeling sorry for someone'. Rather, compassion is to 'get inside the skin' of the one who hurts, to experience with him or her the pain that is there; to sense a kinship with the one who is suffering.

Before we can be compassionate with others we must first enter our own suffering and extend loving kindness to ourselves.

True compassion insists that we enter into the sufferings of others. Yet we cannot become so absorbed by someone else's pain that we cease to have a life of our own. There is a delicate balance between these two dimensions, and sometimes life is such that this delicate balance is shattered. The intensity of someone's painful situation can be so demanding that it swallows our emotional life for a time.'

Your sorrow is my sorrow, Joyce Rubb.

Further reading

Books

Doyle D., Hanks G., Cherny N., Calman K. (2004) *Oxford Textbook of Palliative Medicine*, 3rd edn. Oxford: Oxford University Press.

Green, J. (1991) *Death with dignity*. London: Macmillan Magazines.

Green, J. (1993) *Death with dignity, volume II*. London: Emap Healthcare.

Lloyd-Williams M. (ed.) (2003) *Psychosocial Issues in Palliative Care*. Oxford: Oxford University Press.

Neuburger J. (2004) *Caring for Dying People of Different Faiths*, 3rd edn. Oxford: Radcliffe Medical Press.

Speck P. (1988) *Being There*. London: SPCK.

Stanworth R. *Recognizing Spiritual Needs in People who are Dying*. Oxford: Oxford University Press.

Wilcock P. (1996) *Spiritual Care of Dying and Bereaved People*. London SPCK.

The contribution to palliative care of allied health professions

Palliative care has been very successful at taking ideas, values, and techniques from other disciplines in health care. Such borrowing of ideas has nearly always included considerable adaptation from the parent discipline. However, the notion of cross-boundary, interdisciplinary working is now highly developed in palliative care. Some disciplines such as medicine and nursing have become core parts of the specialist team, whereas others such as speech and language therapy and dietetics have been accessed on an as-required basis. Increasingly, individual allied health professions (AHPs) have seen the need to evolve palliative care specialism within the generic discipline. Example of such AHPs include occupational therapy, physiotherapy, social work, and chaplaincy.

Rehabilitation

Palliative rehabilitation improves the quality of survival, so that patients' lives will be as comfortable and productive as possible with a minimum level of dependency, regardless of life expectancy.

The length of survival for most patients with cancer and other chronic progressive cardiac, respiratory and neurological illnesses has increased over the past 25 years. In some patients this is associated with prolonged disability due to the disease itself and/or the side-effects of treatment.

In general medicine, rehabilitative techniques are generally associated with chronic benign disease and disability and aim to *restore* a person's ability to live and work as normally as possible. In palliative medicine, rehabilitation shares the same principles of maximizing a person's potential but aims to help patients to *adapt* to their clinical situation.

Most patients are fearful of being dependent on others. Regardless of life expectancy, patients can be helped to be as independent as possible and to live a fulfilled life within the constraints of their illness. This not only helps patients but also relieves the stress of caregivers. Patients within palliative care settings are deteriorating and techniques need to be individually tailored to the rate of clinical deterioration. Techniques include setting realistic and achievable goals which are determined in conjunction with the multidisciplinary team. These goals must be reassessed continually in parallel with exacerbations and remissions of disease and symptoms. At different stages of the illness goals may vary. It may be appropriate for a patient with a prognosis of weeks/months to set goals for mobilizing with comfort in order to get away for a holiday or to attend an important family event. For patients with days/weeks prognosis, goals may include providing physical, emotional, social and spiritual support to both patient and carers to manage a home death with confidence.

Palliative rehabilitation helps patients to gain opportunity, control, independence, and dignity.

Assessment of potential for successful palliative rehabilitation

Biological/medical status

A careful medical assessment of the underlying disease, and other disease pathologies which may be contributing to morbidity, needs to be undertaken in order to direct treatment to optimize the control of symptoms (e.g. correction of anaemia or congestive heart failure). In the absence of reversible pathology the empirical control of symptoms is paramount. Consideration should also be given to prognosis. In this way, patients will be in the best position to be able to achieve their own realistic goals.

Psychological status

Patients experience many losses as their illness progresses. These include loss of mobility, self-esteem, position or role in the family and expectation for the future. These factors, together with loss of control over their lives, may intensify their feelings of anger, apathy, depression and hopelessness, which will have a negative impact on rehabilitation.

A lack of motivation may need to be explored, to ensure that there are no reversible factors such as clinical depression which may impede their ability to think in any positive way about the future. A competent unwillingness to participate in rehabilitation, on the other hand, should be respected. Palliative rehabilitation offers positive psychological support to overcome lack of confidence, providing goals to stimulate motivation to maintain activity.

- **Decreased cognition:** patients must be able to follow instructions and retain information in order to benefit maximally from palliative rehabilitation. However, limited functional goals can still be met despite limited cognition
- **Social factors** such as family and social support, both emotional (and sometimes financial), impact on a patient's confidence in goal-setting and achievement

Successful palliative rehabilitation depends on:-
- Speed of team response
- Setting of realistic goals
- Adapting constantly to changing circumstances
- Supporting patients and carers through change

Rehabilitation team
- The patient, family and carers
- Medical staff
- Nursing staff
- Occupational therapist
- Physiotherapist
- Social worker
- Chaplain
- Psychologist
- Complementary therapists
- Nutritionists
- Other specialists, according to need

Further reading

Eva G., Lord S. (2003) Rehabilitation in malignant spinal cord compression. *European Journal of Palliative Care*, **10, 4**: 148–50.

Fialka-Moser V., Crevenna R., Korpan M., Quittan M. (2003) Cancer rehabilitation: particularly with aspects on physical impairments. *Journal of Rehabilitation Medicine*, **35, 4**: 153–62.

Hopkins K. F., Tookman A. J. (2000) Rehabilitation and specialist palliative care. *International Journal of Palliative Nursing*, **6, 3**: 123–30.

Montagnini M., Lodhi M., Born W. (2003) The utilization of physical therapy in a palliative care unit. *Journal of Palliative Medicine*, **6, 1**: 11–17.

Watson P. G. (1990) Cancer rehabilitation: the evolution of a concept. *Cancer Nursing*, **13, 1**: 2–12.

Wells R. J. (1990) Rehabilitation: making the most of time. *Oncology Nursing Forum*, **17, 4**: 503–7.

Occupational therapy

Occupational therapy is the treatment of people with physical and psychiatric illness or disability, through specific selected activities, for the purpose of enabling individuals to reach their maximum level of function and independence in all aspects of life (World Federation of Occupational Therapists).

The occupational therapist (OT) uses a symptom-led rather than a disease- or diagnosis-led approach to treatment, concentrating on dysfunction as it presents while anticipating and preparing for further problems that may arise. The occupational therapist assesses various factors prior to advising on a useful strategy.

Occupational history

A profile of the patient is built up based on family history, past self-care abilities, work experience and leisure and recreational patterns. A functional assessment is then made which includes:
- **Self-maintenance** (looking after oneself)
- **Productivity** (productive to life, either in the form of domestic activities or earning a living)
- **Leisure**

Self-esteem

A degree of social equilibrium and homeostasis is needed for a peaceful life, in harmony with all that life brings. When patients are diagnosed with a life-threatening illness and are changing from being totally independent to becoming dependent, chaotic feelings emerge. The natural protective reactions to this assault on self-esteem include anger, resentment, bitterness and hostility.

These feelings are energy wasting, serve no useful purpose and can lead to withdrawal, apathy and depression. Furthermore, carers are inevitably entrenched in this vicious circle of trying to cope not only with their own feelings but those of the patient, who may be continuing to verbalize that their present life is unacceptable. This extra burden and stress can trigger feelings of helplessness, hopelessness, and uselessness in both patients and carers.

People are only able to feel self-worth if they are in a position to contribute, as a result of which they can engender respect in others. The rôle of the OT is to help identify and analyse the cause of these feelings and reactions and to redirect them towards an attitude of positivism and control.

Physical systems

An analysis of the patient's physical capabilities will depend on the diagnosis and the course of the illness. The OT will need to have an understanding of the likely prognosis in order to advise realistically, sensitively and appropriately.

The OT assesses physical dysfunction as it relates to muscle strength and endurance, assessing the degree to which disuse may have affected this and to what extent some rehabilitative potential might exist. The OT will need to be aware of muscle spasms and other pain and what factors trigger them. They will also assess ambulation and balance. The impact of cognitive abilities will also be relevant and techniques will be found to compensate for these.

Locus of control

An OT will need to gain insight into the personal effectiveness of the individual and how they normally respond and adapt in everyday life situations.

The internal profile is characterized by the person who seeks out environmental opportunities and pays attention to feedback as a way of correcting performance. These individuals take a moderate amount of risk, have a basic belief in their skills and a measure of expectancy of success or failure.

The external profile is characterized by the person who does not seek out opportunities and pays no attention to feedback to correct performance. These individuals do not engage in moderate risk taking and do not believe they have skills or ability to control what happens to them.

Quality of life

Quality of life is defined by the individual. As professionals, we can see potential and give advice that we believe might improve satisfaction (subjectively) in the patient and carer and from which achievement can be measured (objectively). However, it is ultimately the choice of the individual, which must be valued and respected, to take or reject advice. A patient may, for example, feel that they gain more by not fighting physically or mentally to retain any vestige of their independence.

Goals

With the full cooperative involvement of the patient, the OT can help to set realistic goals. The goals must be feasible, and structured in such a way that they can be achieved dependently and ultimately independently according to the goal in question. If a patient has always been very independent and is 'internally motivated', it may be very difficult for them to accept having to adapt to different methods of performance and what they perceive as unacceptably low goals yet still maintain their pride and dignity.

Carers may find pursuing goals a burden. They may worry about hurting the patient or themselves. They should not be asked or be required to do more than they are physically or emotionally capable of doing. They are often reassured by being told that they will be taught what to do. They need support from health professionals and other support groups, and advice for the often unspoken, unrecognized and unrewarded burden of care.

Treatment planning

Patients and families are vulnerable and often fearful of the uncertain future. They may vacillate chaotically between objective, logical thought and subjective, emotional despair. The aim is to work alongside these feelings and to raise the level of functioning by helping independence. A semblance of order, structure, purpose and control can hopefully be regained.

Examples of occupational therapy interventions
- Home assessments and modification to enable independence. Retraining in personal activities which include toileting, feeding, bathing and dressing. Retraining in domestic activities with the use of appropriate equipment, e.g. kitchen activities
- Ensuring a safe environment: this relates particularly to hoists and other equipment adapted for use by the individual
- Liaison with appropriate organizations in the community for packages of care
- Encouraging increasing engagement in purposeful activity. Teaching time management and the usefulness of daily routines. Redeveloping a sense of purpose and accomplishment to increase self-esteem
- Facilitating lifestyle management with continued engagement in hobbies and leisure pursuits. Promoting therapeutic activity programmes, such as involvement in creative activities and socialization, while achieving individual treatment goals is encouraged
- Relaxation training and stress management. Training in energy conservation and work simplification techniques to cope with fatigue
- Supporting and educating carers
- Facilitating psychological adjustment to loss of function. Retraining in cognitive and perceptual dysfunction, e.g. learning compensatory techniques to improve procedural memory during domestic tasks
- Assessment for and prescription of wheelchairs, pressure relief posture management and seating. Assessment of muscle flexibility and positioning. Splints made where necessary and transfers aided. Both indoor and outdoor needs are incorporated

Occupational Therapists define a clear, structured plan of action with the patient and carers to provide strength of purpose and dignity. Life is a delicate balance: a matter of coping and adapting to a situation in which being productive and feeling valued are paramount. The OT is critical to facilitating a person's sense of mastery and competence and re-instilling substance and control into the quality of living.

Further reading

Armitage K., Crowther L. (1999) The rôle of the occupational therapist in palliative care. *European Journal of Palliative Care*, **6, 5**: 154–7.

Bye R. (1998) When clients are dying: occupational therapists' perspectives. *Occupational Therapy Journal of Research*, **18, 1**: 3–24.

Cooper J. (ed.) (1997) *Occupational Therapy in Oncology and Palliative Care*. London: Whurr.

Ewer-Smith C., Patterson S. (2002) The use of an occupational therapy programme within a palliative care setting. *European Journal of Palliative Care*, **9**: 30–3.

Dietetics and nutrition

'Laughter is brightest where food is best.'

Nutrition is not solely concerned with refuelling the body, but has profound emotional and cultural significance. Food preparation symbolizes tangible care and affection and, as far as possible, should continue to be part of daily social interaction. For carers, a good intake is often thought of as a hopeful sign whereas a decreasing intake, particularly as the patient deteriorates, often causes much conflict and distress. The patient may feel guilty for not eating and often forces him/herself to eat in order to please the family.

You must eat up if you want to get better.

Good assessment of factors affecting nutritional status is important. Nutritional intervention focuses on ensuring that symptoms of disease or side-effects of treatment are managed well and initiating appropriate dietary advice and strategies to prevent further morbidity. The aims of nutritional support in palliative care will change as disease progresses. In the earlier stages of illness *aggressive nutritional intervention* is needed, allowing the patient to cope with:
- Metabolic demands of illness and treatment
- Repair of tissue and prevention of infection
- Maintaining well-being and quality of life

Palliative nutritional care, on the other hand, concentrates on symptom control and targetted nutritional intervention later in the disease process, in order to enhance quality of life.

Anorexia (see Chapter 6c)
Anorexia is the absence or loss of appetite despite obvious nutritional needs. Reversible causes of anorexia must be addressed.

Cachexia
Cachexia is the metabolic inability to use nutrients effectively resulting in weight loss, lipolysis, loss of muscle and visceral protein, anorexia, chronic nausea and weakness.

Role of the dietitian in palliative care
State registered dietitians are experts in nutrition and are able to translate scientific theory into practical advice for patients, carers and other health professionals depending on the patient's needs. They can be accessed within the hospital or the community setting and work closely with other members of the multidisciplinary team. Their role is to enhance quality of life.
Tasks for the professional advising on nutrition:
- Assess a patient's nutritional status
- Elicit the patient's goals regarding nutrition
- Provide specialized nutritional advice at diagnosis, during treatment and in the palliative phase

- Advise on food preparation/fortification/supplementation as appropriate
- Relax dietary restrictions if possible i.e. for diabetics, hypercholesterol states
- Recommend and calculate feeding regimens to suit an individual patient's requirements, using enteral or parenteral access
- Provide psychological and emotional support
- Listen to patients' fears

Dietitians don't just give out nice little boxes of milky supplements!

Dietary management of common symptoms affecting nutritional status

The common symptoms experienced require a multidisciplinary team approach.

Loss of appetite

- Eat small frequent meals or snacks
- Eat slowly and relax after meals
- If unable to manage full meals use nutritious snacks e.g. baked beans, scrambled egg, cheese on toast, or tinned, frozen or convenience meals i.e. macaroni, ravioli, cottage pie
- 'Take-aways' and pre-cooked, delivered meals do not need to be prepared so can be useful to stimulate appetite
- Simple exercise or a glass of alcohol, if permitted, can be useful stimulants
- Consider avoiding soups pre-meals since the volume may prevent further appetite for more nutritious foods

Sore mouth

- Choose foods with plenty of sauce or gravy e.g. casseroles, fish in parsley sauce
- Moisten food with milk, butter, cream
- Choose soft foods e.g. pasta dishes with sauces, creamy soups, egg dishes, milk puddings and mousses
- Avoid irritants such as citrus fruits (or juice), spicy or salty foods and rough, coarse, dry foods such as raw vegetables, toast, crackers
- Cook foods until they are soft and tender and cut into small pieces
- Use a blender or food processor to puree foods
- Sipping fluids is more refreshing than gulping
- Keep the mouth clean—brush teeth, gums and tongue at least three times a day with a soft toothbrush
- Use mouth washes regularly
- Sucking ice before being treated with 5-fluouracil, other than in head and neck cancer, is helpful in preventing mucositis

Nausea and vomiting

- Cold foods may be more acceptable than hot
- Eat small amounts slowly
- For morning sickness, eat prior to getting out of bed e.g. plain biscuits, dry toast, or cracker

- Keep meals dry, do not add gravy or sauces
- Sip fluids after meals
- Keep upright whilst eating and for two h afterwards
- Fizzy drinks—especially ginger ale and soda water—can help with nausea
- Use a fan to direct away odours, especially in hospital
- Fatty foods may make nausea worse, so grill foods instead
- Check for other reversible causes such as opioid medication, constipation, patient anxiety

Taste changes

- If red meat tastes unpleasant, try chicken, fish, milk, cheese, beans or nuts. These foods are bland in taste and may be more acceptable
- Marinate meat in lemon juice or vinegar to improve flavour
- Use herbs and spices to mask the taste of meat
- Oranges, grapefruit, pineapple and lemon fruits or juices will freshen the mouth
- Cold food may taste better than hot food. It may suit the patient to have frequent cold snacks throughout the day rather than a more traditional three meal pattern
- Food may have a bitter taste—avoid food and drink which contains saccharin or other artificial sweeteners
- It is mportant to keep the mouth clean—brush teeth three times a day and use a recommended mouth wash
- Use plastic utensils if the patient experiences a metallic taste

Diarrhoea

- High fibre intake should be discouraged i.e. reduce bran, fruit, vegetable, pulses
- Avoid strong tea and coffee which are gut stimulants
- Avoid spicy foods
- Consider malabsorption
- Certain fats may make diarrhoea worse—reduce greasy, fatty foods
- Check inappropriate laxative use

The above includes only some of the advice available and is a guideline only to the merits of a formal dietetic assessment.

Nutritional supplements

In UK see the *British National Formulary* for a full range and nutritional composition of prescribable products.

Oral supplementation is available to assist rather than replace food, but it will not increase weight or prolong the life of patients with cancer. There are many products on the market which range in nutritional support and can be expensive. They should be ideally recommended after assessment by a state-registered dietitian who will select the most appropriate for the individual, according to preferred taste and perceived need.

The challenge for dietitians working with patients in the palliative care setting is to use their expertise to cater for the particular needs of the individual patient whose requirements and goals may change rapidly.

Oral nutritional supplements can be divided into the following categories:

Oral sip feeds
- Some are nutritionally complete and provide a full range of vitamins and minerals
- Milk, juice or yoghurt options are available
- Good source of protein and energy

Fortified puddings
- Provide protein and calories in small volumes
- Useful for dysphagic patients

Modular supplements
- Concentrated source of carbohydrate/protein fat
- Beneficial only if used in conjunction with a diet plan to ensure a range of nutrients is provided
- Carbohydrate drinks are not suitable for diabetics without supervision
- In powder form they can be incorporated into foods without increasing volumes
- Need to be calculated to patient requirements to maximize use and reduce risk of volume overload

Tube feeding
Tube feeding is generally nasogastric or gastric through a percutaneous endoscopic gastrostomy (PEG) or radiologically inserted gastrostomy (RIG) but rarely may be duodenal or jejunal. The aim of feeding may be to replace normal food intake or to supplement it.

There is some evidence that artificial feeding prior to definitive oncological treatment, including surgery, may assist in stabilizing weight, improving quality of life and contributing to better treatment results. There is no evidence that artificial feeding prolongs life in patients with advanced cancer.

The decision to feed artificially requires clinical judgement within the multidisciplinary team and good understanding of the patient's needs and feelings. If used appropriately (e.g. some neurological conditions when proper counselling and discussion have taken place and occasionally in head and neck cancer), it can be useful and take the pressure off patients and carers when eating has become a burden and food can no longer be tolerated or enjoyed.

Ethical issues
Healthcare professionals working within the palliative care setting are faced with ethical dilemmas daily. Decisions should be made with the support of the team and consideration of the patient and carers. In order to make a justifiable, considered decision, the following questions should be considered prior to commencing artificial feeding:
- What are the patient's wishes?
- What benefit will it bring to the patient?
- How much discomfort is caused by eating and drinking normally?
- How keen is the patient to continue eating and drinking?
- What are the risks and discomforts associated with artificial feeding?

Documents are available to offer guidance on nutrition and hydration to health professionals and some are listed below.

Further reading

British Medical Association (2001) *Withholding and Withdrawing Life-Prolonging Treatment.* 2nd edn. London: BMA.

Lennard-Jones, J. E. (ed.) (1998) *Ethical and Legal Aspects of Clinical Hydration and Nutritional Support.* The British Association for Parenteral and Enteral Nutrition.

National Council for Hospice and Specialist Care Services (1995) *Ethical Decision-Making in Palliative Care: Artificial hydration for people who are terminally ill.* London: NCHSPCS.

Physiotherapy

A physiotherapist is 'a healthcare professional who emphasises the use of physical approaches in the promotion, maintenance and restoration of an individual's physical, psychological and social wellbeing, encompassing variations in health states'.

In palliative care, the rôle of the physiotherapist is to reduce the degree to which disabilities, caused by the disease or the treatment, interfere in everyday life. This is particularly pertinent when the disease trajectory may be short and the patient is deteriorating rapidly.

Physiotherapists are important members of the multidisciplinary palliative care team. They may be involved in all healthcare settings in the treatment of patients with any actively progressive condition which most commonly includes cancer, chronic end-stage respiratory, neurological and cardiac disease.

As part of rehabilitation, the specialist physiotherapist is in a good position to identify the needs and coordinate the responses of colleagues working in a wide variety of complementary fields.

The physiotherapist, with a knowledge of the underlying pathological condition, adopts a problem-solving approach in which goals of treatment are planned jointly with the patient. This gives the patient, who may feel helpless because of a loss of independence, a measure of control. These goals must be realistic and achievable for the phase of the disease and continually reassessed. Goals may be simple (to be able to sit comfortably in bed) or more complex (to attend and enjoy a wedding). This is known as 'active readaptation'.

A physiotherapist has a detailed knowledge of functional anatomy and ergonomics, and is able to analyse movement and posture in its relationship to the environment. For instance, weakness and immobility may lead to poor posture, which places a strain on muscles and ligaments and can cause pain, particularly around joints. These stresses may be relieved by strategic physical positioning.

The physiotherapist may be the first professional to be alerted to the signs and symptoms of spinal cord compression due to malignant disease. Alongside immediate medical treatment, the aim initially will be an attempt to minimize loss of function. Should a more complete picture of motor, sensory and autonomic impairment develop, the physiotherapist will be instrumental in helping the patient cope with adapting to a drastic reduction in functional ability by helping the patient to develop a strategy for the future. This may involve balance training, development of upper body strength, instruction in transfers and the use of a wheelchair. Relatives and carers will also require instruction in passive movement, the positioning of paralysed limbs, the use of wheelchairs, and in moving and handling techniques.

Physiotherapy techniques used

Touch

Massage and exercise therapy are core skills of all physiotherapists. Touch is probably the oldest method of relieving pain and discomfort. Therapeutic massage using stroking and gentle kneading may be used to reduce muscle spasm, relieve pain and aid relaxation. Joints become painful and stiff if not moved regularly, leading to the rapid development of shortening of some muscle groups and contractures. Maintenance of joint range is important in the management of neurodegenerative diseases, and passive movements and active assisted exercises need to be implemented and taught to relatives and carers.

Electrotherapy

Physiotherapists are trained in the safe use of electrotherapy. Bone pain and neuropathic pain due to cancer are notoriously difficult to manage. Relief may be obtained by the use of transcutaneous electrical nerve stimulation (TENS) which they may also use for the control of nausea. Physiotherapists use therapeutic ultrasound, interferential or pulsed short-wave diathermy for the relief of pain and muscle spasm. Local applications of heat and ice are also used for pain relief. Physiotherapists provide and fit splints, collars and various supports for weakened muscles, to correct or reduce deformity and to facilitate improved function.

Symptom management

Breathlessness

Breathlessness is very frightening and distressing for patients and carers, making them feel out of control. All physiotherapists are trained in respiratory care and can teach patients and their carers techniques to reduce the work of breathing, to encourage relaxation, to aid expectoration of secretions and coping strategies to improve breathing control. Physiotherapists often help in the management of patients, using non-invasive ventilation for respiratory failure secondary to neuromuscular disability such as motor neurone disease.

Some physiotherapists are trained in various complementary therapies that can be used to help the control of breathlessness such as acupuncture, reflexology, and aromatherapy.

Lymphoedema

Chronic oedema, which may develop in an arm following treatment for breast cancer or as a manifestation of recurrent axillary lymph node disease, or in the legs secondary to impedance of lymphatic drainage from disease in the pelvis, is often managed by physiotherapists. A swollen limb is heavy and affects posture and mobility, placing stresses on weakened muscles and joints.

Gravitational oedema may develop in an immobile, dependent limb, causing discomfort, functional disability, and nursing management problems.

Management of lymphoedema includes using exercise, correct positioning, hosiery, bandaging and manual lymph drainage techniques and skin care. See page 309.

Psychological issues

The physiotherapist works on a one to one basis with patients. Patients often discuss their hopes and fears with a sensitive listener. They feel safe to ask searching questions in these situations, and the physiotherapist needs to be adequately prepared and informed to deal with these issues and to communicate relevant issues with the team, within the bounds of confidentiality.

Walking aids

A physiotherapist can give advice on the use of walking sticks. However, many patients will start using a walking stick without guidance, and the following simple advice can help ensure appropriate use:

- A walking stick should usually be used on the *opposite* side from the affected leg if painful on weight bearing (to halve the weight carried through the affected leg)
- Use on the *same* side if neurological or muscle leg weakness, for extra support
- To check the correct height, the handle of the walking stick should be level with the wrist joint when the arm is resting beside the body
- A rubber cap on the end of the stick will help prevent it slipping

Further reading

Doyle D., Hanks G., Cherny N. and Calman K. (2004) *Oxford Textbook of Palliative Medicine*. 3rd edn. Oxford: Oxford University Press.

Robinson D. (2000) The contribution of physiotherapy to palliative care. *European Journal of Palliative Care*, **7, 3**: 95–8.

Speech and language therapy

Speech and language therapy (SALT) should be available to palliative care teams as patients often have difficulties in communication (particularly verbal) and swallowing. These factors are integral to the patient's feeling of worth, their contribution to and place in society and are a significant contributing factor to their quality of life. SALT plays a pivotal rôle not only in palliative rehabilitation but also in the terminal stages of illness. The aim of therapy is to help the patient compensate for deficits rather than to restore original function.

Communication difficulties

Expressive dysphasia (difficulty in finding and expressing words) interferes with communication. It is seen frequently in palliative care as a result of cerebrovascular accident or intracerebral disease commonly due to primary or secondary cerebral tumours.

The patient should be able to cooperate fully with and benefit from the SALT, if there are no receptive difficulties in understanding what is being said or significant cognitive impairment.

Dysarthria (difficulty in articulating) commonly occurs in chronic neurological conditions such as motor neurone disease, in which cognition is usually preserved, and in multiple sclerosis. It is also a problem for those with cancers in the region of the throat and mouth.

Impairment in comprehension and expressive language skills is not uncommon in the terminally ill, for a variety of different reasons. Patients may have difficulty in understanding long or complex sentences, and may have poor memory retention, poor recall of new information and word finding difficulties. Furthermore, poor breath support and motor control of speech because of general weakness may lead to dysarthria or weakened voice projection, which may contribute further to impairing their communication skills.

However mild, these communication difficulties cause stress not only for the patients themselves but also for the carers. It is frustrating for the patient to be unable to express what would normally be considered as trivial such as 'I am hungry', and emotionally draining if they wish to convey more complex thoughts and wishes such as 'I need to write a will'.

As speech deteriorates, it is not uncommon for patients to insist on trying to continue to try to speak 'normally', delaying having to resort to other means. Understanding what is said may be relatively easy and efficient for the main carer who has become attuned, but difficult for friends who are unaccustomed to the deteriorating speech.

Friends may have to concentrate very hard to pick up a mixture of words, non-verbal clues and nuances only to have to admit finally, when the patient has become exhausted, that they have not understood what is being said. The embarrassment may result in friends visiting less frequently to avoid their own feelings of guilt and inadequacy, leaving the patient feeling ever more embittered, isolated, withdrawn and a burden on others. Communication in these situations often takes a considerable amount of time and perseverance.

In general, patients prefer carers to be honest and to admit that they have not understood, with a willingness to try again, rather than to mislead them by encouraging the 'conversation' to continue when there has been little understanding.

The speech and language therapist can offer advice to carers on facilitating communication. This can include giving patients extra time to understand what is being said to them and allowing the patient time to formulate a response.

- Patients who feel under time pressure to communicate will feel anxious and even less able to make themselves understood
- If it is difficult for the patient to understand complex sentences, these can be separated into simpler sentences
- Reduction of background noise and distractions is essential to aid communication

The therapist may teach compensatory techniques. It may be important to establish a consistent 'yes/no' response before communication can successfully take place. Strategies for 'word finding' difficulties include talking around the subject (circumlocution), the use of gesture, focussing on the initial sound of a target word and writing this down or thinking of a substitute word.

Patients with severe breathing difficulties can be trained to make optimal use of the available breath support by speaking at a slower pace and in manageable segments.

If speech is unclear, picture charts can be used for efficient communication of general needs. These are available from the speech and language therapist, or a simple chart can be devised until a more formally robust one is available. An alphabet chart to which the patient can point may also be useful to spell the first letter of the word or spell out the word.

The therapist assesses the patient for the most suitable communication aid for his unique difficulties. Communication aids such as voice amplifiers, lightwriters with visual displays or electronic speech and other computerized equipment may be appropriate.

Speech problems in head and neck cancer (☐ see Chapter 6h)

Swallowing difficulties

There are numerous causes of swallowing difficulties in palliative care. A speech and language therapist is necessary in the situation in which the reflex mechanism of swallowing has become impaired to such a degree that the larynx and airways are no longer adequately protected from oral contents.

In palliative care, the majority of patients who need specialist input from SALT are those with bulbar symptoms in motor neurone disease and late Parkinson's disease, benign or malignant cerebral disease, head and neck tumours or malignant invasion of the base of the skull directly involving the cranial nerves.

The ability to swallow is inherent in maintaining life naturally. It is very frightening to lose the ability to swallow with ease. Mealtimes may become an anxious time when attempts to eat result in episodes of, or fear of, choking. The SALT, through analysing the unique difficulties of the patient, may be able to recommend a strategy to improve the situation.

- The act of ingesting food begins as the food enters the mouth. The patient may be unable to hold food in the mouth because of a difficulty in lip closure. This can be helped by teaching the patient to carry out exercises to strengthen the lips
- The food, once in the mouth, is chewed and an assessment of any correctible features to improve chewing are analysed
- A food bolus is then formed by the action of the tongue, which may not be functioning adequately
- The bolus is then propelled over the posterior aspect of the tongue, which may be difficult if the tongue is spastic: this may occur in motor neurone disease
- The tongue may be encouraged to relax by placing ice chips in the mouth or applying a cold object around the front of the neck
- If there is a chance of aspiration of contents into the larynx, patients may be advised to cough before and after swallowing

In some cases, if one side of the palate is paralysed, the patient will be advised to turn the neck to the paralysed side, effectively 'blocking' the non-functioning side of the pharynx to make maximum use of the fully functioning side.

The SALT might also suggest other helpful postural tips for patients, and will advise on consistency of food in conjunction with a nutritionist.

The SALT will also advise on meticulous mouthcare, in particular the routine of mouth cleaning after eating, to ensure that no debris collects which could result in an unpredictable and frightening episode of choking.

There may come a point at which the patient is at severe risk of aspirating through inadequate swallowing technique. This needs to be discussed fully with the patient and family and, if strategies to improve swallowing fail, the patient may want to opt for another method of receiving nutritional intake, such as a percutaneous endoscopic gastrostomy (PEG).

The speech and language therapist, conversant in the philosophy of palliative care and the clinical situation and prognosis of the patient, may be very helpful in discussing the merits and burdens of these methods of feeding.

Further reading

Logemann J. (1998) *Evaluation and Treatment of Swallowing Disorders*, 2nd edn. Austin, Texas: PRO-ED.

Salt N. et al. (1999) The contribution of speech and language therapy to palliative care. *European Journal of Palliative Care*, **6, 4**: 126–9.

Clinical psychology

Clinical psychologists are concerned with the psychological well-being of the patient and family and others in the provision of general emotional care and support. They are not the only professionals able to provide this care, but they are specifically trained to work with all individuals 'across the lifespan' with problems from mild to severe.

Experiencing loss through the death of close family members may be the most stressful event in a person's life. Dealing with patients and their families facing the end of life and the loss of important relationships is a central part of the work of psychologists working in palliative care.

Palliative care has traditionally been associated with cancer, but this remit is changing to encompass patients with chronic diseases. These patients, who are often elderly, may be dying over longer periods of time. This is interspersed with acute episodes of care and partial recovery, requiring physical and psychological rehabilitation, as the illness progresses. This gradual change in emphasis will challenge the Multidisciplinary Team (MDT) to help patients and their families adjust to progressively limited functional—and sometimes cognitive—abilities. The specialist palliative care psychologist is becoming a core component of the MDT, facilitating the understanding of the psychological effects of chronic progressive disease.

Theoretical models and understanding of human behaviour

A wide range of theories are used to explain how people respond cognitively, emotionally and behaviourally to issues related to illness. These are based on the assumption that there are normal patterns in human life cycles which inescapably include life and death. One theory is that changes or transitions may be considered as *normal*, permitting psychosocial development and growth as people learn how to cope successfully with change and loss or, alternatively, to consider bereavement and loss as *stressors*, to which individuals are required to adapt.

Another theoretical model, known as restoration-focused coping, suggests that people oscillate in their styles of coping between focusing on the emotional expression of grief and the need to continue with everyday living; the dying and bereaved can be helped to achieve the balance between being overwhelmed by loss and being able to function on a daily basis.

Direct psychological interventions

Sadness and depression are relatively common in palliative care. It may not be clear whether a patient or family member is displaying an appropriate adjustment reaction to loss or change, or whether they have become clinically anxious or depressed. Furthermore, professionals may be reluctant to refer to other specialists for assessment and management of these problems, fearing that their patients will be labelled with the stigma of mental illness. Psychologists are trained in understanding human behaviour and in recognizing psychopathology; whereas professionals, other than psychologists, are relatively poor at detecting psychological morbidity, particularly in palliative care. They have the skills to encourage expression of thought and emotion in a safe, supportive and reassuring environment and, through counselling and skilled communication, to provide resources for coping. They are trained in the objective measurement of psychological functioning and morbidity, which could form part of routine palliative care assessment (forming baseline and change measures). This would be in line with holistic palliative care and good clinical governance in addition to recent[1] National Institute for Clinical Excellence (NICE) guidance.

Psychologists address a variety of clinical issues including:

- Complex grief reactions, such as prolonged grieving
- Adjustment disorders, such as fear of leaving the hospice/hospital
- Psychological morbidity, such as anxiety and depression
- Relationship and communication problems, such as excessive dependency
- Symptom management, such as control of anticipatory nausea or pain by means of relaxation and other techniques (eg cognitive behavioural interventions)
- Anxiety-reducing techniques such as relaxation training, guided imagery and systematic desensitization
- Psychological distress detection and appropriate management

Working with teams and organizations

Palliative care professionals work in MDTs, believing this to be the best model for the holistic management of patients. However, MDT working is not always straightforward. Psychologists are trained in understanding complex interpersonal and interdisciplinary relationships and the difficulties encountered. They can, therefore, facilitate the process of working as a team. Their understanding of group dynamics can help support and further improve patient-focused care.

Psychologists have a rôle in helping staff to support and contain their distress when a clinical issue has been challenging. They may work constructively in groups, reflecting on the difficult issues in an interactive, confidential, non-judgemental manner. This form of support is commonly used following a difficult death, which may have strained the team to its limits. Critical incident learning and learning from the patient, their family and others are aspects of good clinical governance which can both improve care and staff learning.

Psychologists have an important rôle in clinical supervision, because the psychological elements of care are essential to the protection, maintenance and development of the skills of the caregivers. A forum for teaching psychological skills and providing some quality control over these skills can avoid staff 'burn out', which is high in this area of care delivery.

All professionals should have a basic understanding of good psychological care in order to practise in a way that is not damaging to patients, relatives and colleagues. This is particularly pertinent in palliative care. Psychologists provide high-level communication skills supported by their theoretical knowledge and experience of complex human interactions. The basic counselling skills of the MDT may enable patients and families to find their own solutions to concerns, but a minority may lack the necessary insight or psychological coping resources to resolve their difficulties. Families overwhelmed by loss will be helped by the specialist skills and unique perspective of the psychologist.

Research

Psychologists have research skills, often using tools to measure attitude, mood, personality, cognitive and neurological functioning and change generally. Psychometric tools and other techniques are used to assess the usefulness of interventions.

Psychologists may help to bridge the gap between biomedical research and social science research. Substantial practical and ethical problems surround research with the frail and vulnerable. Qualitative research techniques which circumvent some of these problems are becoming increasingly popular, but can also usefully be combined with quantitative techniques. When the taboos of research in the dying lessen, the prospect of action research in which patients and carers lead the research show promise for gaining future palliative care knowledge.

Further reading

Books

Lloyd-Williams M. (2003) *Psychosocial Issues in Palliative Care*. Oxford: Oxford University Press.

Whitaker D. S. (2001) *Using Groups to Help People*, 2nd edn. London: Routledge.

Articles

Brennan et al. (2001) Adjustment to cancer-coping of personal transition? *Psycho-oncology*, **10**: 1–18.

Payne S., Haines R. (2002) Doing our bit to ease the pain. *Psychologist*, **15, 11**: 564–7.

Payne S., Haines R. (2002) The contribution of psychologists to specialist palliative care. *International Journal of Palliative Nursing*, **8, 8**: 401–6.

[1] NICE (2004) *Improving supportive and palliative care for adults with cancer*. London: NICE.

Social work

Social workers are an integral component of the palliative care team, and address many of the non-physical issues so crucial to the holistic care of patients and their families. It is relatively easy to recognize physical problems such as shortness of breath, but healthcare professionals often make assumptions about what they think is important to the patient. Social workers usually approach clinical problems from a different angle, being guided first and foremost by the patient and family, empowering them to identify and express what they feel are their most important needs.

Patients with terminal illness have emotional, spiritual and practical needs which may not always be revealed until distressing physical symptoms are managed. All members of the multidisciplinary team broadly address some of these needs, but patients may not want to talk about their emotional feelings to the professionals who are giving them physical care. The social worker's focus is on the effects of life-threatening illness on the family system: he or she is therefore often in the best position to allow patients to express emotional issues, helping them to reduce fear and anguish and to re-enable them to feel in touch with friends and family.

Friends, family and partners also need help to cope with their fear and anger at the situation. They need to feel involved in care and decision-making, which is essential in order to avoid a complicated bereavement. Patients, families, partners and friends can be helped to say their goodbyes, to be given the opportunity to heal rifts and to complete unfinished business. At-risk families will be recognized by the social work team following full assessment and offered appropriate support.

A full assessment is often aided by constructing the family genogram, finding out who is important to the patient and highlighting relationship issues. The social network may include ethnic and cultural issues that need understanding in order to facilitate family communication. Strong, unfamiliar and often conflicting feelings can be a barrier to open communication. Rifts within families may emerge and will need managing sensitively, often allowing reconciliation and rebonding of relationships. Barriers to communication can also occur when families want to protect each other from the pain of bad news and the limited future. Families may need help so that they feel more confident about knowing how to tell and involve their children.

Spiritual pain can also be addressed, helping to relieve isolation and giving comfort, knowing that concerns, even if unanswered, are taken seriously and recognized as being important and valid. Difficulties such as body image, sexuality and intimacy may need discussion. Patients rarely volunteer these problems and may need prompting to see if they want to talk about them. Appropriate guidance is needed to help patients and families cope with the changing circumstances.

Practical help involves enabling patients to make decisions and exercise choice, both for practical reasons and also to promote a sense of worth and dignity. They may need basic assistance in paying bills or getting a telephone in the house, or to execute more complicated tasks such as preparing a will and thinking about the future of dependants. It is important to ensure that patients receive benefits to which they are entitled, such as Attendance Allowance and Disability Living Allowance. Similarly carers may be entitled to Carers Allowance. Carers themselves may need support at such a distressing time and can have their own needs assessed to ensure they receive appropriate help. The patient and family may want to know about the law and other social institutions, family and mental health legislation and community services according to their particular situation. Ensuring that patients receive packages of care and help with decisions around placement, if required, are part of the social work rôle.

Social workers seek to enable patients and families retain or regain control and promote empowerment and choice, to help people find inner strength and confidence. Realistic goal plans can be set, to stop families feeling so powerless and enable them to plan for and enjoy the important time that is left.

After death, bereavement support is fundamental to the rôle of palliative care social workers, who commonly work with bereavement counsellors within the team. Families are offered one to one, family or group counselling. Special bereavement sessions for children may also be available.

Financial and practical help in the UK

Attendance Allowance
This provides financial help with personal care for people over 65 years. It is paid at variable rates according to dependency. People with a terminal illness (prognosis of six months or less) can receive the benefit faster and the formalities are simpler.

Disability Living Allowance
This provides financial help for personal care and/or mobility for people under the age of 65 years. The same rules apply for dependency and terminal illness (see above).

Other possible benefits
- Council Tax benefit
- Housing benefit
- Statutory Sick Pay
- Disability working allowance
- Funeral payments (social fund)
- Bereavement payment
- Bereavement allowance
- Widowed parents allowance
- Severe disablement allowance
- Income support
- Invalid care allowance
- Incapacity benefit

Social Services may be able to provide:
- Home care for personal care
- Help with housework
- Occupational therapy aids
- Meals on wheels or frozen meals
- Residential/nursing care
- Dial a ride access to community transport

The chaplain

Training levels
There is no current universally required palliative care chaplaincy qualification, though there are masters degrees in healthcare chaplaincy, training courses for new chaplains, and recommendations from the Association of Hospice and Palliative Care Chaplains. Most chaplains will be trained for ordination or other ministry in the church or other religious body. In-service training is expected.

Denominations and faiths
The religious affiliations of chaplains are intended to reflect proportionally the affiliations of the patient group. A chaplain will know how to access minority religious groups not represented on the chaplaincy staff, and will be able to provide information about the usual needs of religious minorities.

Ethos
Respect for religious positions of first, patients and second, relatives is paramount. Chaplains should cater for spiritual needs and must not create them.

Multidisciplinary working
The chaplain expects to be treated as part of the multidisciplinary team. Communication should occur both ways, and chaplains should be involved as far as possible in multidisciplinary meetings.

Availability
Chaplaincy staffing levels depend upon the healthcare setting in the unit, though provision is a requirement. Most units have 24-hour cover from chaplains, and possibly from local clergy; chaplaincy time with patients will be variable. Some units have teams of chaplains.

Bereavement caseloads
Some chaplains are centrally involved in bereavement.

Chapel space
There may be a dedicated chapel, or a multipurpose space. However it is constituted, as far as possible provision that respects both the sensibilities and needs of all religious groups must be made.

Assessment
Patients' spiritual needs must be assessed initially and then on a continuing basis. Spiritual assessment may be undertaken by any member of the multidisciplinary team. There are a number of assessment models available.

Patient and family care
This includes listening, life review, prayer and sacraments. There may be some hostility from patients towards organized religion, which chaplains should accept. The chaplain's rôle must be non-judgemental.

Families may have technical questions about funerals, access to services and beliefs.

Healing

A ministry of healing is now normative in all mainline Christian churches, with new formal services being both devised and adopted. Healing in these terms is not usually presented as a full physical cure, but as the divine having an effect upon both the human spirit and the human body, and may describe death as healing.

Some 'charismatic' believers will encourage belief in the possibility of miracles up to the point of death. Spiritual healers may or may not be aligned to any religious faith; most have been involved in training by one of the professional associations in this country. Healing and prayer for healing are central to most religious traditions. 📖 See Spiritual healing, p. 693.

Marriage

Institutional chapels may be used for marriages of those who cannot be moved elsewhere, and registrars normally come at very short notice *in extremis*. Those who have been divorced have to take special care to present all necessary documents to the registrar. Church of England clergy may not marry the divorced except in a church to which one of the couple marrying belongs by residence or attendance, and therefore cannot do this in hospitals etc.

Funerals

Hospital or hospice chaplains may be requested to take funerals for those patients with whom they have developed a special relationship. Practice varies between always, sometimes or never acceding to requests. Reasons why the chaplain might conduct a funeral are to continue an established pastoral relationship, to personalize the funeral, and to encourage a more open attitude to funeral liturgy. Reasons for not doing so include avoiding the subversion of community-based provision of bereavement and pastoral aftercare.

Remembrance services

These may be included in the bereavement service events, or be free-standing. In many hospice units there is an annual remembrance event at Christmas-time.

Staff support

Chaplains invariably have a rôle in staff support in the organization.

Education

Chaplains teach, but subjects will vary according to the interests and experience of the individual.

Awareness of different faiths

When caring for a terminally ill patient, it is important to obtain a general outline and understanding of their philosophy of life, religious beliefs and expectations of the continuity of life after death. Such knowledge is valuable if a dying patient is to be sensitively and efficiently cared for. The best way of obtaining this information is by talking tactfully to the patient and family.

Spiritual beliefs, even without a particular religious discipline, vary enormously, and a religious label noted down on a hospital form may have little to do with the patient's past or current ways of thinking. Moreover the behaviour and beliefs of an individual enjoying full health may change dramatically when they become terminally ill and reach the threshold of a previously unconsidered period of life.

Most religions provide both ritual procedures and pastoral (or existential) care. Although a Christian priest will administer both, this may not be the case in other religions. Existential care and comfort may well be provided by lay groups.

In this chapter brief guidelines are set out regarding the care of dying patients of the most commonly encountered faiths.

Denominationalism

Buddhism, Christianity, Islam, Judaism and Hinduism all have a wide range of denominations or variations. They all contain fundamentalist groups for whom the correct procedures are most important and liberal groups who are unlikely to take offence provided sensitivity and openness are displayed.

Religious demands and taboos are frequently found with relation to the following subjects:
1 Food
2 Alcohol
3 Privacy
4 Washing
5 Cross-gender care
6 Touching/preparing the body after death
7 Religious objects.

There are two rules:-
1 **Always check** with the patient (and/or family) as to their beliefs and affiliations even if these are many years past.
2 **When in doubt**, follow the more orthodox procedures.

Faiths, preferences and demands

Buddhism

Preferences
- Buddhists may want a Buddhist (or even a Christian!) priest to help with prayer and meditation. With regard to food, Buddhists are commonly vegetarian. It is also usual that Buddhists may prefer cremation to burial
- Buddhists may wish to avoid palliative treatments that lessen either the experience of pain, mental control, or awareness of the moment of death

Demands
- None, except to inform a Buddhist priest of his/her persuasion after death

Christianity

Preferences
- Christians may want a priest/minister of their persuasion for confession (formal or informal), prayers, communion or annointing. In many denominations, lay people fulfil these functions adequately

Demands
• None.

Islam
Preferences
• Muslims may have special dietary requests and strict Muslims will not accept even medicines if they contain alcohol
• There are special fasting times during the year but an ill patient is allowed to eat as necessary. During festivals, routine medical examinations and tests should be avoided
• Women may want to be seen by a female doctor

Demands
• Muslims require plenty of facilities for washing, which is an essential part of worship. The family should be consulted to ensure that the body is specially prepared for burial. Disposable gloves must be used if a body is to be touched. The eyes should be closed and the limbs straightened; the head should be turned towards Mecca and the body wrapped in a plain sheet. The family may wish to wash the body themselves. Muslims are always buried and this should/must be arranged as soon as possible. Post-mortem examinations or any operation on the body is forbidden unless ordered by the coroner, in which case it must be carried out as soon as possible
• Traditional demands for burial within 24 h of death and in the deceased's native country need sensitive handling and explanation

Judaism
Preferences
• Jewish people may want 'Kosher' meals or vegetarian food
• They will probably want a Rabbi and women may want to remain fully clothed and have their hair covered. The religious emphasis on life may mean that the family or patient will question any treatment that could be seen to weaken the fight for life

Demands
• Orthodox Jews have strict dietary laws, and the family or Rabbi should be consulted for advice. At death the body must be handled as little as possible and even then only by his/her children and then covered
• The family, or in their absence a Jewish undertaker, should be informed immediately and a funeral held within 24 h. The exception is during the Sabbath (Friday dusk to Saturday dusk)

Further reading

Cassidy, S. (1988) *Sharing the Darkness. The spirituality of caring.* London: DLT.

Complementary therapies in palliative care

Complementary therapies are based on the belief that mind, body and spirit are interconnected and that health depends on wholeness and balance between them. This is often called the 'holistic' approach.

Definitions
- **Alternative** cancer treatments claim to reduce tumour burden, or to prolong the life of a patient and generally replace conventional treatments.
- **Complementary** treatments, in contrast, can be used alongside mainstream (orthodox, conventional) medicine; this is the *integrated* approach. However, there is no absolute distinction between what is a 'complementary' therapy and what is a 'conventional' one.

The primary aim of complementary therapies is to provide comfort and to increase quality of life by promoting relaxation, improving sleep, reducing stress and anxiety, relieving pain and other symptoms and by reducing the adverse effects of conventional treatments. Some complementary therapies also claim a direct anti-cancer effect.

Types of therapy
A comprehensive list of all the complementary therapies is not appropriate here, but the following are among the most widely practised, particularly within oncology and palliative care: homeopathy, acupuncture, herbalism, spiritual healing, relaxation, aromatherapy, reflexology and hypnotherapy.

For convenience, the individual therapies to be described in this chapter will be considered under four headings: therapies involving direct bodily contact, therapies involving ingestion of substances, mind–body therapies and creative therapies.

Principles and philosophy
A central tenet of complementary and alternative medicine (CAM) is the strong belief in the uniqueness of the individual and the power of the body to heal itself. The body will always strive to establish homeostasis, thereby maintaining good health: hence the logic that the whole person should be treated and not just the area of the body affected. Individuals are encouraged to adopt a way of life that is in harmony with nature, a view supported by Hippocrates who advocated eating simple, good quality nutritious food, exercise, rest, and fresh air, as well as clean water and sunlight.

People who consult complementary practitioners usually have long-standing conditions or illnesses that are difficult to manage such as HIV infection, multiple sclerosis, psoriasis, rheumatological conditions and, in particular, cancer. The interest in complementary therapies in the palliative care setting is perhaps not surprising given the inherent need for the terminally ill to feel supported holistically, with regard to physical, psychosocial, emotional and spiritual domains, in achieving an acceptable quality of their remaining life.

Prevalence

Prevalence studies in the USA show that 30–50 per cent of the general population use complementary therapies either in health maintenance or for illness or symptoms.[1] United Kingdom (UK) surveys, although fraught with methodological inconsistencies, have produced similar results.[2]

A systematic review revealed that a third of all patients with cancer consult complementary therapists.[3] Seventy per cent of all departments of oncology in Britain employ at least one type of complementary therapy practitioner in the palliative care setting. Most hospices now offer a range of complementary therapies for their patients. Therapists are largely volunteers, although some units are beginning to recognize complementary therapies as part of basic and expected care, and salaried posts are emerging.

There are estimated to be 50,000 complementary and alternative practitioners in the UK.

Reasons for seeking complementary therapies

Many years ago, having a paucity of effective treatments, doctors concentrated on the relief of physical and spiritual suffering. The last 50 years have seen unprecedented technical advances, which have encouraged a paternalistic approach to patients and a perceived decrease in respect for them as individuals. The disillusioned patient body is now recognizing that longer survival from cancer is often obtained at the expense of suffering due to orthodox treatments. Patients now demand more involvement in their care and open, honest, empathic communication with their healthcare advisers. The complementary therapies provide some of these needs, making patients feel better recognized as entire individuals and not just as scientific statistics.

There are multiple reasons why patients with terminal illnesses might seek complementary therapies. It is natural for patients to hope for cure or prolongation of life which, even if unrealistic, may be a motivational factor. Patients hope that complementary therapy will improve control of their symptoms, including stress and anxiety, and facilitate their emotional adjustment to the advancing illness.

In addition, complementary therapies provide patients with a greater sense of choice and control than they might achieve with conventional medicine alone.

Motivation for using CAM

Positive

- Perceived effectiveness
- Perceived safety
- Philosophical/spiritual/holistic/natural concepts
- Control over treatment
- High touch/low tech
- Good patient/therapist relationship with time and empathy
- Non-invasive
- Accessibility
- Pleasant therapeutic experience
- Affluence

Negative
- Dissatisfaction with conventional healthcare and its adverse effects
- Rejection of science and technology
- Rejection of the establishment
- Desperation
- False hopes of cure

Evaluation

Relatively little good research into complementary therapies has been conducted, largely because they have developed without a research tradition, organized infrastructure or financial backing. Furthermore, there are those who argue that scientific measurement or clinical validation is not needed since patients feel better after therapy (even if it is not proven significantly better than placebo in a formal research study).

The negative attitudes towards research in the palliative care setting, which encompass ethical and methodological issues, particularly when patients are reaching their last few weeks of life, are pertinent in this regard. However, this attitude, and the lack of research evidence, has been a barrier to collaboration between conventional and complementary practitioners.

The view that we do have a responsibility to investigate the cost-effectiveness, potential future value and adverse effects of complementary therapies is gaining ground. The provision of complementary therapies in mainstream medicine can only be justified with research backing.

From the available literature, there is no compelling evidence to support 'alternative' medicine (which includes diets, herbal medicines and supplements), as an effective treatment for reducing tumour burden or prolonging the life of patients with cancer. Some patients, however, choose to start or continue with this approach in preference to orthodox treatment. This is their choice. The place of complementary medicine, on the other hand, working alongside orthodox medicine is less controversial. It can be very difficult to design studies appropriate for a population of terminally ill patients and many studies are flawed. However, some well-conducted studies using different therapies in palliative care show statistical improvement in various parameters. For instance, a randomized trial of aromatherapy massage using essential oils showed significant benefits in psychological, physical and global quality of life.

Relaxation techniques, used to manage breathlessness in lung cancer patients, demonstrated a reduction in physical and emotional distress combined with improved coping strategies, despite a deteriorating performance status.[4] A retrospective survey of patients receiving hypnotherapy suggested improved coping as a positive outcome.

1 Astin J.A. *et al.* (1998) A review of the incorporation of complementary and alternative medicine by mainstream physicians. *Archives of Internal Medicine*, **158, 21**: 2303–10.

2 Zollman C., Vickers A. (1999). ABC of complementary medicine: users and practitioners of complementary medicine. *BMJ*, **319, 7213**: 836–38.

3 Ernst E., Cassileth B. R. (1998) The prevalence of complementary/alternative medicine in cancer: a systematic review. *Cancer*, **83, 4**: 777–82.

4 Bredin M. *et al.* (1998) Multicentre randomised controlled trial of a nursing intervention for breathlessness in patients with lung cancer. *Palliative Medicine*, **12, 6**: 470 (research abstract).

However, patients diagnosed with a terminal illness are vulnerable and can be exploited easily, and every effort should be made to ensure that they are making a fully informed decision about CAM. They should be made aware of the lack of evidence of efficacy compared with conventional treatment, the possibility that their hopes might be unrealistically raised and the chance that treatment may be a financial burden and a source of stress for the family.

Adverse effects

There is no formal register for monitoring adverse events associated with alternative and complementary therapies. However, reports in the literature confirm that they are not without risk. A report on acupuncture citing 30,000 needle insertions described minor local reactions, tiredness, drowsiness, infection and several cases of pneumothorax. Hypnosis may be associated with negative physiological and psychological effects. Some herbal or dietary additives are known to have side-effects and to interact with conventional medication.

Emotional turmoil in already distressed families can be compounded by patients who either adhere too rigidly or too haphazardly to a therapy or regime that is thought to be beneficial. This is particularly relevant if a patient becomes too unwell to continue with the treatment. Either situation can leading to feelings of anger, blame and guilt for both patient and family which may interfere adversely with family life and relationships.

Practitioner accountability

There is no legislation that restricts the practice of complementary and alternative therapies in the UK. Concerns over this lack of regulation of standards and training together with a paucity of research data prompted the establishment of the Foundation for Integrated Medicine in 1993. This organization is pivotal in the encouragement of research, development, education, regulation and delivery in the UK.

Conclusion

The use of complementary therapies alongside conventional medicine may have advantages in terms of improved symptom control, well-being, satisfaction and cost-effectiveness. This is now seen as an essential component of best practice in cancer care and is supported by the National Cancer Strategy, and the NICE Guidance on Support and Palliative Care for Adults with Cancer[5].

Foundation for Integrated Medicine
13 Sherwood Street
London W1F 7DR
Tel: 020 7439 7332

British Holistic Medical Association
59 Lansdowne Place
Hove
East Sussex BN3 1FL
Tel: 01273 725951

5 NICE (2004) Improving Supportive and Palliative Care for Adults with Cancer. London: NICE.

Bristol Cancer Help Centre
Grove House
Cornwallis Grove
Bristol BS8 4PG
Confidential helpline: 0845 123 2310
Switchboard: 0117 980 9500

Further reading

Books

Mitchell A., Cormack M. (1998) *The Therapeutic Relationship in Complementary Health Care.* Edinburgh: Churchill Livingstone.

Novey D. (2000) *Clinicians Complete Reference to Complementary and Alternative Medicine.* St Louis: Mosby.

Articles

Astin J. A. *et al.* (1998) A review of the incorporation of complementary and alternative medicine by mainstream physicians. *Archives of Internal Medicine*, **158**, 21: 2303–10.

Biley F. C. (2002) Primum non nocere: thoughts on the need to develop an 'adverse events' register for complementary and alternative therapies. *Complementary Therapies in Nursing and Midwifery*, **8, 2**: 57–61.

Bredin M. *et al.* (1998) Multicentre randomised controlled trial of a nursing intervention for breathlessness in patients with lung cancer. *Palliative Medicine*, **12**,6: 470 (research abstract).

Clover C., Kassab S. (1998) Complementary medicine for patients with cancer. *European Journal of Palliative Care*, **5, 3**: 73–6.

Ernst E. (2000) The rôle of complementary and alternative medicine in cancer. *Lancet Oncology*, **1**, 3: 176–80.

Ernst E. (2001) Complementary therapies in palliative cancer care (review). *Cancer*, **91, 11**: 2181–5.

Ernst E., Cassileth B. R. (1998) The prevalence of complementary/alternative medicine in cancer: a systematic review. *Cancer*, **83**, 4: 777–82.

Finlay I. G., Jones O. L. (1996) Hypnotherapy in palliative care. *Journal of the Royal Society of Medicine*, **89, 9**: 493–6.

Jacobson J. S. *et al.* (2000) Research on complementary/alternative medicine for patients with breast cancer: a review of the biomedical literature. *Journal of Clinical Oncology*, **18, 3**: 668–83.

Kainz K. (2003) Avoiding patient self-blame. *Complementary Therapies in Medicine*, **11**,1: 46–8.

Lewith G., Holgate S. (2000) CAM research and development. *Complementary Therapies in Nursing and Midwifery*, **6, 1**: 19–24.

Mason S. *et al.* (2002) Evaluating complementary medicine: methodological challenges of randomised controlled trials. *BMJ*, **325, 7368**: 832–4.

NICE (2004) Improving Supportive and Palliative Care for Adults with Cancer. London: NICE.

Pan C. X. *et al.* (2000) Complementary and alternative medicine in the management of pain, dyspnea, and nausea and vomiting near the end-of-life: a systematic review. *Journal of Pain and Symptom Management*, **20, 5**: 374–87.

Penson J. (1998) Complementary therapies: making a difference in palliative care. *Complementary Therapies in Nursing and Midwifery*, **4, 3**: 77–81.

Vickers A. (1996) Complementary therapies in palliative care. *European Journal of Palliative Care*, **3, 4**: 150–3.

Vickers A. (2000) Recent advances: complementary medicine. *BMJ*, **321, 7262**: 683–6.

Vincent C., Furnham A. (1999) Complementary medicine: state of the evidence. *Journal of the Royal Society of Medicine*, **92**: 170–7.

Walker L. A., Budd S. (2002) UK: the current state of regulation of complementary and alternative medicine. *Complementary Therapies in Medicine*, **10, 1**: 8–13.

White P. (1998) Complementary medicine treatment of cancer: a survey of provision. *Complementary Therapies in Medicine*, **6, 1**: 10–13.

Wilkinson S. (1995) Aromatherapy and massage in palliative care. *International Journal of Palliative Nursing*, **1, 1**: 21–30.

Wilkinson I. (2002) The House of Lords Select Committee for Science and Technology. Their report on complementary and alternative medicine and its implications for reflexology. *Complementary Therapies in Nursing and Midwifery*, **8, 2**: 91–100.

Zollman C. Vickers A. (1999) ABC of complementary medicine: users and practitioners of complementary medicine. *BMJ*, **319, 7213**: 836–8.

Group 1: Therapies involving direct body contact

Acupuncture

Background and theory

The history of acupuncture dates back 2000 years and it is an integral part of and based on the principles of traditional Chinese medicine (TCM). *Acupuncture* involves the stimulation of certain points in the body by the insertion of fine needles, whereas *acupressure* involves firm manual pressure on these selected points.

The workings of the human body are thought to be controlled by a vital force or energy called Qi (pronounced *shee*) which circulates between organs along channels called meridians. There are 12 main meridians, corresponding loosely to 12 major functions or organs of the body. On these meridians, more than 350 acupuncture points have been defined. Qi energy must flow in the correct strength and quality through each of the meridians and organs for health to be maintained. The acupuncture points are situated along the meridians and through these the flow of Qi can be altered. Traditional acupuncture theory is based on the concept of yin and yang, which should be in balance: any imbalance (particularly blockage or deficiency) in the continuous flow of energy causes illness. Acupuncture redresses this balance, allowing the healthy unimpeded flow of Qi.

There are many different schools of acupuncture. Conventional Western health professionals relate acupuncture points to physiological and anatomical features such as peripheral nerve junctions. The concept of 'trigger points', whereby areas of increased sensitivity within a muscle cause referred pain in relation to a segment of the body, has also been recognized.

There is no evidence to confirm the physical existence of Qi or the meridians. A possible explanation for the points is that they are sites at which nerves can be stimulated. There have been attempts to explain the effects of acupuncture within a conventional physiological framework. It is known that acupuncture stimulates A delta nerve fibres which enter the dorsal horn of the spinal cord and mediate segmental inhibition of pain impulses carried in the slower unmyelinated C fibres. Through connections with the midbrain, descending inhibition of C fibre pain impulses is also enhanced at other levels of the spinal cord. Acupuncture is also known to stimulate the release of endogenous opioids and other neurotransmitters such as serotonin, which are involved in the modulation of pain. It has also been noted that the electrical conductivity of organ-related acupuncture points is altered when the corresponding organ is diseased.

All organs of the body are represented on the helix of the ear in an inverted foetal position. Tender points in the ear have been shown to match sites of chronic pain in corresponding distant parts of the body. Acupuncture needles or studs can be used in these sites (auriculoacupuncture).

Uses

Acupuncture is used, for example, in the management of pain, anxiety, fatigue, breathlessness, dry mouth and digestive disorders.

Practical application

Acupuncture may be delivered in a number of different ways. In the UK, typically between 4 and 10 needlepoints are selected. These points are often located in areas where they represent the relevant local, regional and distant meridians. Needlepoints may also be centred around the area of pain to boost the local 'dose' to the area. This is often referred to as 'surrounding the dragon'.

In the UK, the practice in palliative care is to use sterile disposable needles which are usually inserted to a depth of about 5 millimetres (or more deeply into muscle). Needles are left *in situ* for approximately 15 minutes. Needle sizes differ but typically measure up to about 30 mm long and 0.25 mm in diameter. It is possible that the sensation of 'de Qi' (pronounced *deshee*) which causes feelings of heaviness, soreness or numbness at the point of needling is necessary both to indicate that the anatomically correct site has been needled and that the treatment will work well. However, this is by no means universal, the treatment often being successful even in the absence of de Qi or any sensation at the point of skin puncture.

It is not common in palliative care in the UK to increase the stimulation of the acupuncture point other than by gentle turning/manipulation of the needles, although an increase in dose may be achieved using a small electric current, laser beams or ultrasound. Acupuncture studs remain *in situ* and may be pressed by the patient as necessary to give more sustained stimulation. In moxibustion, points are heated by smouldering a substance called moxa over the points.

Acupuncture treatments are often given once a week for a few weeks and thereafter as necessary.

Safety

Acupuncture is generally considered to be a relatively safe form of treatment with a low incidence of serious side-effects. There is no official reporting mechanism for adverse events. One prospective study of 65,000 treatments from Japan recorded only 94 minor adverse events, the most common being forgotten needles and faintness. No serious events were recorded (Yamashita 1999). The conclusion was that acupuncture is probably safe in skilled hands. However, there have been reports of pneumothorax, infection, spinal injuries and hepatitis B transmission. Acupuncture studs in the ear may result in perichondritis of the underlying cartilage.

Acupuncture should be used with care in any patient in whom there is a risk of infection or bleeding. It should be avoided in patients with valvular heart disease. Deep needling should be avoided in patients with bleeding disorders or taking anticoagulants. Acupuncture to spinal muscles should be safe unless there is an unstable spine, in which case it is contraindicated. Extra care should be exercised in patients receiving their first acupuncture treatment as they may react strongly, with dizziness and drowsiness. The initial treatment should be given supine and patients should be advised not to drive or to operate machinery for a few hours.

Further reading

Books

Filshie J., White A. (eds) (1998) *Medical Acupuncture*. Edinburgh: Churchill Livingstone.

Articles

Dibble S. L. *et al.* (2000) Acupressure for nausea: results of a pilot study. *Oncology Nursing Forum*, **27, 1**: 41–7.

Dillon M., Lucas C. (1999) Auricular stud acupuncture in palliative care patients. *Palliative Medicine*, **13, 3**: 253–4.

Ezzo J. *et al.* (2000) Is acupuncture effective for the treatment of chronic pain? A systematic review. *Pain*, **86, 3**: 217–25.

Rampes H., James R. (1995) Complications of acupuncture. *Acupuncture in Medicine*, **13, 1**: 26–33.

Vickers A. (2001) Acupuncture. *Effective Health Care* **7**: 2.

Yamashita H. *et al.* (1999) Adverse events in acupuncture and moxibustion treatment: a six year survey at a national clinic in Japan. *Journal of Alternative and Complementary Medicine*, **5, 3**: 229–36.

Massage

Background and theory

Massage is one of the oldest healthcare practices in existence. It is documented in Chinese texts more than 4000 years ago and has been used in Western healthcare since Hippocrates in the fourth century BC. Massage therapy is the scientific manipulation of the soft tissues of the body for the purpose of normalizing these tissues. It consists of manual techniques that include applying moving or fixed pressure, and movement of the body. These techniques affect all body systems, in particular the musculoskeletal, circulatory, lymphatic and nervous systems. The basic philosophy is to help the body to heal itself, in order to achieve or increase well-being. Touch is the fundamental medium of massage therapy. Touch may involve a degree of pressure which is sensitively defined for each individual and concentrated on areas of muscle tension and soft tissue. Touch is also a form of communication, sensitive touch conveying a sense of caring, an essential element in the therapeutic relationship.

Uses

Massage is widely used in a variety of conditions including lymphoedema, stress, anxiety, back and other pain and insomnia. Through the relaxation of muscle tension and relief of anxiety, massage therapy may reduce blood pressure and heart rate. Massage may also enhance the immune system and increase the capacity of cytotoxic agents to work better. Abdominal massage may be useful for constipation.

Practical application

Either the whole body or relevant specific parts may be treated. Practitioners ensure warmth and modesty and may play background music depending on patient preference. Patients may be encouraged to breath steadily and to communicate with the therapist. Oils, including aromatherapy oils, may also be used, depending on the individual patient and the aims of treatment. Massage usually lasts one hour.

Safety

Massage is comparatively safe and there is no evidence that it encourages the spread of cancer, although it would also be contraindicated in any situation where it might damage tumour or frail tissue, particularly in treatment-related areas.

It is generally contraindicated for advanced heart disease, phlebitis, thrombosis and embolism, kidney failure, infectious diseases, contagious skin conditions, acute inflammation, infected injuries, unhealed fractures, conditions prone to haemorrhage and psychosis. It is also contraindicated in the acute flare up of rheumatoid arthritis, eczema, goitre and open skin lesions.

📖 For aromatherapy massage see the Aromatherapy section, p. 684.

Further reading

Books

Rich G. J. (2002) *Massage Therapy: the Evidence for Practice.* Edinburgh: Mosby.

Articles

Vickers A., Zollman C. (1999) ABC of complementary medicine: massage therapy *BMJ*, **319**: 1254–7.

Reflexology

Background and theory

The therapeutic use of hand and foot pressure for the treatment of pain and various illnesses existed in China and India over 5000 years ago.

It is suggested that there are ten longitudinal, bilateral reflexes or zones running along the body which terminate in the hands and feet. All systems and organs are reflected onto the skin surface, particularly that of the palms and soles. By applying gentle pressure to these areas it is possible to relieve the congestion or imbalance along the zone. Specific organs and the interrelationship between organs and bodily systems can be influenced to regain and maintain emotional, physical and spiritual homeostasis. This results in the relief of symptoms and facilitates the prevention of illness and healing, with the aim of promoting good health and well-being.

Malfunction of any organ or part of the body is thought to cause the deposition of tiny crystals of calcium and uric acid in the nerve endings, particularly in the feet. These deposits are then broken down and eliminated by gentle pressure. This is referred to as 'detoxification' which may lead to a 'healing crisis' including 'flu-like symptoms, a feeling of being light headed and lethargic, feeling cold 3–4 days post-treatment, reduction in blood pressure, increase in excretory functions and alteration in sleep pattern. Following this, healing can then begin.

Uses

Treatment may be used for a variety of clinical problems. Of particular relevance to palliative care are control of pain and anxiety (Stephenson *et al.* 2000), induction of deep relaxation and improvement in sleep.

Practical application

There are different schools of teaching in the application of reflexology, although the underlying principles are consistent.

The foot is treated by applying gentle pressure along each zone systematically until the dorsum, sides and sole have been covered. The practitioner then repeats the treatment on the other foot. Initially gentle massage and stroking movements are used followed by deep thumb and finger pressure. The reflex areas on the foot may feel tender or painful if 'blocked', but this is relieved as the treatment works and the 'blockage' is removed. Treatment may take up to an hour and be repeated weekly as necessary, effects being apparent within a few sessions depending on the individual.

Safety

Contraindications to reflexology include the first trimester of pregnancy. Care should be taken in depressive and manic states, epilepsy and acute conditions. Reflexology practitioners should work closely with medical colleagues, particularly where they are integrally involved in a patient's ongoing medical management.

Patients receiving reflexology may notice an increase in urination and body discharges, leading to fears that medicinal drugs such as chemotherapy agents might be eliminated more quickly from the body and thus be less effective. There is no evidence for this.

Further reading

Article

Stephenson N. L. N. *et al.* (2000) The effects of foot reflexology on anxiety and pain in patients with breast and lung cancer. *Oncology Nursing Forum*, **27, 1**: 67–72.

Group 2: Therapies involving ingestion of substances

Aromatherapy

Background and theory

Aromatic plants, and infusions prepared from them, have been employed in medicines and cosmetics for thousands of years. Aromatherapy uses oils extracted from plants, which are usually referred to as 'essential oils'. These are the pure, concentrated essences of plants, flowers (e.g. rose), leaves (e.g. peppermint), barks (e.g. cinnamon), fruits (e.g. lemon) and seeds (e.g. fennel), grasses (e.g. lemongrass) and bulbs (e.g. garlic) and other plant substances. Fresh plant material usually yields 1–2 per cent by weight of essential oil on distillation. A typical essential oil is a complex mixture of over 100 different chemical compounds which give the oil its smell, therapeutic properties and in some cases its toxicity.

Essential oils are considered to act not only on the body, by stimulating physiological processes, but also on the emotions and the mind. Odour stimulates the olfactory senses and these relay to the limbic system, which is central to the emotions and memory. The limbic system in turn is associated with the hypophyseal–pituitary axis which regulates the endocrine system, affecting reactions to fear, anger, metabolism and sexual stimulus. Pure essential oils exert a positive influence on these reactions. Some oils have an affinity for a particular organ whilst others have a more general effect, promoting homeostasis and well-being. The body uses what it needs and excretes the remainder via the lungs and excretory organs.

Practical application

Aromatherapy oils can be used in the bath and can also be inhaled once vapourized. Essential oils for use on the skin are always diluted by mixing them in an inert unperfumed vegetable carrier such as almond oil, or in lotion or cream. A typical dilution would be two drops of essential oil to 10ml of carrier oil (i.e. 1–5 per cent dilution) for external use and 0.5–2.5ml (10–50 drops) daily for oral use, although this may be diluted further as necessary.

Oils may be light, stimulating, energizing and uplifting e.g. eucalyptus, or try: levelling, balancing and calming e.g. lavender, or calming, sedative and relaxing e.g. benzoin. These three broad types of oil are often mixed, the exact oil depending on the symptoms. For instance:

- Treatment for influenza might include a mixture of eucalyptus (for sore throat/blocked sinuses), lavender (for headache/insomnia) and benzoin (for aching joints)
- Aching muscles and back pain might benefit from a mixture of juniper, rosemary and lavender
- Constipation may usefully be managed with lemon, rosemary and mandarin
- An irritable bowel may benefit from a mixture of peppermint, chamomile and lavender
- Nausea may respond to peppermint and ginger

Safety
The total quantity of oil absorbed into the body from an aromatherapy massage varies according to the percentage dilution of the oil, the total quantity applied and the total area of skin to which the oil is applied. Warmth, massage and applying the oil to hydrated skin increases the amount absorbed. The amount absorbed orally may be 8–10 times greater than that received in a massage. It is possible for small regular amounts to lead to unrecognized chronic toxicity.

Skin reactions can include irritation, sensitisation and phototoxicity. It is potentially dangerous to apply undiluted essential oils to damaged, diseased or inflamed skin and patch testing should therefore always be carried out prior to treatment.

The oils used in clinical aromatherapy are not considered to be carcinogenic or toxic. Potentially carcinogenic oils found in camphor oil, tarragon oil, sassafras oil and methyluegent are not usually found in the range of oils used by aromatherapists.

Patients with cancer are often highly sensitive to the sense of smell, which may have altered due to chemotherapy. Certain smells can be very nauseating, and this should be assessed with the patient before therapy.

Certain oils should be avoided in specific situations. For example, Cade, Ravensara anisata, basil, sassafras, camphor and tarragon shoud be avoided in patients with cancer and anise and fennel should be avoided in those with oestrogen-dependent tumours such as carcinoma of the breast.

Further reading

Books

Tisserand R., Balacs T. (1995) *Essential Oil Safety: A Guide for Health Care Professionals*. Edinburgh: Churchill Livingstone.

Vickers A. (1996) *Massage and Aromatherapy: A Guide for Health Professionals*. London: Chapman & Hall.

Articles

Corner J. *et al.* (1995) An evaluation of the use of massage and essential oils on the well-being of cancer patients. *International Journal of Palliative Nursing*, **1, 2**: 67–73.

Kite S. M. *et al.* (1998) Development of an aromatherapy service at a Cancer Centre. *Palliative Medicine*, **12, 3**: 171–80.

Soden K. (2004) A randomised controlled trial of aromatherapy massage in a hospice setting. *Palliative Medicine*, **18**: 87–92.

Wilkinson S. (1995) Aromatherapy and massage in palliative care. *International Journal of Palliative Nursing*, **1, 1**: 21–30.

Wilkinson S. (1999) An evaluation of aromatherapy massage in palliative care. *Palliative Medicine*, **13, 5**: 409–17.

Dietary therapies and supplements

Background

The rôle of diet in health is of great interest to patients, but has generally been neglected in orthodox medicine. Dietary manipulation, such as decreased consumption of calories, fat, alcohol and smoked or pickled food, has been shown to reduce the incidence of specific adult cancers, while increased dietary fibre appears to have a protective rôle. There are few quality research studies, however, that show that dietary manipulation is influential in altering the prognosis in established cancer.

Theory

The transformation from normal cells to cancer cells is thought to result from successive and cumulative genetic defects. Cancer cells themselves are genetically unstable, defective aspects of malignant DNA metabolism contributing to tumour growth and progression. This genetic instability can be increased through metabolic mechanisms associated with diets high in fat and low in antioxidants (e.g. vitamin E and C).

Radical diets

There are anecdotal reports, although not controlled trials, of dramatic remissions in cancer associated with radical diets, which naturally captures the imagination of patients desperate to find a cure. The Gerson diet is one such example.

Gerson (1996) believes that cancer cells have been pathologically transformed in their ability to digest and exchange proteins and fats, with the result that enzyme metabolism is altered. Proponents believe that most metabolic processes are concentrated in the liver and that treatment therefore needs to detoxify and stimulate the liver.

Detoxification refers to the elimination of any potentially accumulated chemicals including pesticides, hydrocarbons and heavy metals, in addition to the unwelcome products of packaged, processed foods including refined sugars and flours, sweets, caffeinated beverages, dairy products, meats, preservatives and other food additives. It relies on the body's inherent ability to cleanse itself if given the opportunity. Detoxification involves avoiding the intake of toxins, facilitating elimination of waste products and promoting a healthier diet and lifestyle while building the body's nutrition. Gerson proposes intensive detoxification, which is the basis of coffee enemas which are believed to stimulate the enzyme systems of the liver, thereby effectively eliminating the toxins.

Many diets, including the Gerson diet, encourage the drinking of quantities of fresh raw juice, including carrot and celery. Strict diets may include organically grown fruit, vegetables and whole grains with supplements which include potassium, thyroid hormone, vitamins and pancreatic enzymes from organic materials. Salt, fat, coffee, berries, nuts and all bottled, canned, refined, preserved and frozen foods are not permitted.

Dietary burden

Strict adherence to diets may become a burden to the patient and family and for this reason only a minority of patients choose this option. Great effort and determination is needed to adhere to a strict diet, especially if it is not enjoyed. Patients may take the diet willingly or may be under pressure to start or continue, feeling that they will let the family down if they do not do everything in their power to try to fight the cancer.

The family may feel uncomfortably committed to supporting the patient's belief that the diet is imperative to control the cancer. The organization and preparation of the food and associated practices may involve a considerable part of each day and become a burden for families who see that, despite their efforts, the patient is continuing to deteriorate.

Shared family meals may no longer take place, leading to breaks in family cohesion. The diet may begin to dominate family life, altering family dynamics unhealthily at a time when all members need to support each other. Conflict may develop at a time when attention should be turned to quality of life and allowing patients to eat and drink what they feel like. Furthermore, special diets and supplements are often very expensive and may also lead to side-effects from high dose supplements and nutritional deficiencies, adding to further burden.

Since the 1980s, The Bristol Cancer Help Centre have moved away from an emphasis on strict diet and metabolic therapies to a more gentle, caring approach empowering patients to concentrate on self healing and to live with cancer. Greater importance is now afforded to psychological care and integration of transpersonal psychology supporting the holistic complementary approach to patient care. Relaxation and the permission for free expression of emotion and feelings enhances the healing experience and promotes the enjoyment of life by reducing negative influences and increasing positive inputs, while still recognizing the importance of diet.

Guidelines for healthy eating

The tumour host environment depends on a number of factors, including diet. It seems sensible therefore to recognize the influence that diet can have and to base it on ingredients that are thought to promote health. Healthy diets are characterized by low fat, moderate protein (chiefly from vegetarian sources), high vegetable/fruit and whole grain cereals, bread and pasta and other essential nutrients. Other influences may include phytochemicals (e.g. soy products) with known anticancer and detoxification properties and biologically active agents including, among others, vitamin E, A and eicosapentaenoic acid (EPA), all of which demonstrate antitumour effects.

Further reading

Articles

Bloch A. (1999) Alternative nutritional regimens targeted to persons with cancer. *Cancer Practice*, **7, 3**: 151–3.

Weir M. W. (1993) Bristol Cancer Help Centre: success and setbacks but the journey continues. *Complementary Therapies in Medicine*, **1, 1**: 42–5.

Weitzman S. (1998) Alternative nutritional cancer therapies. *International Journal of Cancer Supplement*, **11**: 69–72.

Homeopathy

Background and theory

Practitioners of homeopathy treat disease using highly diluted preparations of a variety of different substances. The principle of homeopathy is that 'like should be cured with like'. Patients are given preparations that will produce the symptom that the patient is presenting with. For instance, hayfever which presents with lacrimation, stinging and irritation around the eyes and nose might be treated with the remedy Allium cepa, derived from the common onion.

Remedies are prepared by a process of serial dilution and succussion (vigorous shaking). The greater the number of times this process of dilution and succussion is performed, the greater the potency of the remedy.

Prescribing strategies vary considerably. In 'classical' homeopathy, practitioners aim to identify a single medicine that is needed to treat a patient holistically, taking into account current illness, medical history, personality and behaviour. 'Complex' homeopathy involves the prescription of combinations of medicine.

Common homeopathic medicines include those made from plants (such as belladonna, arnica and chamomile), minerals (such as mercury and sulphur), animal products (such as sepia (squid ink) and lachesis (snake venom), and more rarely, biochemical substances (such as histamine or human growth factor).

About 10–20 per cent of the UK population have bought homeopathic medication over the counter and it is even more popular in Europe.

Homeopathic medicines are diluted to such a degree that not even a single molecule of the original solute is likely to be present. Conventional scientists remain sceptical about its efficacy although it is possible that some, as yet undefined, biophysical mechanism may exist. One possible explanation, currently being investigated, is that during serial dilution the complex interactions between the solvent (water) molecules are altered to retain a 'memory' of the original solute material. Some laboratory studies have reported biological effects on animals, plants and cells at ultramolecular dilutions.

Uses

Many different, often chronic and recurring conditions are treated with homeopathic medication. Self prescription for various conditions such as the common cold, bruising, hayfever and joint sprains is common.

Practical application

A detailed history is taken paying attention to the 'modalities' of presenting symptoms such as whether they change according to the weather, time of day, season and so on.

Information is also gathered about mood and behaviour, likes and dislikes, responses to stress, personality and reactions to food. A 'symptom' picture is thus built up and matched to a 'drug picture' described in the homeopathic *Materia medica*. One or more homeopathic medicines are then prescribed, usually in pill form, either as one or two doses or on a more regular basis.

A patient's initial symptom picture commonly matches more than one drug picture. Follow-up allows the practitioner to define the best medication for a particular patient.

Safety
Serious, unexpected adverse effects of homeopathic medicines are rare. Symptoms may become acutely and transiently worse (aggravation reactions) after starting treatment and patients should be warned of this possibility. The occurrence of an aggravation reaction may be a sign that the treatment will be beneficial.

The more serious issue is the view of some practitioners who adamantly believe that conventional medication reduces the efficacy of homeopathic remedies. Serious adverse effects have occurred when patients have failed to comply with conventional medication. For instance, some practitioners feel that vaccination can do more harm than good.

Further reading

Book

Swayne J. (1998) *The Homeopathic Method: Implications for Clinical Practice and Medical Science.* Edinburgh: Churchill Livingstone.

Articles

Kleijnen J. *et al.* (1991) Trials of homeopathy. *BMJ*, **302, 6782**: 960.

Linde K. *et al.* (1997) Are the clinical effects of homeopathy placebo effects? A meta-analysis of placebo-controlled trials. *Lancet*, **350, 9081**: 834–43.

O'Meara S. *et al.* (2002) Homeopathy. *Effective Health Care*, **7, 3**: 1–12.

Ramakrishnan A. U. (1997) The treatment of cancer with homeopathic medicine part 2: case studies. *Journal of the American Institute of Homeopathy*, **90, 3**: 126–31.

Thompson E. A. (1999) Using homeopathy to offer supportive cancer care in a National Health Service outpatient setting. *Complementary Therapies in Nursing and Midwifery*, **5, 2**: 37–41.

Thompson E. A., Reilly D. (2002) The homeopathic approach to symptom control in the cancer patient: a prospective observational study. *Palliative Medicine*, **16, 3**: 227–33.

Vickers A., Zollman C. (1999) Homeopathy. *BMJ*, **319**: 1115–18.

Group 3: Mind–body therapies

Relaxation

Relaxation aims to release tension from both body and mind. There are many different methods of relaxation, one of the most used being the progressive clenching followed by conscious relaxation of all the muscles in the body in parallel with concentration on the control of breathing. It can be quickly learnt in groups or classes or by listening to tapes or reading guides. One study used relaxation techniques to manage breathlessness in patients with lung cancer, demonstrating significant reduction in physical and emotional distress combined with improved coping strategies, despite deteriorating performance status.

Hypnotherapy

Background and theory

Hypnotherapy involves the induction of deep physical and mental relaxation, leading to an altered state of consciousness. In simple terms, the individual becomes able to concentrate more and more on less and less, which leads to a greatly increased susceptibility to suggestion. We store much more memory than we can consciously remember. Once guided into a hypnotic trance, patients may recall data not easily accessed by the conscious mind. The dissociation between the conscious and unconscious mind can be used to give therapeutic suggestions, thereby encouraging changes in behaviour and the relief of symptoms. Hypnotherapy can be a powerful, non-invasive tool which can be used for relaxation and also for psychotherapeutic purposes.

Hypnotherapy induces a unique behavioural state with a demonstrable neurophysiological basis. Electroencephalogram (EEG) studies reveal that hypnosis induces an altered state of consciousness in which the subject is in a state of relaxation but not sleep.

Uses

Hypnotherapy is more commonly used for anxiety, for disorders with a strong psychological component (such as asthma and irritable bowel syndrome) and for conditions that are modulated by levels of arousal, such as pain. There is good evidence that hypnotherapy reduces anxiety related to stressful situations such as chemotherapy. It also helps in panic disorder and insomnia. There is evidence that it is effective in reducing cancer-related anxiety, pain, nausea and vomiting in adults and in children.

Practical application

Patients often see a practitioner on a one to one basis for a course of treatments which may last up to an hour or so, although hypnotherapy may also be carried out in groups of up to 12 patients. It is possible to teach patients self-hypnosis. Ninety per cent of the population can be hypnotized to varying degrees, the depth of trance determining the potential success of treatment.

Safety

Hypnosis can sometimes exacerbate psychological problems. Patients with post-traumatic stress disorder who are re-traumatized through revival of memories may be particularly affected. False memories may be induced in the psychologically vulnerable. Hypnosis may be implicated in bringing on latent psychosis, and is therefore best avoided in established or borderline psychosis and personality disorders.

Guided imagery and visualization

This makes use of the imagination in order to focus the mind and induce relaxation through pleasant thoughts. Words create a picture for the mind of some pleasant scene, special to the patient, which is revisitable at any time. All the senses are called upon to make the mind-picture come alive with descriptions of pleasant warmth, smells, sounds, taste and associated feelings. Relaxation tapes may contain music or sounds such as the sea or birdsong. Relaxation training combined with imagery may help reduce side-effects from cancer treatments, and enhance patients' well-being and sense of control.

The underlying hypothesis is that physical processes in the body are affected by what the imagination creates and that, with training, an individual can learn to develop powers of imagination and use them to combat cancer. People with cancer who are interested in these techniques are helped to visualize their cancer being attacked by their immune system. The actual images are chosen by the patient, the cancer being represented by a weak and feeble opponent and the immune system by a strong powerful force. Patients are encouraged to see themselves as healthy and active in the future. The image is used for a short period once or twice a day and is combined with techniques of relaxation. Feelings of regaining control are experienced and this is seen as a positive step to counteracting the negativity of the disease.

Meditation

Meditation aims to quieten the body and the mind. This can be achieved by learning to concentrate, perhaps on an object such as a candle or a word that is special to the individual, their own mantra. Concentration on breathing helps achieve this peaceful state. Patients can then let go of the incessant busyness of life and relentless speed of thoughts, letting them come and go until they reach a state of inner quiet, a silent space. The skill of meditation takes time to learn but books, tapes and classes are available.

Spiritual healing

Background

Spiritual healing is one of the oldest known therapies and is used in every culture around the world. It has been largely rejected by Western medicine because it is alien to conventional ways of relating to health and illness. However, since the 1950s, its benefits have become more recognized. Healers work to a standard code of conduct and medical practitioners now accept this form of treatment within conventional healthcare settings.

Uses

Healing can alleviate symptoms and recovery in a variety of clinical situations such as headache, backache, arthritis, wound healing, anxiety

Palliative care in the home

The significance of community palliative care—Why is it important?

The major part of continuing care for palliative patients is provided by the primary healthcare team, whether with malignant or non-malignant diagnoses: such continuing care cannot realistically be the responsibility of specialist palliative care. The reality is that primary care and the generic hospital services currently provide, and will continue to provide the great majority of palliative care.[1]

Palliative care in the community is important. Primary care contributes a vital rôle, which is greatly appreciated by patients and carers, and has a significant impact on other services. Many general practitioners (GPs) and district nurses feel that palliative care represents the best of all medical care, bringing together the clinical, holistic and human dimensions of primary care. They know their patients well, and are in a key position to provide best support for them and their families at this most crucial stage, with the backing of specialist palliative care and hospice expertise, advice and resources. GPs and district nurses often prioritize care of the dying, some claiming that it reconnects them with their reasons for entering healthcare and affects their standing in a community. However, care at home can break down or become suboptimal, for a variety of reasons: poor communication, limited round-the-clock coordination, difficulties in symptom control, inadequate support for carers, etc.

Good palliative care is appreciated by our patients and their families, and is at the core of good primary care, and in many ways is probably the best thing we do.
(Northern Ireland GP)

First paradox of community palliative care[2]

Most dying people would prefer to remain at home, but most of them die in institutions.

Second paradox of community palliative care

Most of the final year of life is spent at home, but most people are admitted to hospital to die.

Despite most patients expressing a preference to remain at home and to die there if adequately supported, most patients die in institutions. Disturbingly, most are not even formally consulted as to their wishes. 'Home is the place that reminds us of living as well as dying and is where we feel more fully ourselves.'

1 Barclay S. (2001) Palliative care for non-cancer patients: a UK perspective from primary care. In J. Addington-Hall, I. Higginson (eds) *Palliative Care for Non-cancer Patients*. Oxford: Oxford University Press.

2 Thorpe G. (1993) Enabling more dying people to remain at home. *BMJ*, **307**: 915–8.

Community provision of palliative care services is therefore a vital part of the jigsaw, and affects hospital and hospice admission rates and capacity, particularly for non-cancer patients. As many cancer patients die in care homes as in hospices, so good palliative care here is also essential. Many hospice-based hospice-at-home services successfully supplement generic services. The original principles espoused and modelled by Dame Cicely Saunders, the founder of the modern hospice movement, and others, are being mainstreamed into standard healthcare across the world. From the early days of the movement there was discouragement for the proliferation of hospices, in favour of broad dissemination of 'terminal care' principles throughout the health service, including acute hospital and community services.

Ideally, there should be a means to optimize generalist palliative care at home, so that regardless of the setting, the diagnosis and the possible disease timescale, patients should receive the highest standard of palliative care at all times, i.e. the '…care of the dying should be raised to the level of the best' (NHS Cancer Plan England 2000). 'Palliative care at home embraces what is most noble in medicine: sometimes curing, always relieving, supporting right to the end.'[3]

> I think that terminal care is probably if not the most important then certainly one of the most important things that GPs can become involved in. I feel it's that personal involvement that is often the most important thing.[4]

Community palliative care key facts

- Ninety per cent of the final year of life for most patients is spent at home
- People are now living longer with serious illnesses, and mainly in the community
- GPs have always been, and will continue to be the main providers of palliative care for the majority of patients

Patients especially appreciate:
- continuity of relationship
- being listened to
- an opportunity to ventilate feelings
- being accessible
- effective symptom control
- GPs' palliative care rôle can be optimized by specialist support, especially if there is some formalized engagement.[5] 'It is better to help a colleague with a difficult case than to tell him he is wrong, and that he should make way for the expert' (Pugsley and Pardoe 1986).[6]
- On average, each GP will look after 30–40 patients with cancer at any one time, or about 200 patients per practice team of 10,000 patients, or 3,500 for every Primary Care Trust (PCT)
- On average there will be 8 patients newly diagnosed with cancer/GP/year, 50 per practice and 750 per PCT
- The 'average' UK GP will have about 20 patient deaths/year, of which about five will be from cancer, five from organ failure e.g. heart failure or COPD, 7–8 from multiple pathology, dementia and decline, and 2–3 from sudden death e.g. myocardial infarction, road traffic accident etc

- Palliative care occupies a greater proportion of a district nurse's time, including out-of-hours care, than patient numbers would indicate
- There is less support available for patients and carers with non-malignant end-stage illness, and limited support for GPs managing such patients
- There is a steady shift in the place of care for many patients with palliative care needs, away from the hospital setting into the community, for the majority of the last year of life
- Hospital death is more likely if patients are poor, elderly, have no carers, are far from other services or have a long illness trajectory
- The home death rate in England is low (23 per cent for cancer patients and 19 per cent for all deaths)
- The hospital death rate in England is high (55 per cent cancer patients and 66 per cent of all deaths)
- There is a clear preference from most patients and carers for a home death and an increasing choice of hospice death
- For hospitals, improving community palliative care services will help reduce patients with palliative care needs occupying acute beds, improve capacity and waiting lists, and reduce the standard hospital mortality ratio
- It is estimated that 4000 patients a day could be discharged from hospital if there were adequate community places for them according to the National Audit Office
- Gaps are apparent in community care e.g. symptom control management, 24h nursing care, night sitters, access to equipment, out-of-hours support, and there are concerns that this picture may worsen in future with changes in out-of-hours provision
- Specialist palliative care has raised standards of care and symptom control
- Hospice care is changing: with the average length of stay now reduced to two weeks
- Fifty per cent of patients admitted to hospices will be discharged back to the community
- Improved palliative care services can have a very positive effect on a family's bereavement journey
- GPs and district nurses repeatedly demonstrate they are keen to improve the quality of the palliative service they provide, and they regard palliative care as important and intrinsic to primary care
- In England national directives emphasize the vital rôle of community palliative care

'The care of the dying is a test of a successful NHS' (NHS Chief Executive Sir Nigel Crisp March 2003).

3 Gomas J.-M. (1993) Palliative care at home: a reality or 'mission impossible'? *Palliative Medicine*, **7 (Suppl. 1)**: 45–59

4 Jeffrey D. (2000) *Cancer from Cure to Care*. Hochland and Hochland.

5 Mitchell G. (2002) How well do general practitioners deliver palliative care? A systematic review. *Palliative Medicine*, **16**: 457–64.

6 Pugsley R., Pardoe J. (1986) The specialist contribution to the care of the terminally ill patient. *Journal of Royal College of General Practitioners*, **36**: 347–8.

Patients' needs

The user viewpoint

You matter because you are you. You matter to the last moment of your life and we will do all we can not only to help you die peacefully but to live until you die.

Dame Cicely Saunders

John had wanted to stay at home as he became weaker. But suddenly one weekend it all went badly wrong and he went into hospital in the middle of the night. He never came home. I will never forgive myself for this. I will have to live with this feeling of guilt all my life, wishing I could have done more.

Mary, wife of John, a cancer patient

Listening to patients

The care provided both in the provision of day to day clinical care at the bedside and strategically in the planning of services must be based on the needs of patients. Listening to the 'user view' is obvious, increasingly important in both scenarios, yet sometimes still avoided. The importance of the views of the patient and their carers is becoming recognized more formally with the emergence of 'User groups' in cancer networks and elsewhere.

How much do we listen to patients' needs and respond accordingly? Unfortunately the pressure of workload and the daunting task of facing sensitive situations that require good communication skills, can easily deflect from taking time to acquire the patient's view. Some assessment tools have been developed to help facilitate this important task, such as the Problems and Concerns Assessment Tools or Patient/Carer Feedback sheets.

'I think that the most important thing is that we must listen to what the question is and try to hear what is behind the actual words used.'[7]

Truth telling, communication skills and retaining control

Patients and carers cannot be full contributors in decision-making without clear information, and if left uninformed, there will be less sense of retaining autonomy and control. There is a common, well-intentioned but misguided assumption, present at all stages of cancer care, that what people do not know does not harm them.

'Truth may hurt but deceit hurts more.'[8] Healthcare professionals often censor the information they give to patients in an attempt to protect them from potentially hurtful, sad or bad news. However, less than honest disclosure and the desire to shield patients from the reality of the situation often create even greater difficulties for patients, carers and other members of the healthcare team. Although well meant, such a conspiracy of silence often results in a heightened state of fear, anxiety and confusion for patient's who may even feel betrayed by such a process which actually does little to promote patient calm and equanimity. Ambiguous or deliberately misleading information may afford short-term benefits, but denies individuals and their families opportunities to reorganize and adapt their lives towards the attainment of achievable goals, realistic hopes and previously planned-for aspirations. Having said this, breaking bad news is always difficult. Skills in discussing sensitive information can be learned and practised, and most areas run communication skills learning, now an integral part of the Supportive and Palliative Care Guidance in England.

As the Age Concern 12 Principles of a Good Death confirms in 8 out of 12 assertions, retaining control is a vital element for patients, and our rôle should be more to enable than to instruct, ever respectful of the boundaries set by our patients.

Age Concern 12 principles of good death[9]
1 To be able to retain **control** of what happens
2 To have **control** over pain relief and other symptom control
3 To have **choice and control** over where death occurs (at home or elsewhere)
4 To have **access** to hospice care in any location, not only in hospital
5 To have **control** over who is present and who shares the end
6 To be able to issue **Advance Directives** which ensure wishes are respected
7 To know when death is coming, and to understand what can be expected
8 To be afforded dignity and privacy
9 To have **access** to information and expertise of whatever kind is necessary
10 To have **access** to any spiritual or emotional support required
11 To have time to say goodbye, and **control** over other aspects of timing
12 To be able to leave when it is time to go, and not to have life prolonged pointlessly.

Preferred place of death
Asking and noting where patients would like to be cared for in their dying phase is a very significant step towards the tailoring of services to meet patient preferences and needs. This is a key issue in developing a real sense of choice, maintaining some control and self-determination in a world seemingly turned upside down for patients and their carers. The literature confirms that where someone has been asked about preference for place of care it is more likely to be attained, and choice of place of death is increasingly seen now as a patient's right. However, many may express a preference for home or hospice care, but are currently unable to achieve this. Carers are our patients in primary care and also have their own needs, as the toll of caring for the dying patient may be considerable.[10]

Patient needs
We all have needs, whether acknowledged or not. In 1943[11] Maslow proposed that we are all motivated by our wish continually to satisfy our needs. He commented that there were at least five sets of goals which he called basic needs. Briefly, these are:
1 Physiological (food, sleep, warmth, health)
2 Safety (security, protection from threats)

7 Clark D. (2002) *Cicely Saunders, Founder of the Hospice Movement—selected letters 1959–1999.* Oxford: Oxford University Press.

8 Fallowfield L. J., Jenkins V. A., Beveridge H. A. (2002) Truth may hurt but deceit hurts more: communication in palliative care. *Palliative Medicine.* **16**: 297–303.

9 Henwood M. (1999) *The Future of Health and Care of Older People.* London: Age Concern.

10 Simon C. (2001) Informal carers and the primary care team. *British Journal of General Practice,* **51**: 920–3.

11 Maslow A. H. (1943) A theory of human motivation. *Psychological Review,* **50**: 370–96.

Table 12.1 Summary of suggested needs-based care—for the Gold Standards Framework

Need	Outcome	Process	Structure
Hierarchy of need of patient (after Maslow)	Patient feeling—'inner' dimension	Provision—'outer' determinant	Practical measure—examples of suggested means or intervention
1 Physiological	Comfort Health Functioning body	Symptom relief—free of physical symptoms	Assessment-physical Specialist advice out-of-hours palliative care and access to 24h DNs SC Register—identification
2 Safety	Security and support Lack of fear + anxiety Protected from threats	Emotional support Information Continuity of care Practical support Anticipatory care Financial help	Assessment—psychosocial/holistic Information out-of-hours Protocol access to key person Equal access to resources+equipment SC Register—identification PHCT planning and co-ordination Financial + benefits advice

3 Social	Love Belonging Acceptance Harmonious relationships	Supportive, loving relationships Dealing with emotions	Active listening Communication skills Information Family dynamics and carer support
4 Esteem	Dignity Self respect Feeling good about themselves	Control, choice, confidentiality Respect Humane treatment Empowerment Being valued Truth and honesty	Consultation Information e.g. Home pack Agenda-sharing Patient Review sheets in Home Pack
5 Self-actualization	Spiritual peace Personal growth Inner calm	Acceptance Finding meaning Hope, wisdom Dealing with inner fears and all of the above	Time, prayer Supportive relationship Spiritual needs addressed, religious support and all of the above

SC = Supportive Care
PHCT = Primary Healthcare Team

Barriers to community palliative care

The care of all dying patients must improve to the level of the best.
                                        The NHS Cancer Plan, DOH, September 2000

Palliative care is a barometer for all our other care... and we only have one chance
to get it right.
                                                                    DN Liverpool

Several studies confirm that GPs, district nurses and other community
professionals prioritize care of the dying. Yet, despite this high priority,
service provision can be less than optimal. This may be due to lack of communication, poor team working, out-of-hours factors, limited carer
support or difficulties with symptom control. But commonly the major
problem is that the different instruments in the orchestra are not playing
together.

> The challenge is to orchestrate the service so that the patient and carers
> feel enveloped in professional, seamless, supportive care allowing them
> 'a good death' in the place of their choice.

Current gaps in community palliative care provision include (key factors
in **bold**):

1 Clinical competence
  • Assessment of symptoms and diagnostic skills
  • **Symptom control** and drug usage
  • When to refer or seek help
2 Organizational
  • Communication and information transfer
  • Access to other support—social care and **carer support**
  • Continuity including **out-of-hours**
  • Primary care issues—workforce, time and workload
  • **Teamwork** and co-working with specialists
3 Human dimension
  • Patient **control**, autonomy and choice
  • **Supportive care**
  • Listening to deeper underlying needs and spiritual reflections

Specific issues

• **Rôle of the primary healthcare teams.** Primary care teams play a
  pivotal rôle in the delivery and coordination of care. Using a framework
  to increase consistency of standards and formalize good practice
  ensures fewer patients 'slip through the net'. District nurses play a
  crucial rôle in needs assessment, the development of a therapeutic
  relationship and are well placed to liaise across the boundaries of care
  between community and inpatient services
• The main barriers to effective community palliative care however, are
  lack of an organized system or plan of care, communication and team
  working issues, out-of-hours care, carer support, good symptom
  control and effective involvement of specialists

- **Out-of-hours palliative care and 24h district nurses.** The out-of-hours gap in provision can cause significant breakdown in home care and inappropriate crisis admissions to hospitals. Anticipatory planning along with better access to information (e.g. via a handover form), drugs left in the home or carried by the on-call provider (as in palliative care bags held by GP cooperatives) and better access to support at home and specialist advise, can prevent many crises. Lack of out-of-hours district nursing is an important issue and is a first step to improving community palliative care. More terminally ill patients are kept at home where there is 24h district nursing availability
- **The social care of patient and carer at home** is seen consistently as one of the key factors that will prevent institutionalized care, as confirmed in the literature and the experience of professionals. So the availability and coordination of night sitters, Marie Curie nurses, social services input, rapid response teams etc. play a vital rôle in maintaining home care. This is sometimes overlooked in the strategic planning of services. Well functioning co-operation between healthcare and social services is crucial, with continuing care funds or their equivalent, carer assessments, non-medical support, respite care, carer support groups, grants and financial advice being of vital importance
- **Preferred place of care.** Care customized to patient need is another crucial factor, and one vital element of this is choice over where a person wishes to be in their final days. Most people would chose to remain at home to die but this is less likely to occur with some groups of patients, particularly the poor, the elderly, women etc. *Asking and recording the patient's preferred place of death/care has been shown to makes this more likely to be fulfilled. This requires time, good communication skills and a trusting relationship with the patient and carers.* Good use of assessment tools, discussion with the patient and family of their management plans (a 'death plan' in a similar manner to a 'birth plan' in obstetrics), Advance Directives, discussion of 'Do Not Resuscitate' (DNR) decisions (and informing of ambulance staff), route-maps of likely options. These all help to involve patients and families in decisions, enabling some retention of control and self-determination. With better planning and communication, this may also prevent some disasters e.g. emergency calls, failed attempted resuscitations in the ambulance or inappropriate coroner's cases
- **Specialist palliative care and effective symptom control.** There is a need for specialists to work effectively with generalists and there are many good examples of this working well in the UK. Clear referral criteria and regular formalized contact at primary care team meetings, plus availability of telephone advice, can enable more effective working relationships. Symptom control in the community can be difficult, so supportive relationships with specialists helps, along with targeted education programmes, better assessment tools, and agreed guidelines
- **Communication and transfer of information.** Poor organization in this area can create an unbridgeable chasm for all involved, reducing patients' confidence in their professional carers and adding stress to staff. Several factors have been shown to improve information transfer:
  - Using practice registers
  - Handover forms for out-of-hours providers

- Patient held records or medication cards, electronic transfer of information
- Ensuring patients and carers have written information at home to consult when problems arise
- Home packs (potentially needed medication and equipment)

- **Non-cancer patients.** There is less access to services for patents with non-malignant disease than that for cancer patients. GPs will have as many patients dying from organ failure, e.g. heart failure or COPD, as from cancer and yet the disease trajectory is less predictable and the end-stages harder to recognize. Crisis hospital admissions are more frequent, yet there is less specialist involvement or access to supportive cancer-related services such as Marie Curie or Macmillan nurses. Those dying from chronic 'multiple pathology' illnesses causing general decline or dementia may be disadvantaged further. The learning gained from cancer patients may be transferred to care for other end-stage illnesses (as in the Gold Standards Framework) and there is increasing recognition that patients with other end-stage illnesses should be able to benefit from palliative care symptom control, advice, and services

- **Other care settings.** Some patients dying in other settings may be significantly disadvantaged, as they currently do not benefit from specialist palliative care services or even from the generic skills of generalists within the primary care teams. Provision for good palliative care in other settings therefore needs to be included in the area-wide strategic plan, e.g. in care homes, private hospitals, prisons and community hospitals

Specific issues in community palliative care

Out-of-hours palliative care

'It was awfull—just panicked! My husband was in agony. It was three o'clock in the morning. We were at home all alone. It was dark and frightening and we didn't know what to do or who to turn to. Things all came together to make his pain seem much worse than it really was.'

Reducing the burden of symptoms suffered by patients and their carers at home remains a challenging round-the-clock priority. For this to be addressed we need to plan for out-of-hours palliative care services in the community, dovetailing generalist palliative care from GPs, district nurses and their out-of-hours providers with the available specialist palliative care skills and resources.[20] Several protocols have been developed[21]—one such four point plan has been shown to improve care as judged by practitioners' experience.[22]

Suggestions to improve out-of-hours palliative care in the UK

1 **Develop a local protocol**—coordinate a meeting of all out-of-hours health professionals involved in care of the seriously or terminally ill. This would include the GP cooperative, the deputizing service, PCT or health authority, district nurses and specialist doctors. Improve anticipatory care and proactive planning by the PHCT.

2 Look at **communication** and efficient transfer of information between those working in hours and out-of-hours. Use a paper or electronic handover form which is kept by the patient/the district nurse and out-of-hours service. Make sure the patient and the carer know what to do in an emergency.

3 Ensure 24h **carer support**, including 24h access to nursing care. Night sitters and respite care should also be easily available. Preventing a breakdown in the carer system is key to avoiding inappropriate crisis admissions.

4 Make best use of the **specialist advice** out-of-hours and expertise available through the local hospice/SPC service.

5 Keep in the patient's home an adequate supply of **drugs** (including a range for dose increases) and p.r.n. drugs for predictable symptoms, such as hyoscine, midazolam, diamorphine and cyclizine/haloperidol. Coordinate equipment access. On-call cars or out-of-hours centres could hold special palliative care bags.

See the five recommendations of the Macmillan Out of hours Palliative Care report—www.macmillan.org.uk or gsf@macmillan.org.uk

Improving access to palliative care drugs

1 Suggested list of drugs to be left in the home of every palliative care patient Diamorphine, cyclizine, midazolam, hyoscine butylbromide
2 Suggested drug list in palliative care bags carried by out-of-hours provider to be locally agreed
 • Midazolam, haloperidol, cyclizine, hyoscine butylbromide, levomepromazine, rectal diazepam, dexamethasone, metoclopramide, ?glycopyrronium, ?diclofenac, controlled drugs used with special CD measures—diamorphine, oral morphine solution

Summary of four point plan for out-of-hours palliative care
From Calderdale and Kirklees Health Authority West Yorkshire

1 Communication:
 • use handover form—GP/DN to write and fax to on-call service, keep in DN notes
 • inform others e.g. hospice
 • does the carer know what to do in a crisis?
2 Carer support:
 • coordinate pre-emptive care e.g. nightsitters, 24h district nursing service
 • give written information to carers
 • emergency support e.g. Rapid Response Team
3 Medical support:
 • anticipated management in handover form
 • crisis pack, guidelines etc and ongoing teaching
 • 24h specialist advice available from hospice
4 Drugs/equipment:
 • leave anticipated drugs in home
 • Special palliative care bag with drugs and information available on-call
 • on-call stocked pharmacists

Communication—handover form
The handover form has two important functions:
1 To improve information transfer
2 To build in anticipatory care.

The process of completing such a form is part of the benefit—if you think that a patient might become agitated or develop a 'rattly chest' over a weekend, leave some midazolam or hyoscine in the home, for administration either by the on-call doctor or district nurse. If the on-call doctor presented with the handover form notes that the patient has stated a preference to remain at home, there is more chance that they will be enabled to do so. Many are developed electronically and being used by central

20 Thomas K. (2000) Out-of-hours palliative care—bridging the gap. *Eur J Pall Care*, **7**: 22–5.

21 Munday D. (2002) Out-of-hours and emergency palliative care. In R. Charlton (ed.) *Primary Palliative Care.* Oxford: Radcliffe Medical Press.

22 King N., Bell D., Thomas K. (2003) An out-of-hours protocol for community palliative care. *International Journal of Palliative Nursing*, **9**, 7: 277–82

- Ensure staff are informed about the needs and problems of informal carers
- Respond quickly and sympathetically to crisis situations
- Training—e.g. in lifting, giving medication etc
- Confiding in and being listened to, needs expressed and supported, often outside the home
- Coping strategies, both internal (faith, positive attitude etc) and external (social networks)
- Development of a bereavement protocol and raising awareness of bereaved patients in practice teams. Assemble a list of local contacts for bereavement support

---

I was terrified at first when they said they would discharge him home—I didn't think I could cope. But in looking after Peter dying at home, I felt I was fulfilling his wishes and we were a real family—this really helps me now. Our GPs and district nurses were really caring and professional and kept pace with us at every stage—we felt very grateful to them. Although it was so sad, it was also in some ways a very good and satisfying experience, etched forever on our minds. The children and I are glad that we were able to look after him at home, where he wanted to be, with the help of our marvellous team.

Maureen, wife of Peter, a cancer patient

The vast majority of care in the last year of life is not provided by professionals, but by relatives and friends, especially wives and daughters. The support provided by a family caregiver may make all the difference for the dying person in their place of death: some have reported that up to 90 per cent of terminal admissions to hospice are due to the stress of caring on the relatives, or lack of resources available to support the patient at home. The relationship between carers and professionals is often an ambiguous one. For over half the carers, the only supportive service that they are in touch with is their GP.[28]

Bereavement (📖 see Chapter 14)

The loss of a loved person is one of the most intensely painful experiences any human being can suffer, not only is it painful to experience, but it is also painful to witness.[29]

There is a significant increase in morbidity and mortality in grief, making dying of a broken heart a reality for some. The main causes of bereavement associated death are heart disease, alcohol-induced cirrhosis, suicide, road accidents or other violent death. Bereavement is the greatest psychological trauma people can go through, and yet in some cases the carers are not given the 'preventative care' that could ameliorate future problems. The immediate bereavement visit straight after a death is much appreciated but will not in itself constitute the kind of help that heals. Initiating regular support and contact, actively listening, planning even brief follow-up care, tagging notes, awareness of risk factors etc. as well as referral to specialist groups are all proactive means of caring for carers and preventing the feeling of desertion at this most vulnerable time. Recognizing the sense of loss that staff may feel is also important and is where the development of a team approach through shared meetings can be of benefit, especially when there is a sense of guilt of less than perfect care. Care of dying patients, though very rewarding, is also an area of care that many professionals find stressful and challenging, so support for staff is essential.

Other providers of community palliative care

Specialist palliative care services

Clinical nurse specialists, Macmillan and Marie Curie nurses, hospice general staff and home care teams and Hospice at Home initiatives have long been involved in bringing quality palliative care services into patients' homes.

This can only be successfully achieved *in partnership* with generalists from the patient's usual primary care team.

Care homes

Care homes provide important nursing and residential care especially for the frail and alone, although numbers of beds are limited. More people die in care homes than in hospices and, although the palliative care provided in such homes can vary in quality, there is great interest in palliative care education and use of protocols to improve standards of care.

Community hospitals

Particularly in rural areas, community hospitals are a valuable and greatly appreciated resource, allowing continuity of care from GPs and nurses in a more localized environment. Guidelines and protocols exist to maintain high standards.

The 'key worker' rôle

User and patient groups consistently emphasize the value of having one person, a key worker, to relate to, as advocate, advisor and supporter. Some primary care teams have developed this rôle within the practice team, allowing continuity of support from diagnosis, through treatment to bereavement care. For others, a hospital clinical nurse specialist, hospice staff member or other professional may take on this rôle for part of the time and a trusting relationship may develop. Support at the life-changing time of diagnosis and also for the carer are crucial, and may otherwise be overlooked. This person may also be able to reduce inappropriate hospital admissions, unwanted interventions or appointments, thus improving hospital capacity.

Marie Curie staff

Marie Curie community nurses and sitters in the UK work usually through the night to enable patients to remain at home in the final days of illness *and support* carers. Their rôle is acknowledged and appreciated at this critical time.

Allied health professionals and others in the community

There are many others who contribute considerably—pharmacists, physiotherapists, occupational therapists, chaplains, clergy and other religious leaders, voluntary groups, bereavement services and mobilizers of local resources can all play crucial roles in providing quality holistic care.

28 Barclay S. (2001) Palliative care for non-cancer patients: a UK perspective from primary care. In J. Addington-Hall, I. Higginson (eds) *Palliative Care for Non-cancer Patients*. Oxford: Oxford University Press.

29 Bowlby J. (1969) *Attachment and Loss, Vol. 1*. Harmondsworth: Penguin.

Different GPs—GP facilitators, primary care cancer leads and GPs with a special onterest (GPwSIs)

Macmillan GP facilitators have the rôle of:

- educating their colleagues within primary care
- enhancing local service provision for patients in the community

Primary Care Organization (PCO) cancer leads in England focus on improving the strategic planning of services for cancer patients.

GPs with a special interest (GPwSIs) include some with extra clinical training in palliative care and are a new initiative, especially useful in areas short of palliative medicine specialists.

Supportive care guidance

Supportive care is defined as care designed to help patients and families cope. The Supportive and Palliative Care Guidance,[30] commissioned in England as part of the NHS Cancer Plan, makes recommendations to improve the vital areas of care not directly related to curative treatment, i.e. that of palliative care (generalist and specialist), psychological, social and family care, rehabilitation, coordination, communication, information, spiritual support etc. underpinned throughout by user involvement. This guidance is likely to be used in the future planning and commissioning of services, including those in the community, for patients throughout their cancer journey.

---

30 National Institute for Clinical Excellence (2004) *Guidance on Cancer Services: improving supportive and palliative care for adults with cancer: the manual.* London: NICE.

Working partnerships with palliative care specialists

Good effective partnerships with palliative care specialists will ensure best care for patients and their families. Involvement of specialists in primary palliative care can be very fruitful e.g. in local education and training programmes, targeted teaching on individual patient case histories, invitations to team meetings, agreed use of assessment tools and templates, out-of-hours protocols and advice, strategic planning of services and hospice outreach etc. With good relationships and lines of communication, and with roles and responsibilities clarified, there can be excellent dovetailing of generalist and specialist skills, for the benefit of all.

Referral to specialist palliative care services

Eligibility criteria for specialist palliative care help clarify what is expected of both generalist and specialist palliative care providers.[31] By attempting to crystallize and improve 'generalist' palliative care, and better integration with the 'specialist' services available a more comprehensive, and equitable service for those in the last stages of life could be provided.

> ### Eligibility criteria for referrals to specialist palliative care services[32]
> *Eligible patients have:*
> 1 Any active progressive and potentially *life-threatening* disease.
> 2 *Anticipated or actual unresolved*, complex needs that cannot be met by the caring team ie physical, psychological, social, spiritual needs e.g. complicated symptoms, specialist nursing needs, difficult family situations, ethical issues regarding treatment decisions.
> 3 Been recently *assessed* by a member of one of the specialist palliative care teams.

31 Ellershaw J. E., Boyes L.M Peat S. (1995) Assessing the effectiveness of a hospital palliative care team. *Pall Med*, **9**: 145–52.

32 Bennett M., Adam J., Alison D., Hicks F., Stockton M. (2000) Leeds Eligibility Criteria for specialist palliative care services. *Pall Med*, **14, 2**: 157–8.

Further reading

Addington-Hall J., Higginson I. (2001) *Palliative Care for Non-cancer Patients*. Oxford: Oxford University Press.

Charlton R. (ed.) (2003) *Primary Palliative Care*. Oxford: Radcliffe Medical Press.

Cooper J. (ed.) (2000) *Stepping into Palliative Care: a handbook for community professionals*. Oxford: Radcliffe Medical Press.

Doyle D., Jeffrey D. (2000) *Palliative Care in the Home*. Oxford: Oxford University Press.

Ellershaw J., Wilkinson S. (2003) *Care of the Dying: A pathway to excellence*. Oxford: Oxford University Press.

Lee E. (2002) *In Your Own Time: A guide for patients and their carers facing a last illness at home*. Oxford: Oxford University Press.

Lynn J. (2000) *Improving Care for End of Life: A sourcebook for health managers and clinicians*. New York: Oxford University Press.

Thomas K. (2003) *Caring for the Dying at Home: Companions on the journey*. Oxford: Radcliffe Medical Press.

Useful web sites are:
www.goldstandardswframework.nhs.uk/gsf
www.hospice-spc-council.org.uk
www.macmillan.org.uk
www.modern.nhs.uk/cancer
www.palliativedrugs.com
www.palliative-medicine.org

Further reading

The terminal phase

The terminal phase is defined as the period when day to day deterioration, particularly of strength, appetite and awareness, are occurring.

Prognosis

Patients frequently ask, 'How long have I got?' It is notoriously difficult to predict when death will occur, and it is wise to avoid the trap of predicting or making an incorrect guess. If pushed to do so, it should be made clear that any predictions are only a guide. It is best to talk in terms of 'days', or 'weeks' or 'months', as appropriate.

For example:

'When we see someone deteriorating from week to week we are often talking in terms of weeks, when that deterioration is from day to day then we are usually talking in terms of days, but everyone is different.'

Research has shown that nurses, relatives and domestic assistants in hospices are often better at predicting the approach of death than medical staff.

Signs and symptoms of death approaching[1]
The clearest signs of approaching death are picked up by the day by day assessment of deterioration.

Profound weakness	Bed-bound
	Needs assistance with all care
Diminished intake of food and fluids	
Drowsy or reduced cognition	May be disorientated in time and place
	Difficulty concentrating
	Scarcely able to co-operate with carers
Gaunt appearance	
Difficulty swallowing medicine	

Should such symptoms develop suddenly over a matter of days instead of the usual weeks, it is important to exclude a reversible cause of deterioration such as infection, hypercalcaemia, or medication changes.

Goals for the last 24 h
- Ensure the patient's comfort physically, emotionally and spiritually
- Make the end-of-life peaceful and dignified
- By care and support given to the dying patient and their carers make the memory of the dying process as positive as possible

[1] National Council for Hospice and Specialist Palliative Care Services (1997) *Changing Gear— Guidelines for Managing the Last Days of Life in Adults.* London: NCHSPCS 7.

It is very important to continually seek the patient's views on, and feelings about treatment while they remain conscious, even when the weakening state makes communication difficult. Relatives also need to be given time to have their questions, concerns, and requests for information listened to and answered as clearly as possible. As the patient deteriorates, the family's advocate rôle becomes more important, though their wishes need to be balanced with the palliative care team's understanding of the patient's needs.

Where possible, families and carers should be offered the opportunity to participate in the physical care of patients. Carers should be invited to stay, if they want to, while nursing and medical procedures are carried out. Very occasionally relatives would like to participate in laying out the body after death, and this can be a very important part of their last 'duty' on behalf of their dead loved one.

The events and the atmosphere which are present at the time of a patient's death can great influence the grieving process of those left behind.

Cardiopulmonary resuscitation
The issue of cardiopulmonary resuscitation (CPR) has again come to the fore with stories of patients learning that doctors had written 'Not for Resuscitation' in a patient's notes without them being consulted. The response from the medical profession has been to advise that 'Not for Resuscitation' should only be written into the notes after a full discussion with the patient and family has taken place. Nurses can face very difficult situations if they are unsure what their response should be if a particular patient suddenly deteriorates.

1 Many hospices have a policy that they do not carry out CPR and patients have to 'opt in' rather than 'opt out' of resuscitation.
2 Ultimately it is the doctor's decision whether it is in the patient's best interest for a resuscitation attempt to be made.
3 Frank and open discussion with the patient and the family, before admission, about the hospice's resuscitation policy can be a great help, provided that the information is recorded clearly in the medical records.

Different cultures
Different religious and cultural groupings have divergent approaches to the dying process. It is important to be sensitive to their possible beliefs. If in doubt, ask a family member. Offence is more likely to be caused by not asking than by asking.

The patient's wishes
Dying is a very special event for each individual. Helping to explore patients' wishes about death and dying should, if possible, take place before they reach the final 24 h. Important discussions can still, however, take place even at this late phase and professionals should encourage this dialogue. The family gain great comfort in knowing that they have made the most of pre-cious moments and that they have the answers to issues that are important to both of them. Some of these questions can include preferred place of death or burial/cremation and financial or 'unfinished' business issues. Time

to say last goodbyes to close family members, children and dependents and time to forgive and bury guilt can be crucial to enable a normal bereavement.

Collaborative multidisciplinary approach

Effective terminal care needs a team approach. No single member of the palliative care team, no matter how committed or gifted, can meet all the palliative care needs of a patient and their family.

Effective multidisciplinary working depends on:
- Recognising the centrality of patient and family needs
- Good communication
- Clear understanding and respect for the value, importance and rôle of other professionals
- Early referral to specialist palliative services if needed

Referral to Specialist Palliative Care services is appropriate when:
- One or more distressing symptoms prove difficult to control
- There is severe emotional distress associated with the patient's condition
- There are dependent children and or elderly vulnerable relatives

Assessment of patients' needs

The focus in assessment in the last 48 h is to discover what, apart from dying itself, the patient is most concerned about and which concerns need to be addressed. Patients may under-report their symptoms which distresses families. Families may be very helpful in interpreting non-verbal clues but, in their own distress, may also misperceive and exaggerate the patient's symptoms which needs careful handling.

Physical needs

Common problems that need to be addressed are nausea, pain, oral problems, sleep disturbance, weakness, feeling confused (and sometimes hallucinating), pressure sores and the burden of having to take medication. Patients rarely worry about nutritional and fluid intake, but this may be a major concern for the family.

Psychological needs

The key to psychological assessment is finding out what the patient wants to know. Gently assessing how the patient feels about their disease and situation can shed light on their needs and distress. How the patient interprets their disease and its symptoms may be a cause of suffering itself. Deep probing at this stage, however, is inappropriate as the goal is psychological comfort and peace, NOW.

Anxiety and agitation may need to be managed with medication. Patients are more often concerned about the family at this stage than about themselves.

Fears associated with symptoms	e.g. the pain will escalate to agony, breathing will stop if I fall asleep.
Other emotional distress	e.g. dependence on family, ('I am a burden and it would be better if I was out of the way').
Past experience	e.g. past contact with patients who died in unpleasant circumstances.
Preferences about treatment or withholding treatment	e.g. 'What if nobody listens to me or takes my wishes seriously?'
Fears about morphine	e.g. 'If I use morphine now, it will not work when I really need it.'
Death and dying	e.g. Patients frequently adapt to the fact that they will die, but are fearful of the process leading up to death.

Dignity

The palliative care team need to have as a goal the maintenance of the patient's dignity in a manner which is appropriate to that particular patient. What is dignified for one patient may not be for another, which is one of the reasons why many hospices have both single rooms and small wards.

Spiritual needs

There may be particular religious tasks to be accomplished such as absolution, confession, or other forms of religious preparation. Spiritual disquiet or pain may be relieved by allowing expression of feelings and thoughts, particularly fear and loss of control. Patients are more often concerned about the family at this stage than about themselves and may need to address unresolved conflict or guilt.

Families often want to know that the patient is comfortable and not suffering. If appropriate, it may be helpful for them to be aware of the experiences of people who have had near death experiences which are described as tranquil and peaceful. Many mechanisms have been used to explain this phenomenon including the release of endorphins (natural analgesics), retinal hypoxia with resultant neuronal discharge (particularly in the fovea where there are many neurones) so that a bright spot looks like the end of an inviting tunnel. Temporal lobe seizures may also provide an explanation. Whatever the mechanism, nature seems to have a way of allowing dying humans to feel comforted and at peace at the end.

Talking about death and dying

As a taboo subject, few people feel comfortable about discussing death, even though it is natural, certain, and is happening all around us all the time.

Opening up discussion can be very liberating to patients who can feel they have not been given permission to talk about dying as this would be admitting defeat.

Sometimes the direct question 'Are you worried about dying?' is most appropriate.

Often a patient's biggest fears are groundless and reassurances can be given. Where reassurance cannot be given it is helpful to break the fear down into constituent parts and try to deal with the aspects of the fear which can be dealt with.

Physical examination

Examination at this stage is kept to the minimum to avoid unnecessary distress. Examine:

- Any site of potential pain. Patients may be comfortable at rest but in pain on being turned, which they may not readily admit
- Any relevant area of the body that might be causing discomfort as suggested by history or non-verbal signs
- Mouth

Investigations

Any investigation at the end-of-life should have a clear and justifiable purpose, such as excluding reversible conditions, where treatment would make the patient more comfortable. There is little need for investigations in the terminal stages.

Review of medication

At this stage comfort is the priority. Unnecessary medication should be stopped but analgesics, anti-emetics, anxiolytics/antipsychotics and anticonvulsants will need to be continued. Diabetes can be managed with a short-acting insulin as needed. If the patient is unable to swallow essential medicines, an alternative route of administration is necessary. These changes needs to be explained to relatives, who may become anxious that tablets which the patient has had to take for years have now suddenly stopped.

Treatment of symptoms

Dying patients tolerate symptoms very poorly because of their weakness. Important factors:

- Excellence in nursing care
- Prevention of new problems developing by e.g. using appropriate mattresses, thereby preventing bed sores
- Treating specific symptoms such as a dry mouth
- Anticipating the probable needs of the patients so that immediate response can be made when the time comes

Routes for Medicine in the Terminal Phase

The **intramuscular** route for injections should be avoided as it is too painful.

If **buccal** medicines are given it is important that the mouth is kept moist.

The **rectal** route can be very useful for certain patients though is more or less accepted in different cultures.

Topical Fentanyl patches should be avoided in the terminal stage unless they have been used before this time, since it takes too long to titrate against a patient's pain.

In many instances a **syringe driver** containing diamorphine is used so that adjustments can be made more finely in accord with the patient's changing state.

Even when patients are dying, it is often possible to communicate with them and to get their consent for certain treatment, such as subcutaneous medication. As the patient becomes less aware, however, it is the relatives and the nursing staff who become the patient's advocate. At this point a clear plan of goals needs to be agreed between the doctors, nurses and family members.

- The potentially sedative side-effects of analgesia needs to be explained
- The use of alternative routes of medication need to be discussed, as the oral route may be more difficult
- The treatment plan should define clearly what should be done in the event of a symptom breakthrough

Common problems in last 48 h
- Noisy, moist breathing
- Pain
- Restlessness/agitation
- Breathlessness
- Nausea/vomiting
- Myoclonic twitching

Noisy, moist breathing (death rattle)

This is very distressing to relatives, and should be treated prophylactically as it is easier to prevent secretions forming than removing secretions that have gathered in the upper airways or oropharynx.

Management

General measures include re-positioning the patient and giving reassurance to the relatives. It should be explained that the noise is due to secretions collecting which are no longer being coughed or cleared as normal. They should also know that the secretions are not causing suffocation, choking or distress.

Specific measures

These specific guidelines are for patients who are imminently dying and develop 'rattling' or 'bubbly' breathing (the death rattle). The following guidelines should be used with caution, particularly if the patient is still aware enough to be distressed by the dry mouth that will result from treatment.

Acute pulmonary oedema should be excluded, or treated with furosemide.

- Give hyoscine hydrobromide 400mcg stat subcutaneously, and start hyoscine hydrobromide 1.2–1.6mg/24h CSCI
- Wait for half an hour and reassess the patient. If there is still an unacceptable rattle, and there has not been a marked improvement:
- Give a further dose of hyoscine hydrobromide 400mcg stat SC
- Wait for half an hour and reassess
- If the noise has been relieved, but recurs later, give repeat doses of hyoscine hydrobromide 400mcg to a maximum of 800mcg in any 4h
- Increase CSCI to 2.4mg/24h
  NB Hyoscine hydrobromide can cause sedation and confusion

If the patient is conscious, and respiratory secretions are not too distressing, it may be adequate to use a transdermal patch (Scopaderm 1.5mg over three days or sublingual tablets (Kwells).

If the noise of secretions is not relieved:

1 Try an alternative, e.g:
  - Glycopyrronium bromide 0.2mg stat. or CSCI 0.6–1.2mg/24h
  - Glycopyrronium does not cause sedation or confusion. It is useful for the patient who is still conscious and wishes to remain as alert as possible
  - Hyoscine butylbromide (buscopan) 20mg SC stat. and 60–90mg CSCI. Since it does not cross the blood—brain barrier, buscopan is less sedating than hyoscine hydrobromide

2 If the respiratory rate is >20 breaths per minute, the noise may be reduced by slowing the respiratory rate: give diamorphine 2.5–5mg SC (or a sixth of the 24h dose if already on CSCI) and repeat after 30 minutes if respiratory rate still above 20 per minute.

3 If the noise appears to be coming from the back of the pharynx, try tipping the bed 30 degrees 'head-up', allowing the secretions to drain back into the lungs from the throat or trachea.

4 If the patient is deeply unconscious, try using gentle suction.

5 Ensure that the patient is not distressed, using sedative drugs such as midazolam if necessary.

The Liverpool Care Pathway for the dying patient

The preceeding section detailing the last 48 h of life, practical issues and bereavement in this handbook clearly outline good practice for care of the dying. The Liverpool Integrated Care Pathway for the Dying Patient (LCP) aims to translate such best practice into a template of care to guide healthcare professionals with limited or infrequent experience of caring for dying patients. The next section will explain how this best practice can be incorporated into a care pathway which can be used both as an educational tool and to provide a template of care within practice.

There are three sections of the Liverpool Care Pathway for the dying patient:

1 Initial assessment and care of the dying patient
2 Ongoing care of the dying patient
3 Care of the family and carers after death of the patient.

Initiating the Liverpool Care Pathway for the dying patient (LCP)—diagnosing dying

Before a patient is commenced on the Liverpool Care Pathway it is important that the multidisciplinary team have agreed that the patient is in the dying phase. This decision in itself can sometimes lead to conflict within the team, but it is important to make a clear diagnosis if appropriate care and communication is to be achieved.

In cancer patients, if the patient's condition has been deteriorating over a period of time, i.e. the last weeks/days, and two of the following four criteria apply:

- The patient is bed bound
- Semi-comatose
- Only able to take sips of fluid
- Unable to take tablets

it is likely that the patient is entering the dying phase. *These criteria may not be appropriate in a non-cancer population.* It is important to highlight that a patient who is clinically in the dying phase may occasionally recover and stabilize for a period of time. However, this should not prevent the clinical team from using the LCP to provide the appropriate physical, psychological, social and spiritual care.

The three sections of the Liverpool Care Pathway for the dying patient

Section 1—Initial assessment and care of the dying patient

This section identifies the key goals that should be achieved when a patient enters the dying phase. These goals are directly related to and support the guidance given in the chapter on the last 48 h of life regarding the terminal phase. A key component of the LCP is the supporting guidelines for the symptoms of pain, agitation and respiratory tract secretions. These are shown in Figure 13.1. These guidelines ensure that appropriate oral medication is converted to a subcutaneous regimen and that patients have p.r.n. (as required) medication available should they develop

COMFORT MEASURES	**Goal 1: Current medication assessed and non essentials discontinued** Yes ❏ No ❏ Appropriate oral drugs converted to subcutaneous route and syringe driver commenced if appropriate Inappropriate medication discontinued
	Goal 2: PRN subcutaneous medication written up for list below as per protocol *(see blue sheets at back of ICP for guidance)* Pain Analgesia **Yes ❏ No ❏** Nausea and vomiting Antiemetic **Yes ❏ No ❏** Agitation Sedative **Yes ❏ No ❏** Respiratory tract secretions Anticholinergic **Yes ❏ No ❏**
	Goal 3: Discontinue inappropriate interventions Blood test **Yes ❏ No ❏ N/A ❏** Antibiotics **Yes ❏ No ❏ N/A ❏** i V's (fluids/medications) **Yes ❏ No ❏ N/A ❏** Not for cardiopulmonary resuscitation **Yes ❏ No ❏** *(Please record below & complete appropriate associated documentation–policy/ procedure)*
	Goal 3a: Decisions to discontinue inappropriate nursing interventions taken Yes ❏ No ❏ Routine turning regime – reposition for comfort only – consider pressure relieving mattress–and appropriate assessments re skin integrity–Taking Vital Signs
	Goal 3b: Syringe driver set up within 4 h of Doctor's order Yes ❏ No ❏ N/A ❏
PSYCHOLOGICAL/ INSIGHT	**Goal 4: Ability to communicate in English assessed as adequate** a) Patient **Yes ❏ No ❏ Comatosed ❏** b) Family/other **Yes ❏ No ❏**

	Goal 5: Insight into condition assessed
	Aware of diagnosis a) Patient **Yes ❏ No ❏ Comatosed ❏**
	                b) Family/other **Yes ❏ No ❏**
	Recognition of dying c) Patient **Yes ❏ No ❏ Comatosed ❏**
	                d) Family/other **Yes ❏ No ❏**

RELIGIOUS/ SPIRITUAL SUPPORT	**Goal 6: a) Religious/spiritual needs assessed with patient** Yes ❏ No ❏ Comatosed ❏ **b) Religious/spiritual needs assessed with family/other** Yes ❏ No ❏ Patient/other may be anxious for self/others Consider support of chaplaincy team Religious tradition identified, if yes specify:............... **Yes ❏ No ❏ N/A❏** Support of chaplaincy-team offered **Yes ❏ No ❏** In-house support Tel/Bleep No: .... Name .... Date/Time .... External support Tel/Bleep No: .... Name .... Date/Time .... Special needs now, at time of impending death, at death and after death identified:- ....
COMMUNICATION WITH FAMILY/OTHER	**Goal 7: Identify how family/other are to be informed of patient's impending death** **Yes ❏ No ❏** At any time ❏ Not at night-time ❏ Stay overnight at hospital ❏ Primary contact name .... Relationship to patient .... Tel no: .... Secondary contact .... Tel no:.........
	Goal 8: Family/other given hospital information on:- **Yes ❏ No ❏** Concession car parking; accommodation; dining room facilities; payphones; washrooms and toilet facilities on the ward; visiting times. Any other relevant information
COMMUNICATION WITH PRIMARY HEALTHCARE TEAM	**Goal 9: GP Practice is aware of patient's condition** **Yes ❏ No ❏** GP Practice to be contacted if unaware patient is dying
SUMMARY	**Goal 10: Plan of care explained & discussed with:-** a) Patient **Yes ❏ No ❏ Comatosed ❏** b) Family/other **Yes ❏ No ❏**
	Goal 11: Family/other express understanding of plan care. **Yes ❏ No ❏** Family/other aware that LCP commenced and their concerns identified and documented

13.1 Initial Assessment and care of the dying patient

2 Ellershaw J. E., Wilkinson S. (eds) (2003) *Care of the Dying: A pathway to excellence.* Oxford: Oxford University Press. (2003).

symptoms in the dying phase. In care settings where the LCP is not in common usage, healthcare professionals can use the goals of care in Figure 13.1 to guide and inform their practice.

Section 2—Ongoing care of the dying patient
The LCP promotes multidisciplinary working and a joint approach to the care of the patient and their family. In caring for a dying patient, at least four-hourly observations of symptom control, and appropriate action if there are problems identified, should occur. Particular attention is given to pain, agitation, respiratory tract secretions, nausea and vomiting, mouthcare and micturition problems. Support regarding the psychological, social and spiritual aspects of care for the family and patient need to be continued in the dying phase.

Section 3—Care of the family and carers after the death of the patient
The LCP incorporates the certification of death within the document, identifies any special needs for the patient who has died and support for the family and carers immediately after death. It particularly focuses on the information needs of the family at this distressing time and includes a leaflet on bereavement care.

How does using the Liverpool Care Pathway benefit patients?

In providing a template of care for the dying phase, the LCP promotes discussion within the clinical team with regard to the diagnosis of dying, and facilitates the initiation of care which is appropriate for the dying phase. The LCP integrates local and national guidelines into clinical practice. It is a powerful educational tool which can be used to facilitate the rôle of specialist palliative care teams and to empower generic health workers to deliver a model of excellence for care of the dying. The LCP should ensure that patients die a dignified death and that their carers receive appropriate support. Healthcare professionals also benefit by knowing that they have delivered a good standard of care to the patient. In the words of the National Cancer Plan 'The care of all dying patients must be improved to the level of the best.'

Further reading

Books
de Luc K. (2000) *Developing Care Pathways*. Oxford: Radcliffe Medical Press.

Department of Health (2000) *The NHS Cancer Plan—A plan for investment, A plan for reform*. London: DoH.

Ellershaw J. E., Wilkinson S. (eds) (2003) *Care of the Dying: A pathway to excellence*. Oxford: Oxford University Press.

Articles
Campbell H., Hotchkiss R., Bradshaw N., Porteous M. (1998) Integrated care pathways. *BMJ*, **316**: 133–7.

Ellershaw J. E., Smith, C., Overill S., *et al.* (2001) Care of the dying. *Journal of pain & symptom management*, **21**: 12–17.

Elllershaw J. E., Ward C. (2003) Care of the dying patient: the last hours or days of life. *BMJ*, **326**: 30–4.

Bereavement

How small and selfish is sorrow. But it bangs one about until one is quite senseless.

Queen Elizabeth the Queen Mother, in a letter to Edith Sitwell
shortly after the death of King George VI

Grief is a normal reaction to a bereavement or other major loss. Its manifestations will vary from person to person but will often include physical, cognitive, behavioural and emotional elements. For a close personal bereavement, grief is likely to continue for a long time and may recur in a modified form, stimulated by anniversaries, future losses or other reminders. People are likely to be changed by the experience of grieving but most, in time, find that they are able to function well and enjoy life again.

Normal manifestations of grief

Physical manifestations

Symptoms experienced by a bereaved person may include hollowness in the stomach, tightness in the chest or throat, oversensitivity to noise, feeling short of breath, muscle weakness, lack of energy, dry mouth and a sense of depersonalization.

Emotional manifestations

For many, a sense of shock and numbness is the initial emotional response to bereavement. Feelings of anger (directed at family, friends, medical staff, God, the deceased or no one in particular) and feelings of guilt (relating to real or imagined failings) are common, as is a yearning or desire for the return of the deceased. Anxiety and a sense of helplessness and disorganization are also normal responses. Sadness is the most commonly recognized manifestation of grief, but the greatest depth of sadness, something akin to depression, is often not reached until many months after the death. Feelings of relief and freedom may also be present, although people may then feel guilty for having these feelings.

Cognitive manifestations

Disbelief and a sense of unreality are frequently present early in a bereavement. For a while elements of denial may also be present. The bereaved may be preoccupied with thoughts about the deceased. It is also not uncommon for the bereaved to have a sense (visual, auditory etc.) of the presence of the deceased. Short-term memory, the ability to concentrate and sense of purpose are frequently detrimentally affected.

Behavioural manifestations

Appetite and sleep may be disturbed and dreams involving the deceased, with their attendant emotional impact for the bereaved, are not infrequent. The bereaved person may withdraw socially, avoid reminders of the deceased or act in an absent-minded way. They may also engage in restless overactivity, behaviour which suggests that they are at some level searching for the deceased or visit places or carry objects which remind them of the deceased. Some people contemplate rapid and radical changes in their lifestyle (e.g. new relationship or move of house), which may represent a way of avoiding the pain of bereavement. Such rapid changes soon after a bereavement are not normally advisable.

Psychological/psychiatric models

> He was my North, my South, my East and West,
> My working week and my Sunday rest,
> My noon, my midnight, my talk, my song;
> I thought that love would last forever: I was wrong.
>
> W.H.Auden 1907–73: *Funeral Blues* (1936)

Grief and bereavement have been analysed over many years, and it is generally agreed that there are no single 'correct' or 'true' theories that explain the experience of loss or account for the emotions, experiences and cultural practices which characterize grief and mourning. Within broad cultural constraints, individuals manage bereavement in different ways, reflecting the diverse range of human responses. There are no strict rules in the UK about how people should behave, but the importance of ensuring that the bereaved are encouraged to express their emotions, to acknowledge the reality of the loss and to share thoughts and feelings with appropriate others, is recognized.

Theories of grief

Most cultures are aware of what happens after death and have ideas about how the bereaved should feel and behave. The range of beliefs, practices and rituals associated with death is large, particularly in multicultural societies, although many adapt to the customs of the host culture. Most religions support certain behaviours and practices both before and after death, but in an increasingly secular society this may now have less influence.

Psychological models

These are based on developmental notions of change and growth. It is assumed that bereavement is a process in which there is an outcome: individuals need to progress through phases or stages and tasks need to be accomplished. The theory is based on the fact that people have some control over their feelings and thoughts and that these can be accessed through talk. Individuals need to accept the reality of the loss so that the emotional energy can be released and redirected.

The effortful, mental process of withdrawing energy from the lost object is referred to as 'grief work'. It is essential to break relationships with the deceased, and to allow reinvestment of emotional energy and the formation of new relationships with others.

The most influential and earliest theories emerged from psychoanalysts such as Freud (1917), who also described normal and pathological grief. Bowlby (1969) proposed a complex theory of close human relationships in which separation triggers intense distress and behavioural responses.

Parkes (1996) proposed that people progress through phases in coming to terms with their loss and that they have to adapt to changes in relationships, social status and economic circumstances. Kubler Ross (1969) also proposed a staged model of emotional expression of loss described in terms of shock/denial, anger, bargaining, depression and ultimately acceptance.

Worden (1991) based his therapeutic model on phases of grief and tasks of mourning. He suggested that grief was a process, not a state, and that people needed to work through their reactions to loss to achieve a complete adjustment. Tasks that need to be accomplished in order to allow recovery from mourning included:

Task 1—To accept the reality of the loss
Task 2—To experience the pain of grief
Task 3—To adjust to an environment in which the deceased is missing
Task 4—To emotionally relocate the deceased and move on with life.

Stress and coping model

Stroebe and Schut (1999), in their dual process model of coping with grief, suggested that bereaved people tend to oscillate between loss-oriented experiences and restoration-oriented activity and that both are necessary to successfully negotiate the bereavement journey.

Social and relationship-focused models

Walters (1996) and Klass et al. (1996) have explored continuing bonds, emphasizing the importance for the living of interpreting the memory of the dead into their ongoing lives, recognizing the enduring influence of the deceased.

Stress and coping

These ideas are based on an assumption that if certain things, called stressors, are present in sufficient amounts, they trigger a stress response which is both physical and psychological. Humans are able to adapt to most things but things that challenge the adaptation process are considered to be stressful. The transactional model (Lazarus and Folkman 1991) proposed that any event may be seen as threatening and that cognitive appraisal is undertaken to estimate the degree of threat needed to mobilize resources to cope with it. Coping may focus on dealing with the threat directly (problem-focused), or may emphasize the emotional response (emotion-focused). Stroebe and Schut (1999) developed this idea proposing that after death people oscillate between restoration-focused coping (dealing with everyday life) and grief-focused coping (e.g. expressing their distress). People move between these extremes but become more restoration-focused with time. This is known as the dual processing model.

Continuity theory

This is based on an assumption that people wish to maintain feelings of continuity and that even though physical relationships may end at the time of death, relationships become transformed but remain important within the memory of the individual. Walters (1996) explored continuing bonds, emphasizing the importance for the living of interpreting the memory of the dead into their ongoing lives, recognizing their enduring influence.

Bereavement support

In practice, bereavement support whether through GPs or formally trained counsellors helps clients to tell their story. Staged or phased models are recognized, the bereaved being given affirmation that they are progressing satisfactorily along a path over time, even though this progression may not be linear.

It is recognizsed that people may become 'stuck' and unable to move through grief satisfactorily. Various techniques are used to support and encourage people to move forward and to begin engaging in life again.

GPs may become involved in grief counselling, but their main rôle is to screen for people who may be most at risk (📖 see below) from a complicated bereavement.

Specialist palliative care and bereavement

The philosophy of the hospice movement encompasses the care of patients and their families after death and into the bereavement period. The provision of bereavement support is regarded as integral to their services. Most services are based on the assumption that bereavement is a major stressful life event but that a minority experience substantial disruption to physical, psychological and social functioning.

Some argue that offering support to those people who have adequate internal and external resources can be disempowering and detrimental to coping. Bereavement support may include a broad range of activities such as social evenings, befriending, one to one counselling and support groups.

A mutlidisciplinary team including social workers, nurses chaplains, counsellors and doctors are usually involved. Occasionally clients present such difficult and complex problems that psychiatrists, clinical psychologists or other specialist healthcare workers may be required.

Table 14.1 Types of hospice and palliative care bereavement support for adults

Social activities	Supportive activities	Therapeutic activities
Condolence cards	Drop-in centre/coffee mornings	One-to-one counselling with professional or trained volunteer
Anniversary (of death) Cards	Self-help groups	Therapeutic support groups
Bereavement information leaflets	Information support groups	Drama, music or art therapy
Bereavement information resources (videos/books)	Volunteer visiting or befriending	Relaxation classes
Staff attending the funeral		Complementary therapies
Social evenings	Psychotherapy	
Memorial service or other rituals		

From M. Lloyd-Williams (ed.) (2003) *Psychosocial Issues in Palliative Care.* Oxford: Oxford University Press.

Complicated grief

Normal and abnormal responses to bereavement cover a continuum in which intensity of reaction, presence of a range of related grief behaviours, and time course betray the presence of an abnormal grief response.

'Complicated grief involves the presentation of certain grief-related symptoms at a time beyond that which is considered adaptive. We hypothesize that the presence of these symptoms after approximately 6 months puts the bereaved individual at heightened risk for enduring social, psychological and medical impairment.'

Prigerson, et al., 1995

'Complicated mourning means that, given the amount of time since the death, there is some compromise, distortion or failure of one of more of the ...processes of mourning.'

Full realization of the pain of living without the deceased is denied, repressed or avoided The deceased is held on to as though alive. Symptoms do not resolve spontaneously and need active intervention

Rando, 1993

'...is more related to the intensity of a reaction or the duration of a reaction rather than the presence or absence of a specific behavior.'

Worden, 1982

Risk factors for developing complicated grief

Personal
- Markedly angry, ambivalent or dependent relationship with the decesed
- History of multiple loss experiences
- Mental health problems
- Perceived lack of social support

Circumstantial
- Sudden, unexpected death, especially when violent, mutilating or random
- Death from an overly lengthy Illness
- Loss of a child
- Mourner's perception of loss as preventable

Historical
- Previous experience with complicated grief
- Insecurity in childhood attachments

Personality
- Inability to tolerate extremes of emotional distress
- Inability to tolerate dependency feelings
- Self-concept, rôle and value of 'being strong'

Social
- Socially unspeakable loss (e.g. suicide)
- Socially negated loss (e.g. loss of ex-spouse)
- Absence of social support network

Complicated grief includes:
- Symptoms of depression
- Symptoms of anxiety

- Grief specific symptoms of extraordinary intensity and duration that include:
  - Preoccupation with thoughts of the deceased
  - Disbelief
  - Feelings of being stunned
- Lack of acceptance of the death
- Yearning for the deceased
- Searching for the deceased
- Crying

The common psychiatric disorders related to grief include:
- Clinical depression
- Anxiety disorders, alcohol abuse or other substance abuse and dependence
- Psychotic disorders
- Post-traumatic stress disorder (PTSD)

While frank psychiatric disorders following bereavement are reasonably straightforward to diagnose, it is more difficult to pick up complicated grief, in which the pathological nature of the grief response is only distinguishable from normal grief by its character.

Recognition of complicated bereavement calls for an experienced clinical judgement that does not 'rationalize' the distress as understandable.

Warning signs of complicated grief
- Long term functional impairment
- Exaggerated, prolonged and intense grief reactions
- Significant neglect of self-care
- Frequent themes of loss in conversation, activity, behavior
- Idealization of the deceased
- Impulsive decision making
- Mental disorders following loss
- PTSD-like symptoms

Ways of helping a bereaved person
- 'Being there' for them
- Non-judgemental listening
- Encouraging them to talk about the deceased
- Giving permission for the expression of feelings
- Offering reassurance about the normality of feelings and experiences
- Promoting coping with everyday life and self care (eg adequate food intake)
- Screening for damaging behaviours (eg increased alcohol use, smoking, etc)
- Providing information, when requested, about the illness and death of their loved ones—also about the range of grief responses
- Educating others (family members and other support networks) about how best to help the bereaved person
- Becoming familiar with your own feelings about loss and grief
- Offer information about local bereavement support services eg. Hospice services or Cruse

Table 14.2 Clinical presentations of complicated grief

Category	Features
Inhibited or delayed grief	Avoidance postpones expression
Chronic grief	Perpetuation of mourning long-term
Traumatic grief	Unexpected and shocking form of death
Depressive disorders	Both major and minor depressions
Anxiety disorders	Insecurity and relational problems
Alcohol and substance abuse/dependence	Excessive use of substances impairs adaptive coping
Post-traumatic stress disorder	Persistent, intrusive images with cues
Psychotic disorders	Manic, severe depressive states, and schizophrenia

From Doyle, D.H., Hanks, G., Cherny, N. (2004) *Oxford Textbook of Palliative Medicine*, 3rd edn, p. 1140. Oxford: Oxford University Press.

Bereavement involving children

One feature of the grief of most children is that they do not sustain grief over continuing periods of time, but tend rather to dip in and out of grief—jumping in and out of puddles, rather than wading through the river of grief.

Adults should be aware that children will learn what is 'acceptable grief' from the adults around them.

Allowing expression of feelings—children will be helped by knowing that the expression of feelings is acceptable. Children may express their emotions and grief in many ways e.g. through play, artwork, music, drama etc.

Children's understanding, responses and needs will be affected by many factors, including their previous experiences of loss and how these were handled. It is important also to consider the age and the developmental level of the child, although any attempt to consider responses according to age will require flexibility and there is considerable crossover between different children.

Children under the age of 2–3 years may have little concept of death, but will be aware of separation and may protest against this by detachment or regressive behaviour. Children of this age need a consistent caregiver, familiar routines and the meeting of their physical and emotional needs.

Children aged between 3 and 5 years do not see death as irreversible. Their concerns will relate to separation, abandonment and the physical aspects of death and dying. Their response may include aggressive and rejecting behaviour. They may also become withdrawn or demonstrate an increase in clinging or demanding behaviour. There may also be regression to infant needs. Routine, comfort, reassurance and a simple answering of their questions will help a child of this age. They should be allowed to participate in family rituals and to keep mementos of the deceased. Adults should be aware of the words they use since they can be misinterpreted (e.g. do not associate death with sleep or a long journey).

Children age between 6 and 8 years seek causal explanations. A whole range of behaviours may be evidence of their response to grief—withdrawal, sadness, loneliness, depression, acting-out behaviour or becoming a 'perfect' child. Short, honest, concrete explanations will help a child of this age, as will maintaining contact with friends and normal activities. Short-term regression may be allowed and they should be reassured that they will always be cared for. Involvement in the family's grief related rituals will also help.

Pre-teenage children appear to have a calmer, more accepting attitude to death. They often have a good factual understanding of what has happened. The child should be encouraged to talk about the deceased and provided with clear and truthful answers to their questions. The feelings of adults do not need to be hidden, allowing the child to provide mutual help and reassurance.

Teenage years—children of this age are engaged in a search for meaning and purpose in life and for identity. They feel that they have deep and powerful emotions that no one else has experienced. Teenagers may exhibit withdrawal, sadness, loneliness and depression, or they may act-out in an angry, hostile and rejecting way. They may seek to cover up fears with joking and sarcasm. Young people of this age need as much comfort as possible, involvement, boundaries, a sense that their feelings are being taken seriously and reassurance that their feelings are normal. Continuing

---

Risk factors for complicated grief in bereaved children
These may be divided into three groups:

Features of the loss
- Traumatic
- Unexpected

Features of the child
- History of psychiatric disorder
- Multiple losses
- Child less than 5 years old
- Adolescent

Features of the relationship
- Ambivalent/conflicted
- Unsupportive family
- Death of a father (adolescent boys)
- Death of a mother (very young children)
- Mental illness in surviving parent

---

contact with their peers should be encouraged. Young people will often identify for themselves someone with whom they feel comfortable to talk.

Bereavement due to death of a child

The death of a child is a devastating loss, particularly in times where most childhood illness can be prevented or cured. It profoundly affects all those involved—parents, siblings, grandparents, extended family, friends and others involved in caring for the child. As a community we rarely experience the death of a child, which makes it all the more difficult when we do. There is a sense that the natural order of things has been upset.

Principles for working with bereaved parents
1 Make early contact and assess the bereaved parents.
2 Provide assurance that they can survive their loss, but acknowledge the uniqueness of their pain.
3 Allow adequate time for parents to grieve.
4 Facilitate the identification and expression of feelings including negative feelings such as anger, and guilt.
5 Encourage recall of memories of the deceased child.
6 Maintain a professional and realistic perspective—not all pain can be 'fixed'.
7 Allow for individual differences in response relating to gender, age, culture, personality, religion and the characteristics of the death.
8 Assist in finding a source of continuing support.
9 Identify complicated grief reactions and refer to appropriate services.

Interpret recovery to parents, and that 'recovery' is not a betrayal of their child. Health professionals need to recognize the significance they may have in a family's life. Many children are treated over long periods of time and the hospital/hospice may become something of a second home. Health professionals also care for families during the intense highs and lows of serious illness, and may even be present at the time the child dies. The significance of this cannot be overstated. These relationships cannot be abruptly ended and many (but not all) families will want ongoing contact with people they feel truly understand what they have experienced. A follow-up appointment with the child's paediatrician should always be offered to discuss the child's illness and treatment, the results of any outstanding investigations including post-mortem examinations and how the family is coping.

Sibling grief
Siblings almost universally experience distress, but many feel unable to share this for fear of burdening their already fragile parents. One of the many factors which influence sibling grief is developmental level and the impact this has on the child's understanding of illness and death.

Most children learn to recognize when something is dead before they reach three years of age. However, at this early age, death, separation and sleep are almost synonymous in the child's mind. As children develop and experience life, their concept of death becomes more mature. Six sub-concepts are acquired during this process (average age of attainment in brackets):

Separation (age 5)	Dead people do not co-exist with the living
Causality (age 6)	Death is caused by something, be it trauma, disease, or old age
Irreversibility (age 6)	A dead person can not 'come alive' again
Cessation of bodily functions (age 6)	The dead person does not need to eat or breathe
Universality (age 7)	All living things will die
Insensitivity (age 8)	The dead can not feel fear or pain

Supporting bereaved children

- Adjusting to the loss of a loved person does not necessarily require 'letting go' of the relationship. Indeed, bereaved children (and adults) often maintain a connection to the dead person. The relationship is reconstructed over time and maintained by remembering the person, keeping their belongings and sometimes talking to them. Children spend most of their time in the care of their parents. It is therefore important to empower parents to support siblings by equipping them with knowledge and ideas. Staff can encourage the family to:
  - **Provide information** in simple, developmentally appropriate language
  - **Be alert to misunderstandings** which may arise as a consequence of an incomplete death concept
  - Set aside special **time** for the child/young person
  - Openly **express emotion**
  - Recruit family, friends and teachers to help
  - **Allow the child to play** with friends and reassure them that it is OK to have fun
  - Help the child **create memories** e.g. Stories, photos, drawings, memory books
  - **Maintain normal routines and discipline** as much as possible
  - Allow the child/young person opportunities to feel in control
  - Resist any temptation to 'fix their grief'
  - Encourage them to do what feels right for them
  - Be there—to provide love, reassurance and routine
  - **Allow the child time alone.** Private 'space' is important
  - Talk about the death
  - **Answer questions,** no matter how explicit
  - Not be surprised if children use symbolic play, stories and art to make sense of their experience.

School grief

The following is adapted from *A Practical Guide to Paediatric Oncology Palliative Care*, Royal Children's Hospital, Brisbane 1999.

After the family, the school community may contain the people most affected by the death of a child—friends, fellow students, teachers, administrative staff. Parents form part of a wider school community. It may well be the first bereavement experience for the child's peers, their parents and teachers. Close attachments are formed between children and their teachers, so that the death of a child may be a personal as well as a professional loss.

In a school, there will be a range of grief responses. It is anticipated that both staff and students will be vulnerable to stress and may express themselves differently. For the student, the closer they were to the child the more profound will be the consequences. Teachers may notice a change in the other student's behaviour, thought processes, concentration and academic performance. A greater level of support, monitoring and care may be warranted, even for those students who may not be expressing their grief in an obvious way.

People who may be at increased risk are:
- those who have already experienced significant loss in their lives
- those who have a close relationship with the child who has died or the child's siblings, and those who have similar health problems themselves or in their family

The school is in an ideal position to provide opportunities for students to be supported as well as to identify those who may be experiencing difficulty. The child's parents should always be consulted before any information is released so that their privacy and the best interests of any siblings are considered and respected.

Ways in which the school can help include:
- Informing staff and students of the child's death is a priority. Anxiety and misinformation are fuelled by uncertainty and delay
- Senior staff need to acknowledge the sadness of what has happened, perhaps by way of assemblies, class announcements and letters home
- Staff and children need the opportunity to talk about what has happened, to ask questions, and to express their feelings. This is best done in familiar small groups, though it may also be appropriate to set aside a time where people can come and talk together. Students can also be given opportunities to write farewell letters or tributes, and to create artwork as an expression of thoughts and feelings
- A sense of routine provides reassurance to staff and students who have experienced trauma. It is therefore important that the school continues to function as a supportive and stable part of the staff and student's environment
- Staff will need their own support. Staff meetings provide an opportunity to provide information, monitor the reactions of the children and discuss feelings. In some cases, it may be helpful to hold a special meeting facilitated by someone with expertise in this area. Senior staff are usually required to manage the immediate crisis and may experience a 'delayed reaction'
- There are a number of ways in which the school can maintain contact with the family. This may be through friends or formal rituals. Some families welcome the participation of the school in the funeral for example, and may wish to be involved in school memorial services. The child may also have expressed wishes regarding the involvement of their school friends

Assessment of bereavement risk

The assessment of bereavement risk presupposes that some individuals will display a grief reaction that does not fit a 'normal' or expected pattern or level of intensity. Factors that influence complicated bereavement are:
- stage of the life cycle particularly when:
  the bereaved parent is an adolescent and family support is perceived as inadequate. the surviving parent of a deceased child is a single mother/father as a result of divorce or being widowed
- a history of previous losses, particularly if unresolved. Losses may include:
  - loss of a pregnancy
  - loss of a job
  - divorce

- the presence of concurrent or additional stressors such as:
  - family tension
  - compromised financial status
  - dissatisfaction with caregiving
  - reliance on alcohol and psychotropic medications, pre-bereavement
- physical and mental illness particularly:
  - current/past history of mental health problems that have required psychiatric/psychological support
  - family history of psychiatric disorders
- high pre-death distress
- inability or restriction in use of coping strategies such as:
  - maintenance of physical self-care
  - identification of prominent themes of grief
  - attributing meaning to the loss
  - differentiation between letting go of grief and forgetting the bereaved
  - accessing available support
- isolated, alienated individuals
- low levels of internal control beliefs, such as:
  - feeling as if he/she has no control over life
- the availability of social support particularly if:
  - people in the immediate environment are, or are perceived to be, unsupportive
  - support from family and friends immediately prior to death was good and following death it subsided
- the bereaved lack a confidant with whom to share feelings, concerns, doubts, dreams and nightmares
- the bereaved is dissatisfied with the help available during their child's illness

Further Reading

Bowlby, J. (1969) *Attachment and loss: vol. 1*. Harmondsworth: Penguin.

Freud, S. (1961a) Mourning and melancholia. In J. Strachey (ed. and trans.) *The standard edition of the complete psychological works of Sigmund Freud*, vol. 14, pp. 243–58. London: Hogarth Press (original work published 1917).

Klass, D., Silverman, P., Nickman, S. (eds.) (1996) *Continuing bonds*. London: Taylor & Francis.

Kubler-Ross, E. (1969) *On death and dying*. London: Tavistock Publications.

Lazarus, R., Folkman, S. (1991) *Stress and coping*. 3rd edn. New York: Columbia University Press.

Parkes, C. M. (1996) *Bereavement*. 3rd edn. London: Routledge.

Prigerson, H. G., *et al.* (1995) Inventory of complicated grief. *Psychiatry research*, **59**: 65–79.

Rando, T. A. (1993) *Treatment of complicated mourning*. Champaign: Research Press.

Stroebe, M., Schut, H. (1999) The dual process model of coping with bereavement. *Death studies*, **23**: 197–224.

Walters, T. (1996) A new model of grief. *Mortality*, **1**: 7–25.

Winston's Wish. www.winstonswish.org.uk.

Worden, J. W. (1991) *Grief counselling and grief therapy*. 2nd edn. London: Routledge.

A Charter for Bereaved Children

"A child can live through anything provided they are told the truth and allowed to share the natural feelings people have when they are suffering" Eda Le Shan

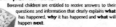

This Charter has been written following our conversations with over 2,000 bereaved children and their families since Winston's Wish began in 1992. Although supporting a bereaved child can seem a daunting challenge, we have found that there are simple and straightforward ways which can make a positive difference to a grieving child. If we live in a society that genuinely wants to enable children and young people to re-build their lives after the death of a family member, then we need to respect their rights to the following:

1. Adequate Information

Bereaved children are entitled to receive answers to their questions and information that clearly explains **what** has happened, **why** it has happened and **what** will happen **next**.

'Daddy died of a tumour, but I don't know what a tumour is.' Alice, age 6, whose father died of stomach cancer.

2. Being Involved

Bereaved children should be asked if they wish to be **involved** in important decisions that have an impact on their lives (such as planning the funeral, remembering anniversaries).

'I helped to choose mum's favourite music which they played at her funeral.' Kim, age 12.

3. Family Involvement

Bereaved children should receive support which **includes their parent(s)** and which also respects each child's confidentiality.

'Meeting other parents in exactly the same situation as me was so helpful.' John whose wife died from a brain haemorrhage.

4. Meeting Others

Bereaved children can benefit from the opportunity of **meeting other children** who have had similar experiences.

'Often I want to break down and cry but I can't do that in front of my school mates... meeting all the other kids who have been through the same thing – I don't feel alone any more.' Colin, age 12, whose mother died.

5. Telling the Story

Bereaved children have the right to **tell their story** in a variety of ways and for those stories to be heard, read or seen by those important to them. For example, through drawing, puppets, letters and words.

'My picture shows the car banged dad on the head, he fell off his bike, hit his head and died later in hospital.' Georgina, age 7, whose father died in a road accident.

6. Expressing Feelings

Bereaved children should feel comfortable expressing **all** feelings associated with grief such as anger, sadness, guilt and anxiety, and to be helped to find appropriate ways to do this.

'It's alright to cry and OK to be happy as well.' James, age 9, whose dad died from a heart attack.

7. Not to Blame

Bereaved children should be helped to understand that they **are not responsible and not to blame** for the death.

'I now understand it wasn't anyone's fault.' Chris, age 12, whose dad died by suicide.

8. Established Routines

Bereaved children should be able to choose to **continue** previously enjoyed activities and interests.

'I went to Brownies after Meg died. I wanted my friends to know.'

9. School Response

Bereaved children can benefit from receiving an appropriate and positive response from their **school or college**.

'My teacher remembers the days which are difficult, like father's Day and dad's birthday.' Alex, age 9.

10. Remembering

Bereaved children have the right to remember the person who has died for the rest of their lives if they wish to do so. This may involve re-living memories (both good and difficult) so that the person becomes a comfortable part of the child's on-going life story.

'I like to show my memory book to people who didn't have the chance to know my dad.' Bethany, age 8, whose father died from cancer.

Winston's Wish

© Winston's Wish 2002. The Clara Burgess Centre, Gloucestershire Royal Hospital, Great Western Road, Gloucester, GL1 3NN. Tel 01452 394377. Fax 01452 395656. Registered Charity – No. 1061359

Fig. 14.1 A charter for bereaved children

Emergencies in palliative care

While this chapter focuses on the common oncological emergencies in palliative practice, other emergencies include a wider range of issues such as:

- An emergency discharge so a patient's wish to die at home can be met
- Emotional emergencies, with high levels of expressed anxiety
- Spiritual/existential/social emergencies with pressure to 'sort things out' before it is too late

It is important to have a clear understanding of the management of emergencies in palliative care as clear thinking is crucial in handling such, thankfully rare, situations. Providing transparent decisiveness to the patient, family and staff can transform a crisis situation filled with anxiety.

The time frame for normal hospice and palliative care interventions are modulated by the need for calmness and patient comfort. There are however several emergency situations which can occur for hospice patients requiring urgent and prompt diagnosis and management. This may create some dissonance among staff and other patients. It is vital that all staff appreciate the nature of these emergencies and the importance of an emergency response.

Sepsis in the neutropaenic patient

All clinical staff should be acutely aware of the serious risk and potential rapid fatality of patients who have become neutropaenic and febrile with oncological treatments.

Patients should be admitted to a unit where essential investigations can be carried out rapidly and where intravenous antibiotics can be given and suitable monitoring maintained. Appropriate facilities are not usually available within a hospice unit. Occasionally patients may develop neutropaenic sepsis while in a palliative care unit, which may create a dilemma. After full discussion of the seriousness of the situation and the high chance of a good response to optimal management in an acute unit, patients may still refuse ambulance transfer, preferring to stay in the hospice and to risk suboptimal care. This should be discussed with their oncologist if possible.

Empirical treatment of a febrile neutropaenic patient should be instigated and an appropriate antibiotic regime started, *with advice from the local bacteriologist since antibiotic regimes vary across the country.*

A regime currently being advocated at The Royal Marsden Hospital is outlined below as an example:

- Tazocin 4.5g q.d.s. + gentamicin 5mg/kg i/v o.d.
- Or, if allergic to penicillin
- Ceftazidime 2g i/v t.d.s. + gentamicin 5mg/kg i/v o.d.
- If still febrile after 48 h:
- Add vancomycin 1g i/v b.d.

- If still febrile after 96–120 h:
- Stop tazocin + gentamicin
- Start ciprofloxacin 400mg i/v b.d.
- Add amphotericin 0.75mg/kg/day i/v (or 1mg/kg/day for haemato-oncology patients)
- Treat for a minimum of seven days and continue until neutrophil count >0.5 × 10^9/l.[1]

Signs of Spinal Cord Compression
- Back pain 90%
- Weak legs
- Increased reflexes
- Sensory level
- Urinary hesitancy (late feature)

Spinal cord compression
Spinal cord compression occurs in 3–5 per cent of patients with cancer, and 10% of patients with spinal metastases develop cord compression,[2] the frequency being highest in multiple myeloma and cancers of the prostate, breast and bronchus.
- Malignant causes:
  - intramedullary metastases
  - intradural metastases
  - extradural compression (80 per cent)—vertebral body metastasis
    - vertebral collapse
    - tumour spread
    - interruption of vascular supply

It is important to have a high index of suspicion for possible cord compression, because of the consequences of paraplegia and urine and faecal incontinence with a delay in diagnosis.

Symptoms and signs
- Back pain, a sensation of weakness in the legs and often vague sensory symptoms in the legs may be early manifestations. Patients may complain of a band-like pain, particularly on coughing or sneezing
- For those presenting with profound weakness, a sensory 'level' and sphincter disturbance, which are relatively late features, the outcome is poor and the compression is much less likely to be reversible

The site of compression is
- thoracic in 70%
- lumbosacral 20%
- cervical 10%

Lesions above L1 (lower end of spinal cord) will produce upper motor neurone signs and often a sensory level, whereas lesions below L1 will produce lower motor neurone signs and peri-anal numbness (cauda equina syndrome). Multiple sites of compression may produce different and confusing neurological signs.

Table 15.1 Neurological signs of upper and lower motor neurone lesions

	Upper motor neurone lesion	Lower motor neurone lesion
Power	Reduced/absent	Reduced/absent
Tone	Increased	Reduced
Sensation	Sensory loss	Sensory loss
Reflexes (plantars)	Increased (upgoing)	Absent/reduced (downgoing)

Management

High dose corticosteroids (dexamethasone 16 mg/day) to relieve peritumoural oedema; urgent referral to oncology centre.

Spinal cord compression is an EMERGENCY and two questions need to be answered urgently.

1 Does this patient have a reasonable likelihood of having spinal cord compression?
2 Would this patient benefit from instituting emergency investigation and treatment?

Does this patient have a reasonable likelihood of having spinal cord compression?

Even the most skilled clinician is unable to diagnose spinal cord compression with absolute certainty. Often by the time clinical signs are 'classic', it is too late for patients to benefit from treatment, as it has a limited rôle in reversing symptoms which are already established. Thus if intervention to prevent paraplegia is to be successful, potential compression needs to be diagnosed early.

The keys to diagnosing Spinal Cord Compression include:

• Having a high index of suspicion in patients with spinal metastases particularly in patients with breast, lung and prostate cancer and with pain and tenderness on palpation or percussion of the vertebra at the level of the suspected lesion
• Taking patients' complaints about back pain, odd sensations in the legs, and difficulties in passing urine seriously

Would this patient benefit from instituting emergency investigation and treatment?

The patient will need to be transferred to a specialized unit where an MRI scan can be carried out and treatment given. In the context of metastatic cancer, radiotherapy is often the most appropriate treatment, but surgery may need considering in specific circumstances.

Deciding whether the particular course of treatment is appropriate for a particular patient involves an overall assessment.

1 The Royal Marsden Drug and Therapeutics Advisory Committee Prescribing Guidelines, including symptom control guidelines, p. 110. London: Royal Marsden NHS Trust.

2 Kaye P. (1999) *Decision-making in Palliative Care*, p. 183. Northampton: EPL Publications.

Key questions in deciding on emergency investigations and management.
- Does the patient want emergency management?
- Is the patient still walking?
- Is the patient suffering from severe back pain?
- Has the patient already established cord compression?
- Has the patient a short prognosis (eg. week by week deterioration.)

Where suspicion of spinal cord compression is high, it is quickest to contact by telephone the oncological team in the cancer centre where the patient has been managed, who can then co-ordinate the necessary scan and appropriate emergency treatment.

Table 15.2 Definitive treatment of spinal cord compression

Indications for surgical decompression	Indications for radiotherapy
1 Uncertain cause—to obtain histology	1 Radiosensitive tumour
2 Radiotherapy has not been effective or symptoms persist despite maximum radiotherapy	2 Multiple levels of compression
3 Radio-resistant tumour e.g. melanoma, sarcoma	3 Unfit for major surgery
4 Unstable spine	4 Patient choice
5 Major structural compression	
6 Cervical cord lesion	
7 Solitary vertebral metastasis	

Patients with spinal cord compression provide great challenges to the multidisciplinary team. These challenges include:
- Mobility management (risk of venous thrombosis)
- Skin management in a patient confined to bed (risk of pressure sores)
- Bowel management
- Urinary system management
- Psychological management.

There is no consensus on the optimum time to start mobilizing patients diagnosed with cord compression. In general principles, if the spine is stable and the pain is relatively well controlled it would seem wise to introduce physiotherapy as soon as possible to maintain muscle tone and motor function as well as possible. The occupational therapist will be crucial in helping with goal-setting and rehabilitative techniques.

Steroids are usually continued at high dose to start with and then tailed off gradually and completely over a few weeks (4–6 weeks or so) or to the lowest dose that maintains stability. Radiation-induced oedema may exacerbate symptoms and the dose of steroids may need to increase temporarily during treatment.

Prognosis

Overall, 30 per cent of patients may survive for one year. A patient who is ambulant after treatment may survive 8–9 months, but the life expectancy for a patient who remains paraplegic is a few weeks only. Function will be retained in 70 per cent of patients who were ambulant prior to treatment but will return in only 5 per cent of those who were paraplegic at the outset. Return of motor function is better in those with incomplete spinal compression and particularly with partial lesions of the cauda equina. Loss of sphincter function is a bad prognostic sign.

In practice, most patients with an established diagnosis are relatively unwell and have multiple metastases, and will be referred for radiotherapy, achieving similar results to those of surgery.

Superior vena cava obstruction

Superior vena cava obstruction (SVCO) is due to external compression of and/or thrombosis of the SVC by mediastinal lymph nodes or tumour in the region of the right main bronchus. It is caused most commonly by carcinoma of the bronchus (75 per cent) and lymphomas (15 per cent). Cancers of the breast, colon, oesophagus and testis account for the remaining 10 per cent.

Symptoms and signs

Symptoms are those of venous hypertension and include breathlessness (laryngeal oedema or tracheal or bronchial obstruction/compression), headache (cerebral oedema), visual changes, dizziness and swelling of the face, neck and arms.

Signs include engorged conjunctivae, peri-orbital oedema, non-pulsatile dilated neck veins and dilated collateral veins (chest and arms). If the latter sign evolves, the symptoms of SVCO may stabilize. Papilloedema is a late feature.

Management

In the palliative care setting, the diagnosis (usually of carcinoma of the bronchus) is established already. SVCO can present acutely, resulting in very distressing symptoms. The patient should be referred to the oncology centre for urgent management.
- Dexamethasone 8–16mg p.o. or i/v. There is no good evidence for the efficacy of steroids but they may be helpful in reducing oedema (if there is associated stridor), or as an anti-tumour agent for lymphoma
- Frusemide 40mg p.o. or i/v
- Consider prophylactic anticonvulsant
- Treatment is the standard oncology treatment for the particular underlying cancer; for instance, chemotherapy for SCLC and lymphoma, radiotherapy for non-small cell carcinoma of the bronchus
- Intraluminal stents can be inserted via the femoral vein and is the treatment of choice for patients with severe symptoms
- Thrombolysis may be considered prior to stenting

Prognosis

Without treatment, SVCO can progress over several days leading to death. Prognosis is poor in a patient presenting with advanced SVCO unless the primary cancer is responsive to radiotherapy or chemotherapy. Generally, the prognosis is that of the underlying tumour.

Haemorrhage

Haemorrhage may be directly related to the underlying tumour or caused by treatments such as steroids or non steroidal anti-inflammatory drugs resulting in gastric/duodenal erosion. A generalized clotting deficiency, seen in thrombocytopaenia, hepatic insufficiency or anti-coagulation with warfarin, are also contributory factors in patients with cancer.

Treatments for *non-acute haemorrhage* include oncological, systemic and local measures. Palliative radiotherapy is very useful for superficial tumours and those of the bronchus and genito-urinary tract. If radiotherapy is not appropriate, coagulation should be enhanced with oral tranexamic acid 1 g t.d.s., but caution is necessary with haematuria since clots may form in the renal tract, resulting in further problems. Local measures for superficial tumours, such as topical tranexamic acid or adrenalin (1:1000) soaks, may be useful. Sucralfate may act as a local astringent to stop stomach mucosal bleeding in addition to a proton pump inhibitor such as lansoprazole.

Erosion of a major artery can cause *acute haemorrhage*, which may be a rapidly terminal event. It may be possible to anticipate such an occurrence, and appropriate medication and a red blanket to reduce the visual impact should be readily available. Relatives or others who witness such an event will need a great deal of support. If the haemorrhage is not immediately fatal, such as with a haematemesis or bleeding from the rectum, vagina or superficially ulcerated wound, the aim of treatment is local control if possible and sedation of a shocked, frightened patient. Rectal or sublingual diazepam (stesolid 10 mg) or midazolam 10 mg SC or buccally act quickly.

The palliative care team need to balance the anxiety of alerting and preparing the family for such an event against the likelihood of it occurring. If the patient chooses to be looked after at home, the issues of managing acute haemorrhage need to be discussed with the family and the home care team and a clear plan worked out.

It may be appropriate to have emergency medication in the home to sedate the acutely bleeding patient. Such a strategy needs lengthy discussion with the family, carers, and the patient's local GP, and clearly documented plans.

Convulsions ▢ see Chapter 6j

Hypercalcaemia

Hypercalcaemia occurs in 10 per cent of patients with cancer. The pathogenesis of hypercalcaemia includes increased bone resorption (osteolysis) and systemic release of humoral hypercalcaemic factors, with or without evidence of metastatic bone disease. Calcium is released from bone and in addition there may be a decrease in excretion of urinary calcium. Calcium release from bone is attributed to locally active substances produced by bone metastases (cytokines, particularly interleukins and tumour necrosis factor, and other factors which stimulate prostaglandin function), or by factors such as ectopic parathyroid hormone related protein (PTHrP). The tumours most commonly associated with hypercalcaemia include squamous cell carcinoma of the bronchus (and other squamous cell tumours), carcinoma of the breast and prostate and multiple myeloma.

A corrected plasma calcium concentration above 2.6 mmol/litre defines hypercalcaemia. It is often mild and asymptomatic and significant symptoms usually only develop with levels above 3.0 mmol/litre. Levels of 4.0 mmol/litre and above will cause death in a few days if left untreated.

Symptoms include drowsiness, confusion, nausea, vomiting, thirst, polyuria, weakness and constipation.

Management

Treatment is only necessary if there are symptoms and may be unnecessary if the patient is very near to death. Patients should be encouraged to mobilize if appropriate. Absorption of calcium from the gut is generally reduced, so patients may eat what they wish regardless of the calcium content of food.

Hypercalcaemia usually responds to specific antitumour therapy if appropriate.

Fluid replacement

Patients are usually dehydrated and need adequate fluid replacement. A high oral intake of fluid should be encouraged as appropriate for the individual clinical situation. Alternatively, extra fluid should be given intravenously. Fluid replacement alone improves symptoms but rarely achieves total control.

Bisphosphonates

Bisphosphonates inhibit osteoclast activity and thereby inhibit bone resorption. Because of poor alimentary absorption, they are usually given intravenously initially. Disodium pamidronate or sodium clodronate are effective in 70–80 per cent of patients for an average of two to three weeks. Zoledronic acid can be given over a shorter period and the effect lasts for longer. Patients receiving bisphoshonates may develop transient fever and bone pains; they may also become hypocalcaemic and need to be monitored.

Give:

- e.g. zoledronic acid 4 mg in 50 ml sodium chloride 0.9 per cent over 15 minutes
- disodium pamidronate 60–90 mg in sodium chloride 0.9 per cent, 500 ml over 2–4 h
- sodium clodronate 1.5 g in sodium chloride 0.9 per cent, 500 ml over 4 h
- Plasma calcium levels start to fall after 48 h and fall progressively for the next six days. Oral bisphosphonates have been reported to delay the recurrence of hypercalcaemia and may be important for maintenance

The introduction of once or twice daily oral bisphosphonates have made complying with the strictures to avoid eating for one hour before and after treatment easier.

Prognosis

Eighty per cent of cancer patients with hypercalcaemia survive less than one year.

Further reading

Books

Doyle D., Hanks G., Cherny N., Calman K. (2004) *Oxford Textbook of Palliative Medicine*, 3 rd edn. Oxford: Oxford University Press.

Regnard C., Tempest S. *A Guide to Symptom Relief in Advanced Disease.*

Twycross R., Wilcock A. (2001) *Symptom Management in Advanced Cancer.* 3rd edn. Oxford: Radcliffe Medical Press.

Handbooks

Back, I. (2001) *Palliative Medicine Handbook.* 3rd edn. Cardiff: BPM Books.

Kaye P. (1999) *Decision-Making in Palliative Care*, pp. 182–3. Northampton: EPL Publications.

The Royal Marsden Hospital (2000) *Prescribing Guidelines*, including symptom and control guidelines p. 110. London: Royal Marsden NHS Trust.

Articles

Falk S., Fallon M. (1997) ABC of palliative care. Emergencies. *BMJ*, **315**, 7121: 1525–8.

Kramer J. A. (1992) Spinal cord compression in malignancy. *Palliative Medicine*, **6**: 202–11.

Hillier R., Wee B. (1997) Palliative management of spinal cord compression. *European Journal of Palliative Care*, **4**: 189–92.

Smith A. M. (1994) Emergencies in palliative care. *Annals of Medicine*, **23**, 2: 186–90.

Miscellaneous

Fitness to drive

In the interest of road safety those who suffer from a medical condition likely to cause a sudden disabling event at the wheel or inability to safely control their vehicle from any other cause should not drive.

Doctors have a duty to inform patients when they are prescribed medication which may impair their driving (GMC guidelines). Patients should be reminded that motor insurance may become invalid if there are changes in medical circumstances.

Many drugs used in palliative care may impair cognitive and motor skills including:-
1 Opioid analgesics
2 Benzodiazepines-e.g. diazepam, lorazepam
3 Antidepressants-e.g. amitriptyline
4 Phenothiazines-e.g. levomepromazine
5 Antihistamines-e.g. cyclizine

It is the duty of the **licence-holder** to notify the DVLA of any medical conditions which may affect safe driving. Most patients are sensible and responsible and with the support of family members are safe on the roads. They will avoid driving when their physical or mental condition begins to affect their judgement and ability to react quickly to unpredictable circumstances.

Driving is often seen as an important factor in maintaining the struggle for independence. It may be very hard for the patient, on both a practical and emotional level, to agree to letting go of the last vestiges of control over their lives. Very sensitive handling is needed.

If a patient is obviously unfit to drive for any reason and refuses to comply, the GMC issues the following guidelines:
1 The DVLA is legally responsible for deciding if a person is medically unfit to drive. They need to know when driving licence holders have a condition which may, now or in the future, affect their safety as a driver.
2 Therefore, where patients have such conditions, the doctor should:
   • Make sure that the patients understand that the condition may impair their ability to drive. If a patient is incapable of understanding this advice, for example because of dementia, you should inform the DVLA immediately.
3 Explain to patients that they have a legal duty to inform the DVLA about the condition. If the patient refuses to accept the diagnosis or the effect of the condition on his/her ability to drive, you can suggest that he/she seeks a second opinion, and make appropriate arrangements for

this. You should advise patients not to drive until the second opinion has been obtained.

4 If patients continue to drive when they are not fit to do so, you should make every reasonable effort to persuade them to stop. This may include telling their next of kin.

5 If you do not manage to persuade patients to stop driving, or you are given or find evidence that a patient is continuing to drive contrary to advice, you should disclose relevant medical information immediately, in confidence, to the medical adviser at DVLA.

6 Before giving information to the DVLA you should inform the patient of your decision to do so. Once the DVLA has been informed, you should also write to the patient, to confirm that a disclosure has been made.

Driving and opioid analgesia

Patients on longer term stable doses of opioids show only minor effects in terms of diminished cognition, perception, coordination or behaviour related to driving.

Patients, however, who are started on opioids or who are prescribed an increase above their 'normal' stable dose may show cognitive impairment for a few weeks or so. These patients should be advised not to drive during this period.

Driving and brain tumours

The diagnosis of a high grade primary or secondary brain tumour, whether or not a convulsion has occurred, must be notified to the DVLA. Patients will not be allowed to drive for at least two years after treatment.

Driving and seat belts

Exemption from having to wear a seat belt may be sought if it is thought to pose a danger to the patient's safety, such as in the situation of significant intra-abdominal disease.

Application forms for a Certificate of Exemption in the UK, may be obtained through the NHS Response telephone line.

Useful contact

The Medical Adviser
Drivers Medical Unit DVLA
Longview Road
Morriston
Swansea SA99 1TU
DVLA At A Glance—Current medical standards of fitness to drive—www.dvla.gov.uk

Tissue donation

The benefits offered by organ and tissue transplantation are now recognized by many, but demand continues to exceed supply. The majority of organs are donated by the relatives of patients who fulfil brainstem death criteria in intensive care units. There is evidence that donation, far from increasing relative's distress, may help in bereavement, families gaining comfort and meaning to the sudden death. Studies have shown that relatives are generally happy to talk about donation and to feel that some good has resulted from the death. Donation of tissues of patients dying from cancer, however, is relatively uncommon, possibly stemming from the relative lack of research in this group of patients.

Some professionals feel that there is a 'duty to ask' for tissue donation and indeed some families have felt cheated by not being given the opportunity to discuss the issue.

The subject of tissue donation may be straight forward if it has been discussed with the patient prior to death and if a donor card is available. Even in this situation, a lack of objection should always be sought from the next of kin.

In practice, it is easiest for corneas to be donated since this can be organized (it must be within 24 h) at the location of death without the need for transfer to a hospital pathologist. The transplant coordinator will arrange for the eyes to be removed. (The sockets are packed to ensure that the body does not appear to have been mutilated.)

A fear in popular culture that mutilation of the body, particularly the eyes, affects the deceased's beauty, identity or personhood and the idea that vision is necessary for the after-life, may be some of the reasons cited for families being reluctant to agree to donation.

Debate continues on presumed consent with an 'opt out' clause. There is evidence that those who consent to donation do so not out of social duty but out of altruism and generosity, with which they gain positive rewards. The subject of tissue donation remains a very individual and sensitive issue which needs careful handling in inevitably vulnerable families.

There are various practical considerations, some are outlined below.

	Cornea	Heart valves and trachea	Kidneys
Max. age of donor	Any age	60 years	70 years
Max. time from asystole to tissue removal	24h	72h	1hr

Contra-indications
The criteria for acceptability of tissues for donation are inevitably becoming more stringent. In the UK, a regional transplant coordinator is available 24 h a day and gives very helpful advice.

Follow up
The transplant team writes an acknowledgement letter to the family informing them of how the tissues have been used. Families usually find this very comforting.

Travelling abroad

It is not uncommon for terminally ill patients to want to travel abroad in order to see family or to die in their home country. A wish to travel by air needs to be balanced against the risk to the individual and the inconvenience and cost to fellow passengers and airlines in the event of unscheduled changes to flight plans. If there is any doubt, the airline medical officer, who will give the final authorization, should be contacted well in advance of travel.

In flight

During flight, changes in air pressure occur and p02 may be reduced. For this reason, patients with marked breathlessness (who are not able to walk more than 50 metres), with Hb less than 7.5g/l, ischaemic heart disease, cardiac failure or those who are oxygen-dependent may have difficulty.

In-flight cabin oxygen is inadequate for such patients. Extra supplies of oxygen may be made available as necessary if the airline is aware in advance.

At lower atmospheric pressures, air expands and for this reason patients with a pneumothorax, large bullae, ear/sinus disease and recent surgery or colonoscopy should not fly without advice. Other conditions to consider carefully are patients with intracranial tumours or confusion.

Patients will be at risk of thromboembolism on long haul flights, especially if they are not able to mobilize adequately; the use of support stockings or foot rocking devices may be appropriate.

Special arrangements

Transport to and from airports is arranged by the patient. If a stretcher is required, nine economy class seats are required, the cost of which is born by the patient.

Cabin staff are not authorized to look after personal care needs, medical treatment or specialized medical equipment.

> **An escort for a patient who is flying will be needed if:**
> - a patient is relatively dependent
> - if a patient has a syringe driver
> - if a patient has surgical drains
> - if emergency management of symptoms may be needed
> - if medication might need to be given by injection
> - if the journey is long and interrupted by several transfers

It is important to remember that all medication or equipment that might be needed during the flight are kept as *hand* luggage. This includes all regular medication including analgesics, antiemetics, anticonvulsants, steroids, insulin, inhalers and any medication such as GTN which might be needed on an 'as required' basis. Syringes, needles, spare batteries and a sharps disposal box, if appropriate, should be remembered.

Medication

All drugs, particularly controlled drugs, should be contained in the original packaging, clearly labelled and in a sturdy shockproof container. A letter from the doctor outlining the medical condition and prescribed med... should also be carried for customs officers. Prior to travelling it is sensible to liaise with medical services in the area of destination, and to check that all medication, especially opioids, are available in that country.

Opioids to an equivalent total dose of morphine 1200mg may be taken abroad legally; however, a Home Office licence needs to be obtained for drugs taken out of the UK in excess of the following amounts:

Total dose allowed:
- Oral morphine 1200mg
- Diamorphine 1350mg
- Oxycodone 900mg
- Hydromorphone 360mg
- Fentanyl 45mg
- Methadone 500mg
- Benzodiazepine 900mg

Useful information address
Home Office Licensing Department
For taking opioids abroad
Tel: 020 7273 3806; 020 7217 8457

Further reading

Books

Doyle D., Hanks G., Cherny N., Calman, K. (2004) *Oxford Textbook of Palliative Medicine*. 3rd edn. Oxford: Oxford University Press.

The Liverpool integrated care pathway for the dying patient

What is an integrated care pathway?

Integrated care pathways (ICP) were originally developed in the North American healthcare system. More recently they have been introduced in Great Britain (1,2). An ICP provides a template of care which outlines best practice for a given clinical situation e.g. chest pain, breast cancer, leg ulceration, care of the dying. It incorporates guidelines and supporting documentation to facilitate the integration of evidence-based practice into care. The ICP is the central organizational tool for documenting patient care and is completed by all healthcare professionals. It replaces all other documentation. ICPs are widely seen as the precursor of the electronic patient record (3).

Developing an ICP

To develop integrated care pathways throughout an organization is an ambitious aim. The process is usually initiated by identifying a particular phase of care from which a pathway can be developed, for example in palliative care, the care of the dying. Following the development and implementation of a care pathway for one phase of care, subsequent ICPs can be developed to include the whole patient journey.

In order to develop an ICP, all professions involved in the care of the patient during the identified phase of care meet to review and identify the key goals of care. Key goals or outcomes of care reflect evidence-based practice and incorporate national and local guidelines. Having identified the key goals, prompts that enable the goal to be achieved or not achieved (i.e. a variance) are identified for each goal. Involvement and ownership of the pathway by all members of the team is crucial at this stage if the document is to be a true reflection of multidisciplinary working. It is therefore essential that when appropriate nurses, doctors, social workers, chaplains, occupational therapists and physiotherapists all participate in the development process and that the perspective of the user is sought.

The use and understanding of *variance* is critical to the success of integrated care pathways. When used in the context of integrated care pathways, a variance can be defined as a deviation from the identified plan of care. These variances should not be viewed as failures, but can be subdivided into those that are avoidable and those that are unavoidable. An example of an avoidable variance in the care of the dying would be an occasion when no member of the team had informed the relatives that the patient was dying. If the patient had no relatives, then this would be an unavoidable variance. By analysing the variance, it is possible to identify potential training and resource needs. In the example given above, a need for training in communication skills would be identified to improve communication with relatives regarding dying patients.

Further reading

Books

de Luc K. (2000) *Developing Care Pathways.* Oxford: Radcliffe Medical Press.

Department of Health (2000) *The NHS Cancer Plan—A plan for investment, A plan for reform.* London: DoH.

Ellershaw J. E., Wilkinson S. (eds) (2003) *Care of the Dying: A pathway to excellence.* Oxford: Oxford University Press.

Articles

Campbell H., Hotchkiss R., Bradshaw N., Porteous M. (1998) Integrated care pathways. *BMJ,* **316**: 133–7.

Elllershaw J. E., Smith, C., Overill S., *et al.* (2001) Care of the dying. *Journal of Pain & Symptom Management,* **21**: 12–17.

Elllershaw J. E., Ward C. (2003) Care of the dying patient: the last hours or days of life. *BMJ,* **326**: 30–4.

Death certification and referral to coroner

In the UK death certification has been a medical obligatory legal procedure since 1874, to provide proof of death and statistics of causes of death. A certificate must be issued by a medical practitioner who has been in attendance during the deceased's last illness. It states the cause of death to the best of the doctors' beliefs and knowledge.

The certificate should be filled in promptly to avoid further distress to the relatives, and clear statements of the disease process should be used, avoiding giving the mode of death as the only entry. Abbreviations should not be used.

The death must then be formally registered (within five days) at the Registration Office for Deaths, Births and Marriages, and arrangements can be made for disposal of the body. The doctor is legally responsible for the delivery of the death certificate but a family member can act as the doctor's agent, (which is usual practice).

It usually less complicated for families to register the death at the registration office in the area where the patient died, although it is possible to register at any registry. The registrar will exchange the doctor's certificate for a certificate for burial or cremation which must be handed to the funeral director involved. Copies of the entries made in the Register of Death by the registrar can be obtained and are needed for probate (wills) or letters of adminstration (if intestate), insurance claims and so on.

- Deaths that cannot be readily certified as due to natural causes should be referred to the coroner
- Once a death has been reported to the coroner, he or she has duty to investigate the cause of death
- The coroner may order a post-mortem to establish a cause of death
- If the family objects to this for religious or other reasons an appeal can be made, but this may delay the funeral
- There is no statutory duty to report any death to the coroner.
- Nevertheless doctors are encouraged to report voluntarily any death where it is judged that the Registrar should refer to the coroner. Such circumstances include:
- Death within 24 h of admission
- Death during detention under the Mental Health Act
- Death where there is a court case pending

In a hospice setting it is not uncommon for a patient to die with a pathological fracture or to die within a short time of arrival at the hospice. The coroner is very helpful in discussion of these cases.

A death should be referred to the coroner if:

- Cause Unknown
- Suspicious or violent circumstances
- Accidental injury
- Industrial diseases e.g. mesothelioma
- Abortion
- Anyone operated on with 48 h of death

- Suicide
- All drug deaths
- Operative or anaesthetic procedures
- Medical procedures/ treatment
- Self neglect/drug abuse
- Police/prison custody

- Septicaemia
- Doctor not attended within 14 days
- Poisoning
- Creutzfeldt Jakob Disease

If in doubt, discuss the situation with the coroner

Doctors have a legal duty to state all they know. However, it is relatively easy for any member of the public to obtain a copy of the death register entry which will include the cause of death. There is therefore the potential for a breach of confidence. The Office of Population Census and Surveys (OPCS) accepts that the present system is unsatisfactory.

The current practice of stating a superficial cause of death rather than the underlying disease process in such cases is widespread. Although it is technically illegal it is condoned by the OPCS—PROVIDED the box on the reverse side of the certificate is ticked stating that additional information may be forthcoming.

This point has yet to be tested in the courts. These comments often apply to patients dying with AIDS-related illnesses.

Cremation

If a body is to be cremated a certificate of medical attendant (Form B) and a confirmatory medical certificate (Form C) should be completed.

In **Form B**, if the doctor has not attended the deceased within 14 days of death, the coroner should be notified. The doctor must see the body after death.

Form C must be completed by a registered medical practitioner of not less than five years standing, who shall not be a relative of the deceased or a relative or partner of the doctor who has given the certificate in Form B.

The doctor must see and examine the body after death. In addition the doctor must have seen and questioned the medical practitioner who completed Form B.

Wills

- If there is a will, the executors named in the will (or if there is no will, the deceased person's representative) is responsible for arranging the funeral and looking after (and subsequently disposing of) the person's assets and property
- If there is a will, the executor should prove this to obtain probate
- If there is no will, the deceased's personal representative should apply for letters of administration

Funeral director

- The funeral director will need to know whether the body is to be buried or cremated (60 per cent of deaths in the UK are followed by cremation)
- They will need to know of any religious customs or rituals that might be necessary
- Bodies may be 'partially' embalmed routinely or this might be discussed with the family
- Traditionally, embalming involves draining blood from body and replacing it with formaldehyde plus a pinkish dye pumped under pressure, which has a hardening and disinfecting effect
- Nowadays the blood is not drained, but a small amount of embalming fluid is infused to help prevent the body smelling and to make the face more presentable
- This is particularly relevant either for hygienic reasons or if the families wish to view

Help and advice for patients

UK national resources

Macmillan Cancer Relief

Funds Macmillan nurses: referral via GP or hospital. Information line; financial help through patient grants. Applications for patient grants through hospital and hospice nurses, social workers and other healthcare professionals. (London)

☎ 0845 601 6161

Cancerline 0808 808 2020

🖥 http://www.macmillan.org.uk/

@ information_line@macmillan.org.uk

Marie Curie Cancer Care

Hands-on palliative nursing care, available through the local district nursing service. Also runs inpatient centres: admission by referral from GP or consultant. Both the services are free of charge. (London)

🖥 http://www.mariecurie.org.uk/

Tenovus Cancer Information Centre (Wales)

Information and support for patients, their families, carer. Helpline staffed by experienced cancer trained nurses, counsellors and social workers. Individual counselling service; free literature.

Velindre Hospital, Whitchurch, Cardiff CF14 2TL

☎ 0808 808 1010

🖥 http://www.tenovus.org.uk/

CancerBACUP

Helps people with cancer, their families and friends live with cancer. Cancer nurses provide information, emotional support and practical advice by telephone or letter. Booklets, factsheets, a newsletter, website and CD-ROM provide information. (London)

☎ 0808 800 1234

🖥 http://www.cancerbacup.org.uk/

Cancerlink

Provides emotional support and information. Register of over 600 cancer support and self-help groups nationwide. Free training and consultancy in setting up and running groups. (London)

Bereavement

Asian Family Counselling Service

Includes bereavement counselling.

☎ 020 8571 3933

CancerBACUP Counselling

☎ 020 7833 2451

🖥 http://www.cancerbacup.org.uk

Cruse

Bereavement counselling

☎ 0870 167 1677

🖥 http://www.cruisebereavementcare.org.uk

The Compassionate Friends
A self-help group of parents whose son or daughter (of any age, including adults) has died from any cause.
🖳 http://www.compassionatefriends.org

Samaritans/Age Concern/Citizens Advice Bureaux
☎ From local directory

Carers
Carers National Association
Information and support to people caring for relatives and friends. Free leaflets and information sheets.
☎ 0345 573369 (Mon–Fri 10am–midday, 2pm–4pm)
☎ 029 2088 0176 (Cardiff)

Crossroads—Caring for Carers
Provide a range of services for carers, including care in the home to enable the carer to have a break.
☎ 0845 450 0350
🖳 http://www.crossroads.org.uk

Children
ACT—Association for Children with Life-threatening or Terminal Conditions and their Families
🖳 http://www.act.org.uk

Complementary therapies
Bristol Cancer Help Centre
☎ 0845 123 2310
🖳 http://www.bristolcancerhelp.org

British Acupuncture Council
☎ 020 8735 0400
🖳 http://www.acupuncture.org.uk

British Homoeopathic Association
☎ 0870 444 3950
🖳 http://www.trusthomeopathy.org

National Federation of Spiritual Healers
☎ 0845 123 2777
🖳 http://www.nfsh.org.uk

Institute for Complementary Medicine
☎ 020 7 237 5165
🖳 http://www.i-c-m.org.uk

Conditions other than cancer
Parkinson's Disease Society
☎ 020 7931 8080
🖳 http://www.parkinsons.org.uk

Stroke Association
☎ 0845 303 3100
🖳 http://www.stroke.org.uk

British Brain and Spine Foundation
Helpline provides information and support about neurological disorders for patients, carers and health professionals.
☎ 0808 808 1000
@ info@bbsf.org.uk
🖥 http://www.bbsf.org.uk/

Alzheimer's Disease Society
☎ 020 7306 0606
🖥 http://www.alzheimers.org.uk

Motor Neurone Disease Association
Professional and general enquiries: 0604 250505
Helpline: 0845 7626 262
🖥 http://www.mndassociation.org

Specific Cancers
Brain Tumour Foundation
☎ 020 8336 2020
🖥 http://www.patient.co.uk/showdoc/26739371

Breast Cancer Care
☎ 0808 800 600
@ information@breastcancercare.org.uk
🖥 http://www.breastcancercare.org.uk/

Lymphoma Association
☎ 0808 808 5555 (Mon–Fri 10am–8pm)
🖥 http://www.lymphoma.org.uk/

Oesophageal Patients' Association
☎ 0121 704 9860
🖥 http://www.opa.org.uk

Ovacome
A support organization for women with ovarian cancer.
☎ 020 7380 9589
@ ovacome@ovacome.org.uk
🖥 http://www.ovacome.org.uk/ovacome

Prostate Cancer Charity
☎ (Mon–Fri 10am–4pm) 0845 300 8383
🖥 http://www.prostate-cancer.org.uk/
@ info@prstate-cancer.org.uk

Prostate Cancer Support Association (PSA)
☎ 0845 601 0766 (10am–8pm)
🖥 http://www.prostatecancersupport.co.uk

The Roy Castle Lung Cancer Foundation
☎ 0800 358 7200
🖥 http://www.roycastle.org/

Specific health problems
Changing Faces
Offers information, social skills training and counselling for people with facial disfigurements.
☎ 0845 4500 275
🖳 http://www.changingfaces.co.uk/

British Colostomy Association
☎ 0118 939 1537
Freephone: 0800 32842 57
🖳 http://www.bcass.org.uk

Impotence Association
☎ 0870 774 3571
🖳 http://www.impotence.org.uk/

Let's Face It
A contact point for people of any age coping with facial disfigurement.
☎ 01843 833 724
Tel/Fax: 020 8 931 2829
🖳 http://www.Letsfaceit.force9.co.uk

Lymphoedema Support Network
☎ 020 7 351 4480
🖳 http://www.lymphoedema.org/
@ ADMINLSN@lymphoedema.freeserve.co.uk

National Association of Laryngectomy Clubs
☎ 020 7 381 9993
🖳 http://www.nalc.ik.com

Urostomy Association
☎ 0870 770 7931
🖳 http://www.uagbi.org

Specific patient groups
Chai
Lifeline Cancer Support and Centre for Health
Emotional, physical, practical and spiritual support to Jewish cancer patients, their families and friends.
🖳 http://www.chailifeline.org.uk
@ info@chai-lifeline.org.uk

Gayscan
Offers completely confidential help and support to gay men living with cancer, their partners and carers.
Helpline: 020 8 368 9027

National Network for Palliative Care of People with Learning Disability
☎ 01284 766 133

Investigations

Blood tests
- Blood tests should never be taken 'routinely'
- Blood tests may be taken to confirm or exclude a treatable/reversible diagnosis such as anaemia or hypercalcaemia
- Blood tests may also help assess disease progression **if** this will in turn:
  - help with management decisions (e.g. deteriorating renal function may make plans for discharge inappropriate), or
  - help the patient understand his/her disease (e.g. demonstrating deteriorating liver function tests may help in explaining to the patient why he/she is not getting better)

Microbiology investigations
Midstream specimen of urine (MSU)
Urinalysis checks will show a positive result to blood and/or protein (largely representing red and white cells in the urine) in >90 per cent of urinary tract infections (UTI). Generally speaking an MSU need only be sent if urinalysis is positive but this has to be judged in relation to the specific clinical situation of the patient.

Urinalysis may not be positive if:
- The patient is immunosuppressed (usually a diabetic/septicaemic patient (only true if neutropaenic (ie no white cells), OR
- The UTI is present in an obstructed urinary tract, in which case the sample of urine will not be representative. For example, in a bladder tumour obstructing a ureter, infection can develop in the obstructed kidney, which is effectively isolated from the rest of the urinary tract

Catheter specimen of urine (CSU)
Up to 5 per cent of healthy people have bacteruria (bacteria found in the urine) without symptoms of a UTI. In patients with a catheter this figure is very much higher.

Attempts to sterilize the urine in patients with catheters by treating with antibiotics are only successful as long as the patient continues to take the drug. Bacteriuria always returns on stopping.

In view of this, patients with urinary catheters are only investigated if they have **symptoms** that might relate to a UTI, and that warrant treatment e.g.
- dysuria, frequency or urgency
- suprapubic pains—'bladder spasms'
- loin pain
- toxic symptoms e.g. confusion, nausea and vomiting especially if associated with fever.
- sludging, bypassing and blocking catheter

Unpleasant-smelling urine indicates infection rather than simple bacteriuria, but does not by itself warrant investigation unless the patient considers it a problem.

Magnetic resonance imaging (MRI)

MRI cannot be performed on patients who have a cardiac pacemaker or ferrous/magnetic metal in their body since the magnetic field may interfere with function. This includes patients with:

- aneurysm clips in the brain
- cochlear implants
- metal fragments in the eye
- shrapnel

Hip replacements are made of non-ferrous metal and do not exclude an MRI.

Intravenous contrast studies

Radiological examinations requiring intravenous contrast to be given (IVP, CT scan etc.) can precipitate lactic acidosis in patients taking metformin. The metformin should be stopped well in advance of the investigation.

Influenza vaccination

Annual immunization with influenza vaccine is recommended for those of all ages with:
- immunosuppression due to disease or treatment
- chronic respiratory or heart disease
- chronic renal failure
- diabetes mellitus
- persons over the age of 65 years
- residents of nursing and residential homes

There is evidence that it is still effective in patients with cancer. The 'flu vaccine is a preparation of inactivated virus, and will not cause influenza in immunosuppressed patients. The main contra-indication is an allergy to eggs.

Needlestick injury and HIV
- The risk of HIV transmission following needlestick injury involving contaminated blood is about 0.4 per cent. Zidovudine treatment reduces the transmission rate by about 80 per cent
- Ideally treatment should start within 1–2h of such exposure
- All needlestick injuries should be reported and prompt advice sought from local infection control advisors

Falls

All patients who have had a fall should have a full history, examination and appropriate investigations looking for reversible causes whether or not they have terminal cancer. The consequences of the fall, e.g. hip fracture, subdural bleed etc. will need managing on an individual basis according to clinical frailty and patient's wishes.

Assessment should include:

Blood pressure

Postural hypotension should be assessed by measuring the blood pressure both lying and standing. If there is a significant blood pressure drop on standing, reversible possibilities should be sought such as medication (e.g. diuretics, antihypertensives, antimuscrinics, beta-blockers, phenothiazines, withdrawal of steroids), anaemia, dehydration, insufficient adreno-cortical function etc. Patients should be advised to rise slowly from a lying/sitting position, to sleep propped up with pillows and to consider support hosiery. If no obviously reversible cause is found, treatment with fludrocortisone 0.05–0.1mg o.d. may be appropriate.

Medication review

- Consider reducing or stopping:
  - Hypotensive drugs: antimuscarinics, beta-blockers, phenothiazines etc.
  - Sedative drugs: benzodiazepines, opioid analgesics etc.
  - Anticonvulsants (ataxia)
  - Corticosteroids (proximal myopathy)
- Neurological assessment for:
  - Spinal cord compression
  - Cerebellar dysfunction
  - Parkinson's disease or extrapyramidal symptoms
  - Long tract signs suggestive of hemiparesis etc.
  - History suggestive of a seizure, TIA etc.
- Physiotherapist assessment for:
  - Balance
  - Transfers
  - Gait

Legal standard of care

All doctors and other health professionals work in an increasingly litigious climate. In palliative medicine, a specialty where doctors are involved at a highly emotional time in patients' and families' lives, and in light of the aftermath of a number of high profile medicolegal/ethical cases, the importance of the shift from the traditional Bolam approach to a new more enquiring approach should be understood.

- In medical litigation, the central question that arises is whether or not a doctor has attained the standard of care that is required by law
- The standard expected is one of 'reasonable care'
- This is judged by taking into account all the circumstances surrounding a particular situation and by balancing the diversity inherent in medical practice against the interests of the patient
- In determining the standard, the court uses the Bolam test
- The Bolam principle, however, has been perceived as being excessively reliant upon medical testimony supporting the defendant
- The judgement given by the House of Lords in the recent case of Bolitho imposes a requirement that the standard proclaimed must be justified on a logical basis and the risks and benefits of competing options must have been considered
- The effect of this case is that the court will take a more enquiring stance to test the medical evidence offered by both parties in litigation in order to reach its conclusions

In 1954, Mr Bolam underwent electroconvulsive therapy (ECT) for clinical depression. At that time medical opinion differed on how best to minimise the risk of injuries possible from convulsions induced by ECT. In Mr Bolam's case the technique of manual restraint was ineffective and as a result he fractured his pelvis. He subsequently argued that the doctor had been in breach of the standard of care in providing treatment and that the hospital had been negligent. The judge in his direction to the jury said that a doctor is not guilty of negligence if he has acted in accordance with the practice accepted as proper by a responsible body of medical opinion skilled in that particular art. If therefore a medical practice is supported by a body of peers, then the Bolam test is satisfied and the practitioner has met the required standard of care in law. This test has been used on numerous occasions in cases of medical litigation.

Wills

- Palliative care involves looking after patients and families in the broadest sense
- Many people delay writing a will for a number of reasons, which often leaves families in a difficult situation, not knowing what the deceased would have wanted
- Palliative care teams are often in contact with patients for several months before death, and are in a good position to encourage the family to discuss important issues and the patient to consider making a will
- This is particularly important if the family dynamics are complicated
- The intestacy rules dictate not only who receives the estate but also who should manage the affairs of the estate
- Unmarried partners may have no claim on the estate unless they are dependent on the deceased
- If the deceased is divorced or separated, the rules will determine who the legal guardians of the children will be

It is not uncommon for patients to wish to make a will in the last few days of life, having not wanted to face up to it before this time. This is a time when patients may have episodes of being distressed or muddled, a situation which lends itself to the possibility of family members contesting what they attest to be an incompetently considered 'death bed' will. Although it is not absolutely necessary, it is best to advise that the will is drawn up by a qualified solicitor who will be in the best position to defend the will if it is ever contested. If a doctor is asked to witness a signature, it would be wise to confirm first that the patient is competent to do so.

Competency for drawing up a will

The legal test for Testamentary Capacity was described by Mr Justice Cockburn in the case of Banks v. Goodfellow in 1879:

> 'It is essential . . . that a testator shall understand the nature of the act and its effects; shall understand the extent of the property of which he is disposing; shall be able to comprehend and appreciate the claims to which he ought to give effect and, with a view to the latter object, that no disorder of the mind shall poison his affections, pervert his sense of right, or prevent the exercise of his natural faculties, that no insane delusion shall influence his will in disposing of his property and bring about a disposal of it which, if the mind had been sound, would not have been made.'

Following death:
- If a will has been written, the executors appointed in the will apply for a grant of probate
- If a will has not been written, the administrators apply for a grant of letters of administration
- When it comes to distributing the estate the nearest relatives in fixed order are entitled to apply for the grant
- If the nearest relative does not wish to apply, he can renounce his right to do so in which case the next-nearest becomes entitled to be administrator and so on down the line of kinship

- There is a hierarchy of those that are legally next of kin and as such entitled to apply for the grant
- The widow or widower is primarily entitled to be the administrator and if there is no surviving spouse or he/she does not apply for a grant, then any of the children can apply
- Grandchildren and other offspring may apply if their parents have died
- In-laws and people related by marriage do not count, only blood relations
- There is no distinction made between natural, adopted or illegitimate relationships
- An adopted child is deemed to be the legal child of his adoptive parents and has exactly the same inheritance right as the adoptive parents' other (natural) children, but loses any rights to his natural parents estate

Enduring Power of Attorney

An Enduring Power of Attorney can continue in force after the maker of the power (donor) becomes mentally incapable of handling his or her affairs. The donor must me competent at the time of appointing an attorney.
   It may give:
- General power—which authorizes the attorney to carry out any transaction on behalf of the donor, or
- Specific power—which authorizes the attorney to deal only with those aspects of the donor's affairs which are specified in the power

When the donor becomes mentally incapable, the attorney must apply to register the Enduring Power of Attorney with the Court of Protection, before it can be undertaken.
   The donor can revoke or cancel it at any time while she or he is mentally capable, but cannot revoke it once it has been registered unless the Court of Protection confirms the revocation.
   Once registered, the attorney has the power to act on behalf of the donor, either in the general or specific way as outlined, but has no power over the 'person' of the donor and cannot make a will on behalf of the donor.

- Most attorneys are honest, decent people. Some, however, abuse their situation
- Financial abuse probably occurs in 10–15 per cent of cases involving registered Enduring Power of Attorney and more often when they are unregistered
- The powers of the Court of Protection and the Public Trust Office (a registration authority only) are limited where the donor is being financially abused
- The court can only intervene when the donor is, or is becoming, mentally incapable
- The court is generally not concerned with unregistered powers.
- The court can revoke the Enduring Power of Attorney (but this is often too late) and can appoint a receiver with authority to investigate but this is often not satisfactory
- Some people believe they have an indefeasible right to inherit another person's estate intact
- In a number of cases, attorneys have disposed of the donor' assets to secure entitlement to public funding for long ter

- The risk is greater if the attorney lives abroad
- Mutual dependency is also a problem, since the donor is dependent on the attorney as the principal or only carer but also the attorney is dependent on the donor, especially when they share living accommodation and financial arrangements
- In cases where a donor comes from an unreliable or dysfunctional family and has a relatively short life expectation, it may be prudent for solicitors to recommend that the donor appoints a receiver and not an attorney

Donors who are more at risk from abuse include those with no immediate family or only one child, those who are moderately affluent (but not extremely rich or extremely poor) and those who suddenly come into additional wealth through inheritance on the death of a relative. An aggravating factor is the expectation of inheritance and the desire to preserve and precipitate it.

Advance Directive (also known as Living Will)

> Where is the wisdom we have lost in Knowledge?
> Where is the knowledge we have lost in information?
>
> T. S. Eliot, *The Rock*, 1934

Medical advances such as cardiopulmonary resuscitation, renal dialysis, artificial ventilation and artificial hydration and nutrition may prolong life. The fear of being kept alive artificially, with no prospect of recovery and no perceived quality of life, has prompted society to discuss and to draw up guidance on the issue of end-of-life care. This is supported by health-care professionals who are concerned about providing non-beneficial, over-burdensome medical interventions to patients with a terminal illness.

> Advance Directives allow a competent patient to express their wishes about treatment decisions in the event of them becoming incompetent and unable to give consent.

The US was the first country to formalize the use of Advance Directives following a case in which a patient, whose previously held wishes for treatment and care and basic values were unknown, lapsed into a permanent vegetative state in 1976. A similar debate on the rôle of Advance Directives took place in the UK following the case of Tony Bland (1993).

A House of Lords select committee on medical ethics discussed the merits of Advance Directives, although it did not consider that legislation was necessary. It encouraged the development of a 'code of practice' which was produced by the British Medical Association in1995, outlining the inherent ethical and legal issues.

The UK government is satisfied for the time being that this BMA document, *Advance Statements about Medical Treatment*, together with case law, provides sufficient clarity and flexibility to enable the validity and applicability of Advance Directives to be decided on a case by case basis.

The idea of patients discussing their wishes is not new, but the aim of the Advance Directive is to provide a more formal, registered means for the patient to continue to exercise autonomy in the event of future mental incapacity.

Advance Directives can encompasses all type of anticipatory decision-making, including oral and written decisions and records of discussion in case notes, of advance refusals or authorisations of treatment. They can be specific, general or list the patient's fundamental values as a guide for others to decide. Legally, no person has a right to accept or decline treatment on behalf of another but a representative, nominated by the patient, may be helpful in communicating the patient's views.

Advance Directives of refusal are only of repute if the patient was;
  competent
  fully informed
  uncoerced at the time of drawing up the Advance Directive
  In addition, it must be valid and clearly applicable to this particular situation

The legality of non-documented verbal advance refusals is debateable.

There should be no reason to suggest that the patient might have changed his/her mind. Others should not be put at potentially serious harm by applying the Advance Directive. Patients are not able to authorize treatment that is not legal (e.g. euthanasia) nor are they able to refuse future basic care.

Any Advance Directive is superseded by a clear and competent contemporaneous decision. An Advance Directive of a patient under the age of 18 years should be taken into account and accommodated if possible but can be overruled by a court or a person with parental responsibility.

If the patient has been detained for compulsory treatment under mental health legislation, any advance refusal of treatment can be overruled.

Advising the person enquiring about creating an Advance Directive

- Ensure that the patient is competent. An Advance Directive should not be made under pressure, particularly if the patient has recently received a poor prognosis. The patient should not be unduly influenced in any way and there should be no question of clinical depression that might affect competence
- Provide the patient with information on Advance Directives (Patients Association 2000)
- Allow for dialogue and openness in discussion with relevant healthcare professionals including doctors and nurses. Patients must be able to make informed choices and will need to be aware of predictable phases of their disease and treatment options, diagnosis, prognosis and rehabilitation potential. They need to know the options considered to be in the patient's best interests although the patient will be the ultimate judge. They will also need to know what will be done if the treatment is not carried out. (Advance Directives are an aid to, and not a substitute for, discussion and communication.)
- Written statements, on firm decisions or general views, should use clear and unambiguous language. Oral statements are equally valid if supported by appropriate evidence
- Advance Directives should be signed by the individual and a witness. The witness should not be a family member since they may stand to gain from the death. If a healthcare professional witnessess, it is implied that assessment of competence has taken place
- Review the Advance Directive regularly
- Encourage the patient to store the document safely. It is the patient's responsibility to ensure its availability. A copy should be sent to the GP, specialist team and stored in the case notes
- In an emergency situation, health professionals should make all reasonable efforts to acquaint themselves with the contents of the Advance Directive if they know or have reason to believe that one is available but should not delay treatment in anticipation of finding one

A guide to core content of an Advance Directive

- Full name
- Address
- Name and address of GP

- Whether advice was sought from health professionals
- Signature of patient
- Date drafted and reviewed
- Witnessed
- Clear statement of the patient's wishes, either general or specific
- Name, address and telephone number of patient's nominated person, if one chosen
- Consider for inclusion:
  - List of the individual's values as a basis for others to reach appropriate decisions
  - Request for all medically reasonable efforts to be made to prolong life or expression of preferences for treatment options
  - Where the patient would like to be cared for
  - Contingency issues for pregnancy where appropriate

Further reading

Travis S., Mason J., Mallett J., Laverty D. (2001) Guidelines in respect of Advance Directives: the position in England. *International Journal of Palliative Nursing*, **7, 10**: 493–500.

BMA (1995) *Advance Statements about Medical Treatment. Code of practice with explanatory notes.* London: BMJ Publishing Group.

Luttrell S. (1996) Living wills do have legal effect provided certain criteria are met. *BMJ*, **313**: 1148.

Dermatomes

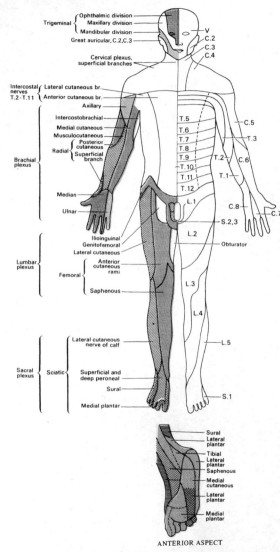

ANTERIOR ASPECT

Dermatomes. Reproduced from the *Oxford Handbook of Clinical Medicine*, ... e et al. Oxford: Oxford University Press. With permission.

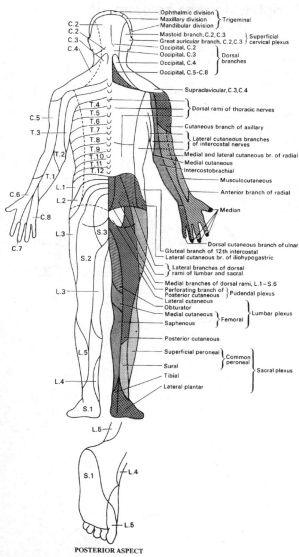

Fig. 16.1 (Continued).

Peripheral nerve assessment

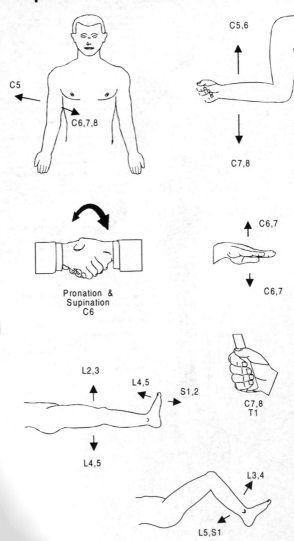

C5,6

C7,8

C5

C6,7,8

Pronation &
Supination
C6

C6,7

C6,7

C7,8
T1

L2,3

L4,5

S1,2

L4,5

L3,4

L5,S1

...rological diagrams.

Drawing a family tree (genogram)

Family Tree

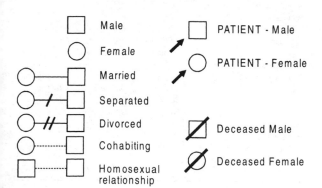

2nd AND 3rd MARRIAGES

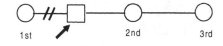

1st   2nd   3rd

PARENTS

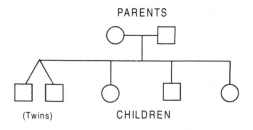

(Twins)   CHILDREN

NB Alternative system: ⊗ for the Patient and ● for Deceased

Fig. 16.3 How to draw up a family tree.

Emergency drug doses

Table 16.1 Emergency drug doses[1]

	Route	Adult	Child
Anaphylaxis/asthma			
Adrenaline 1:1,000			
(epinephrine)	i/m	0.5ml	0.1ml/yr
Aminophylline	i/v 20mins	250–500mg	5mg/kg
	infusion	0.5mg/kg/h	1mg/kg/h
Chlorphenamine			
(chlorpheniramine)	i/v	10mg	200 mcg/kg
Salbutamol	i/v slow	0.25mg	4 mcg/kg
	SC, i/m	0.5mg	
neb	5mg	2.5mg	
Hydrocortisone	i/v	100–300mg	
Fits/sedation			
Diazepam	i/v, PR	10mg	0.25–0.5mg/kg
Diabetes—hypoglycaemia			
Glucagon	i/m	1mg >12yrs	0.5mg <12yrs

1 Back I. (2001). *Palliative Medicine Handbook*. 3rd edn. BPM Books: Cardiff.

Laboratory reference values

These are guides only—different labs use different ranges. Pregnant women and children also have different normal ranges—consult the lab.

Haematology

Measurement	Reference interval
White cell count (WCC)	$4.0–11.0 \times 10^9/l$
Red cell count (RCC)	Men: $4.5–6.5 \times 10^{12}/l$
	Women: $3.9–5.6 \times 10^{12}/l$
Haemoglobin	Men: 13.5–18g/dl
	Women: 11.5–16.0g/dl
Packed cell volume (PCV) or	Men: 38.5–50.1%
haematocrit	Women: 36.0–44.5%
Mean cell volume (MCV)	76–97fl
Mean cell haemoglobin (MCHC)	32.7–34.6 g/dl
Neutrophils	$2.0–7.5 \times 10^9/l$ *40–75% WCC*
Lymphocytes	$1.3–3.5 \times 10^9/l$ *20–45% WCC*
Esoinophils	$0.04–0.44 \times 10^9/l$ *1–6% WCC*
Basophils	$0.0–0.1 \times 10^9/l$ *0–1% WCC*
Monocytes	$0.2–0.8 \times 10^9/l$ *2–10% WCC*
Platelet count	$150–400 \times 10^9/l$
Reticulocyte count	$25–100 \times 10^9/l$ *0.8–2% RCC**
Erythrocyte sedimentation rate (ESR)	Depends on age
International normalized ratio (INR)	0.8–1.2
	Ranges for warfarin therapy depend on indication, 🔲 Chapter 6c
Prothrombin time (PTT) Factors I, II, VII, X	12–17 sec.
Activated partial thromboplastin time Factors VIII, IX, XI, XII	28–40 sec.
Red cell folate	180–300 ng/ml

....

* Only use percentages as reference interval if red cell count is normal. Otherwise use absolute value.

Biochemistry

Substance		Reference interval
Adrenocorticotrophic hormone	P	<80ng/l
Alanine aminotransferase (ALT)	P	5–35iu/l
Albumin	P	35–50g/l
Alkaline phosphatase	P	30–150u/l
α-amylase	P	0–180u/dl
Aspartate transaminase (AST)	P	5–35iu/l
Bicarbonate	P	24–30mmol/l
Bilirubin	P	3–17μmol/l
Calcium (total)	P	2.12–2.65mmol/l
Creatinine kinase (CK)	P	Men: 25–195iu/l
		Women: 25–170iu/l
Creatinine	P	70–≤150μmol/l
Ferritin	P	12–200μg/l
Folate	S	2.1μg/l
Follicle stimulating hormone (FSH)	P/S	2–8u/l >25u/l *post menopause*
Gamma-glutamyl transpeptidase (GGT, γGT)	P	Men: 11–51iu/l
		Women: 7–33iu/l
Glucose (fasting)	P	3.5–5.5mmol/l
Iron	S	Men: 14–31μmol/l
		Women: 11–30μmol/l
Luteinizing hormone (LH)	P	3–16u/l
Osmolality	P	278–305mosmol/kg
Phosphate (inorganic)	P	0.8–1.45mmol/l
Potassium	P	3.5–5.0mmol/l
Prolactin	P	Men: <450u/l
		Women: <600u/l
Prostate specific antigen (PSA)	P	0–4ngrams/ml
Protein (total)	P	60–80g/l
Sodium	P	135–145mmol/l
Thyroxine (T_4)		70–140nmol/l
Total iron binding capacity	S	54–75μmol/l
Triglyceride	P	0.55–1.90mmol/l
Urate	P	Men: 210–480μmol/l
		Women: 150–390μmol/l
Urea	P	2.5–6.7mmol/l
Vitamin B_{12}	S	0.13–0.68nmol/l
		(>150ng/l)

P = plasma (e.g. heparin bottle); S = serum (clotted—no anticoagulant).

Index

Page numbers in *italics* indicate tables and figures.